"When I first wanted to learn about acceptance and commitment therapy (ACT), I started with the excellent first edition of this book, and this second edition is even better. The second edition of *ACT Made Simple* is a perfect introduction to ACT—easy to read, well organized, and filled with examples, strategies, and demonstrations that make the therapy come alive in the mind of the reader. Essential reading for all therapists."

> —**Russell Kolts, PhD**, professor in the department of psychology at
> Eastern Washington University, and author of *CFT Made Simple* and
> *The Compassionate-Mind Guide to Managing Your Anger*

"Russ Harris has completely reworked the new edition of *ACT Made Simple*. This book is essential reading for all trainees and qualified practitioners who want to use the wisdom of ACT ideas in their work. The book has cleverly integrated all the latest advances in the field in an accessible and immediately useable format. It has a lot to offer a newcomer to the area of ACT, but also provides an up-to-date account of the cutting-edge technologies in the area, as well as some innovative new ideas. The examples are easy to identify with, and the exercises well timed. An excellent contribution from arguably the most accessible author in the field."

> —**Louise McHugh**, associate professor in the department of psychology at
> University College Dublin; peer-reviewed ACT trainer; fellow of the Association for
> Contextual Behavioral Science; and coauthor of *The Self and Perspective Taking*

"How do you improve a classic? You distill another ten years of clinical experience and research and write a tour de force. Every page shines with Russ's hallmark humor, compassion, and wonder. Expanded, without being more complicated, the second edition of *ACT Made Simple* is a vital clinician's resource, and an exciting road map for anyone who wants to live life fully."

> —**Chris McCurry, PhD**, clinical child psychologist, and author of
> *Parenting Your Anxious Child with Mindfulness and Acceptance*

"Russ Harris, a premier leader in ACT, has updated his watershed book *ACT Made Simple* with new and vibrant content. His colloquial style makes it a pleasure to read. More importantly, he focuses on fresh content, so that even if you've already read the first edition, this is worth your attention. One of the remarkable new topics in this edition is the way he helps you set up sessions for success with your client. I've supervised hundreds of ACT clinicians, and I reliably recommend Russ's publications, and that will continue to be true for this updated version!"

> —**D.J. Moran, PhD, BCBA-D**, Pickslyde Consulting; coauthor of
> *ACT in Practice* and *Committed Action in Practice*

"For clinicians who are trying to learn the 'how to' of ACT, Russ's humor, clarity, wisdom, and experience makes this one of the most accessible books you will ever read. Weaving the 'choice point' throughout this edition provides structure to the clinical work, and is an effective tool for therapists at every level of experience. Each chapter includes an assortment of scripts, debriefing suggestions, tips, worksheets, and new 'skilling up' exercises to take your learning beyond the pages and into active, experiential practice. If the first edition is already on your bookshelf, don't hesitate to add this to your collection—the fresh new examples and topics make this a worthwhile investment. This book is, quite simply, indispensable for both novice and seasoned ACT clinicians."

—**Sheri Turrell, PhD**, clinical psychologist working with teens and adults in
Toronto, ON, Canada; Association for Contextual Behavioral Science (ACBS)
peer-reviewed ACT trainer; and coauthor of *ACT for Adolescents* and
The Mindfulness and Acceptance Workbook for Teen Anxiety

"The word 'simple' can sometimes be equated to words like 'basic,' 'unsophisticated,' or even 'elementary.' Although the second edition of *ACT Made Simple* can definitely be equated with the words 'easily understood,' make no mistake about it: this book is a thoughtful, entertaining, and comprehensive introduction to the ACT model."

—**Nic Hooper, PhD**, senior lecturer at the University of the West of England,
and coauthor of *The Research Journey of Acceptance and Commitment Therapy*

"There are books in the life of an ACT therapist that really help us to be better clinicians, and the second edition of *ACT Made Simple* is one of them! This book is a vitally important one because it includes the basics of very relevant clinical themes such as exposure, self-compassion, emotion regulation, cognitive flexibility, the 'choice point,' and much more.

"There is no other ACT book that has included all these topics at once, and that is based on years of collecting the most frequent struggles an ACT therapist or ACT coach encounters on a daily basis; I don't have any doubt that this book will transform the way we deliver and live ACT every hour. Here are my last words: read it, try it, track it, and read it again!"

—**Patricia E. Zurita Ona, PsyD**, author of *Parenting a Troubled Teen*
and *Escaping the Emotional Roller Coaster*, and coauthor of *Mind and Emotions*

"The practice of ACT continues to evolve at a rapid pace. In this second edition of *ACT Made Simple*, Russ has managed to delightfully update tried-and-tested content on the six processes of flexibility, while also adding clear and easy-to-follow descriptions of more recent nuances and applications of the model (e.g., 'choice point,' shame, self-compassion, flexible exposure). Russ manages to convey complex ideas and strategies in a way that is both accessible and engaging. This book is definitely the first I recommend for clinicians interested in applying or integrating ACT techniques into their practice."

—**Robert N. Brockman, PhD**, senior research fellow at Australian Catholic University, director of Schema Therapy Sydney, and coauthor of *Contextual Schema Therapy*

"The second edition of *ACT Made Simple* is even better than the first. If you want a clear and entertaining guide to the core elements of ACT and the easiest ways to help clients build psychological flexibility, this is the perfect place to start. Russ is a masterful trainer."

—**Paul Atkins, PhD**, honorary associate professor at Australian National University, and project coordinator for Prosocial

"*ACT Made Simple* is one of my favorite introductions to ACT. It's practical, informative, and fun to read. I've used it for years to teach ACT to social work graduate students and supervisees. It offers great examples of dialogue between practitioners and clients that model how you would facilitate ACT processes in plain language. The second edition is a worthy update, with important additions and updates throughout."

—**Matthew S. Boone, LCSW**, editor of *Mindfulness and Acceptance in Social Work*

"*ACT Made Simple* is more than a classic in the psychotherapy literature, it is *the* introductory text for learning ACT from the ground up. This book is a gateway to a larger world of clinical possibilities. A must-read."

—**Dennis Tirch**, coauthor of *The ACT Practitioner's Guide to the Science of Compassion*

"Does what it says on the tin. This book really does provide a simple way to understand ACT concepts, gives helpful guidance of where to start when you're doing therapy, and at the same time doesn't lose sight of the flexibility or scientific principles required to do therapy well."

—**Ben Sedley**, clinical psychologist, and author of *Stuff that Sucks*

The Mastering ACT Series

Acceptance and commitment therapy (ACT) is a powerful, evidence-based model that has been used successfully in treating an array of disorders such as addiction, depression, anxiety, self-harm, post-traumatic stress, and eating disorders. Written by renowned leaders and researchers in the field of ACT, the *Mastering ACT* series explores each of the six processes of the ACT hexaflex: acceptance, cognitive defusion, being present, self-as-context, values, and committed action.

Based in the latest ACT research, this series is designed to take complex theories and translate them into easy-to-apply skills clinicians can utilize in treatment sessions. Each book examines the theoretical aspects of a core ACT process, details how each process can be seamlessly and effectively introduced into therapy, and offers multiple techniques to enhance treatment outcomes and increase client psychological flexibility—the backbone of ACT. These books are essential tools for clinicians, researchers, students, and anyone interested in ACT.

Visit www.newharbinger.com for more books in this series.

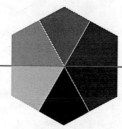

ACT
made simple

SECOND EDITION

**An Easy-to-Read Primer on Acceptance
and Commitment Therapy**

RUSS HARRIS

New Harbinger Publications, Inc.

Publisher's Note

Distributed in Canada by Raincoast Books

Copyright © 2019 by Russ Harris
New Harbinger Publications, Inc.
5674 Shattuck Avenue
Oakland, CA 94609
www.newharbinger.com

Cover design by Amy Shoup

Acquired by Catharine Meyers

Edited by Rona Bernstein

Indexed by James Minkin

Library of Congress Cataloging-in-Publication Data

Names: Harris, Russ, 1938- author.
Title: ACT made simple : an easy-to-read primer on acceptance and commitment therapy / Russ Harris ; foreword by Steven C. Hayes, PhD.
Identifiers: LCCN 2019022143 (print) | LCCN 2019022320 (ebook) | ISBN 9781684033010 (paperback) | ISBN 9781684033027 (pdf e-book) | ISBN 9781684033034 (epub)
Subjects: LCSH: Acceptance and commitment therapy. | BISAC: PSYCHOLOGY / Clinical Psychology. | PSYCHOLOGY / Psychotherapy / Counseling.
Classification: LCC RC489.A32 H37 2019 (print) | LCC RC489.A32 (ebook) | DDC 616.89/1425--dc23
LC record available at https://lccn.loc.gov/2019022143
LC ebook record available at https://lccn.loc.gov/2019022320

Printed in the United States of America.

23   22   21

15   14   13   12   11   10   9   8

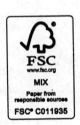
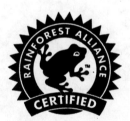

Dedication

To my brother Genghis: for all your love, support, inspiration, and encouragement over the years; for pushing me when I needed pushing; for anchoring me when I needed stability; for showing me the way when I got lost; and for bringing so much light, love, and laughter into my life.

Contents

Part 4: Wrapping Up

Your Choice Point

Acceptance and commitment therapy (ACT) is commonly said to be confusing. This book mentions a couple of reasons why—the basic theory of cognition on which it is based is technically precise, and its methods are nonlinear. But I think there is another reason: The logical mind does not like to be dethroned. It resists changing the mental agenda from problem solving to a vital life.

ACT asks clients to experience the world in a new and meaningful way. In this new world, the core of life is more like appreciating a sunset than it is solving a math problem. A whole list of odd things become possible:

- you can turn toward your pain and life will open up;

- you can consciously embrace contradictory thoughts without declaring a winner and find great coherence and understanding as a result;

- you can consider yourself to be no-thing, and find enormous peace of mind and purpose because you did;

- you find what you deeply care about is lying there in plain sight inside your pain, joy, admiration, or authenticity; and

- choice is possible, even while your mind constantly tries to turn choices into logical syllogisms.

What makes such a journey possible is the vitality of living that psychological flexibility affords. That is a beacon for clients and therapists alike—once you can cut through the mental underbrush enough to see it. Russ Harris has completely reworked this new edition of *ACT Made Simple* around a tool that quickly and effectively helps therapists do just that.

The *choice point* clinical tool that Russ, Joe Ciarrochi, and Ann Bailey developed a few years ago quickly drills down to the essential core of the psychological flexibility model. I have used the tool many times and have been deeply impressed with its elegance, simplicity, and power. Using it, therapists and clients alike can very quickly catch that turning away from pain is not helpful, that workability trumps syllogisms, and that it is possible to choose. In Russ's hands, the choice point tool simplifies, but it is never simplistic; it facilitates understanding, but not by underestimating the reader. It does not dumb down—it drills down.

Russ has a world-renowned skill for clearing away the underbrush. The detailed theory that sits inside ACT is important, but not for everyone on day one. If you are interested in using ACT in practice, it is most important to get started so that you can begin to learn. It is important to find that beacon. In this book, Russ uses his clear voice to get beginners up and moving.

I have seen other efforts to simplify ACT that do so by losing contact with the work, hoping that eventually practitioners will figure it all out. In my experience, that has never happened with Russ. His methods and sentences always ring true. They are filled with clinical wisdom, heart, and skill. Russ understands the work deeply, and he applies and extends it with integrity. In this book, he has brought his considerable talents to bear on the clear presentation and formulation of the ACT model, and he has brought his clinical creativity to new methods, tools, and ways of getting to the heart of these issues with clients. The second edition is filled with helpful extensions in areas that have sometimes not been given adequate attention, such as anger, how to use exposure, and the wisdom that resides inside emotions.

This book does a masterful job of opening up the ACT model for you to explore. If you've looked at the range of books available, you know that ACT now covers a vast landscape. That fact can intimidate therapists new to the model, but don't feel alone in that—I may have initiated ACT, but a large community developed it, and I confess that sometimes I have a similar reaction.

No matter—there is a simple way forward. You are holding it in your hands.

You yourself are at a choice point right now. You picked up this book because you sensed that it was time to turn toward learning ACT. I agree with you, and all you need to do is turn the page and begin.

—Steven C. Hayes, PhD
University of Nevada

What's New in Version Two?

If you've already bought edition one of *ACT Made Simple* (Harris, 2009a), you're probably wondering, *Is it really worth stumping up the cash for edition two?* Well, if you were to ask me, my answer would be "Yes, absolutely. It's great value for the money and probably the single smartest purchase you'll make this year." Of course, I may have a slightly biased opinion, so in order to help you make this tough decision, here's a quick summary of the main differences between edition one and edition two:

A. A massive amount of new material, including exposure, relationship issues, flexible thinking, harnessing the power of emotions, self-compassion, shame, overcoming hopelessness, and much, much more. In fact, over 60 percent of the book is new—and the rest of it has been significantly rewritten. In the ten years since the first edition came out, I've radically changed both the way I do ACT and the way I teach it. (Indeed, I wanted to write a whole new textbook from scratch, called "ACT Made Even Simpler," but the publishers talked me out of it.) So in AMS 2, you'll find plenty of new exercises, metaphors, tools, techniques, transcripts of therapy sessions, bad jokes, and so on (as well as cool abbreviations like "AMS 2").

B. The *choice point*: this is the simplest, easiest, most impactful tool I know for helping people to learn and apply ACT quickly and effectively. Since 2015, it has become the central tool in all my live workshops and online training courses, and I'm currently rewriting all my books to center around it. So if you don't already know it, I trust you'll soon see how effective it is. And if you do know it, I trust you'll learn a whole lot more about how to use it for maximum impact. Having said all that, it's not an essential tool; I'd hate for anyone to think they have to use the choice point to do ACT well. So while it pops up in quite a few chapters, I'll also give you many, many alternatives.

So, are you in? If not, so be it. I tried my best. But if yes…then as we say in Australia, "Good on ya!!" I'm sure you won't regret it.

How to Use This Book

If you're brand new to ACT, I recommend you read this entire book from cover to cover before you start using any of it. This is because the six core processes of ACT are all interdependent, so unless you have a good sense of the entire model and the way these different strands interweave, you may well get confused and head off in the wrong direction.

When you're ready to start using ACT with your clients, you can use this book to loosely guide you, or you might prefer to use a protocol-based ACT textbook that will coach you along in detail, session by session. If, however, you're already doing ACT, then apply each chapter as you go to build on and enhance what you're already doing in your sessions.

The Extra Bits

The hardest part of writing this book was deciding what to leave out. Indeed, by the time I finished writing the second edition, I had gone over my word limit by 40,000 words. But rather than throw all this stuff away, I have compiled it into a free eBook called *ACT Made Simple: The Extra Bits*. You can download this, at no cost, from the "Free Stuff" page at http://www.actmindfully.com.au. There you'll find all the extra bits I wanted to put into each chapter but didn't have space for: Q&As, pitfalls and tips, additional scripts for exercises and metaphors, and downloadable audio recordings. It also includes all the worksheets mentioned or featured throughout this textbook.

In most chapters of this book, you'll find an "Extra Bits" text box toward the end; this will inform you about all the goodies you can find in the corresponding Extra Bits chapter.

"Skilling Up" Sections

The "Skilling Up" sections suggest things for you to do to build your ACT skills. Reading this book is nowhere near enough to learn ACT; you'll also need to actively practice the exercises as you go. After all, you can't learn to drive merely by reading about it; you have to actually get in a car, put your hands on the wheel, and take it for a spin. So I'll repeatedly encourage you to actively practice new skills, at home and in session. You'll find these sections in many but not all chapters; but even where it's not explicitly included, I hope you'll nonetheless practice some combination of filling in the worksheets, reviewing the scripts, rehearsing interventions with an imaginary client, trying techniques on yourself—and then doing it all for real, in session.

"Takeaway" Sections

At the end of each chapter, you'll find a "Takeaway" section, which is a brief summary of key points or messages.

How This Book Is Structured

This book is composed of four sections. In part 1,"What Is ACT?" (chapters 1 through 4), we're going to zip through an overview of the ACT model and the theory underlying it. Then, in part 2, "Getting Started" (chapters 5, 6, and 7), we'll cover the basics of getting started, including how to do experiential therapy, obtain informed consent, and structure your ongoing sessions.

In part 3, "The Nitty Gritty Stuff" (chapters 8 through 28), we'll go step by step through the six core processes of ACT and how to apply them to a wide range of clinical issues. The emphasis in each chapter will be on simplicity and practicality so you can start using this approach straight away. (But please keep in mind: newcomers should first read the whole book, cover to cover, before applying it.)

In part 4, "Wrapping Up" (chapters 30 through 32), we'll cover a wide range of important topics including enhancing the client-therapist relationship, common therapist pitfalls, overcoming barriers to change, dancing around the six core processes, and where to go next on your journey as an ACT therapist.

Adapt and Modify Everything

I made a big mistake in my early days of ACT: I tried to do it word for word, exactly as written in the textbooks. This didn't work very well for me, because the way I naturally speak is just so different from the scripts I found in the books. Then I attended a workshop with Steve Hayes, the founder of ACT, and made another big mistake: I was so impressed with his unique style of doing therapy, I started trying to copy him. This didn't work too well, either. The problem was, I wasn't being authentic; I was just doing a bad impersonation of Steve.

Then one day, I heard this quote from Oscar Wilde: "Be yourself: everyone else is taken." And that's when the lightbulb went on. I moved away from the scripts, let go of impersonating ACT gurus, and found my own way of doing ACT. I developed my own style and my own way of speaking, a manner that felt natural and also suited the clients I work with. That's when ACT truly came to life for me. So I strongly encourage you to do the same. Be yourself. As you go through this book, use your creativity. Feel free to adapt, modify, and reinvent the tools and techniques within these pages (provided you're remaining true to the ACT model) to suit your own personal style. Wherever I present metaphors, scripts, worksheets, or exercises, change the words to fit your way of speaking. And if you have better or different metaphors or exercises that accomplish the same ends, then please use yours rather than the ones in this book. There's enormous room for creativity and innovation within the ACT model, so please do take every advantage of it.

PART 1

What Is ACT?

CHAPTER 1

The Human Challenge

When you're going through hell, keep going!

—Winston Churchill

It Ain't Easy to Be Happy

Life is both amazing and terrible. If we live long enough, we will experience joyful success and spectacular failure, great love and devastating loss, moments of wonder and bliss and moments of darkness and despair. The inconvenient truth is that almost everything that makes our life rich, full, and meaningful comes with a painful downside. And unfortunately, what this means is that it's hard to be happy for long. Heck, it's hard to be happy for *short*. The fact is, life is tough, and it doles out plenty of pain for every one of us. And one of the main reasons for this (as we'll soon explore) is that the human mind has evolved in such a way that it naturally creates psychological suffering. So basically, if we live long enough, we're all going to experience a whole lot of hurt.

Hmmm. I guess that's not the most optimistic of book openings. Is it really that bleak? Is there nothing we can do about this miserable state of affairs? Should we give up on life and throw ourselves into a pit of nihilistic despair?

Well, as you've probably guessed, the answer to all those questions is no. Luckily for us, we have acceptance and commitment therapy (ACT) to show us a way forward in the face of life's many hardships. ACT gets its name because it teaches us how to reduce the impact and influence of painful thoughts and feelings (acceptance) while simultaneously taking action to build a life that's rich, full, and meaningful (commitment). And in the pages that follow, I have one primary aim: to take the complex theory and practice of ACT and make it simple, accessible, and enjoyable.

What Is ACT?

We officially say ACT as the word "act" and not as the initials A-C-T. And there's a good reason for this. At its core, ACT is a behavioral therapy: it's about taking action. But not just any old action. It's about action guided by your core values—behaving like the sort of person you want to be. What do you want to stand for in life? What really matters, deep in your heart? How do you want to treat yourself, others, and the world around you? What do you want to be remembered for at your funeral?

ACT gets you in touch with what really matters in the big picture: your heart's deepest desires for how you want to behave and what you want to do during your brief time on this planet. You then use these values to guide, motivate, and inspire what you do.

And it's also about "mindful" action: action that you take consciously, with full awareness—open to your experience, and engaging in whatever you're doing. The aim of ACT is to increase one's ability for mindful, values-guided action. The technical name for this ability is *psychological flexibility*. We'll explore this term in more depth soon, but first let's look at the aim of ACT in lay terms.

Where Did ACT Come From?

ACT was created by Professor Steven C. Hayes in the mid-1980s. Steve's colleagues Kelly Wilson and Kirk Strosahl developed it further. It evolved from a field of psychology called *behavior analysis* and is based upon a behavioral theory of cognition known as *relational frame theory* (RFT). Now I don't know about you, but when I first discovered ACT, I couldn't believe that such a spiritual, humanistic model came out of *behaviorism*. I thought behaviorists treated humans like robots or rats, that they had no interest in thoughts and feelings. Boy, was I wrong! I soon discovered there are quite a few different schools of behaviorism, and ACT comes from one known as *functional contextualism*. (Just rolls off the tongue, doesn't it?) And in functional contextualism (try saying it ten times very fast), we are extremely interested in people's thoughts and feelings!

ACT is part of the so-called "third wave" of behavioral therapies—along with dialectical behavior therapy (DBT), mindfulness-based cognitive therapy (MBCT), compassion focused therapy (CFT), functional analytic psychotherapy (FAP), and several others—all of which place a major emphasis on acceptance, mindfulness, and compassion, in addition to traditional behavioral interventions.

What Is the Aim of ACT?

In lay terms, the aim of ACT is to maximize human potential for a rich and meaningful life, while effectively handling the pain that inevitably goes with it.

You may be wondering: does life *inevitably* involve pain? In ACT, we assume it does. No matter how wonderful life is, we'll all experience plenty of frustration, disappointment, rejection, loss, and failure. And if we live long enough, there'll be illness, injury, and aging. Eventually, we'll need to face our own death, and before that day comes, we'll witness the deaths of many loved ones. And as if all that's not enough, the fact is that many basic human emotions—normal feelings that each and every one of us will repeatedly experience throughout our lives—are inherently painful: fear, sadness, guilt, anger, shock, disgust, and so on.

But it doesn't stop there. Because on top of all that, we each have a mind that can conjure up pain at any moment. Wherever we go, whatever we do, we can experience pain instantly. In any moment, we can relive a painful memory or get lost in a fearful prediction of the future. Or we can get caught up in unfavorable comparisons (*Her job is better than mine*) or negative self-judgments (*I'm too fat, I'm not smart enough*, and so on).

Thanks to our minds, we can even experience pain on the happiest days of our lives. For example, suppose it's Susan's wedding day, and all of her friends and family are gathered together to honor her joyful new union. She is blissfully happy. And then she has the thought *I wish my father were here*—and she remembers how he committed suicide when she was only sixteen years old. Now, on one of the happiest days of her life, she's in pain.

And we're all in the same boat as Susan. No matter how good our quality of life, no matter how privileged our situation, all we need do is remember a time when something bad happened, or imagine a future where something bad happens, or judge ourselves harshly, or compare our life to someone else's that seems better, and instantly, we're hurting.

Thus, thanks to the sophistication of the human mind, even the most privileged of lives come with plenty of pain. And unfortunately, most of us do not handle pain very effectively. All too often when we experience painful thoughts, feelings, and sensations, we respond in ways that are self-defeating or self-destructive in the long run.

In summary, then, the big challenges we all have to face in life are:

A. Life is difficult.

B. A full human life comes with the full range of emotions, both pleasant and painful.

C. A normal human mind naturally amplifies psychological suffering.

So How Can ACT Help?

ACT aims to maximize human potential for a rich and meaningful life by:

*   helping us to clarify what's truly important and meaningful to us—that is, clarify our values—and use that knowledge to guide, inspire, and motivate us to do those things that will enrich and enhance our life; and

*   teaching us psychological skills ("mindfulness" skills) that enable us to handle difficult thoughts and feelings effectively, engage fully in whatever we are doing, and appreciate and savor the fulfilling aspects of life.

Why Does ACT Get a Bad Rap?

Have you ever been accused of something you weren't guilty of? This happens to ACT all the time. I've heard many people say it's complex and confusing—and even that you need a high IQ to understand it. Well, if I were the defense lawyer for the ACT model, I'd say, "Not guilty, your honor!" I think there are two main reasons why ACT has gained this unfortunate reputation. One is because of the theory that underlies ACT: relational frame theory (RFT). We won't be covering RFT in this book because it's quite technical and takes a fair bit of work to understand, whereas the aim of this book is to welcome you into ACT, simplify the main concepts, and get you off to a quick start.

The good news is you can be an effective ACT therapist without knowing anything about RFT. If ACT is like driving your car, RFT is like knowing how the engine works: you can be an excellent driver while knowing absolutely nothing about the mechanics. (Having said that, many ACT therapists say that when they understand RFT, it improves their clinical effectiveness. Therefore, if you're interested, appendix C will tell you where to go for more information.)

The other big reason why people see ACT as complex is that it is a nonlinear model of therapy. It's based around six core processes, and you can work with any one of them at any time in any session with any client. And if you ever hit a roadblock with one process, you can simply switch to another. This makes ACT very different from linear models of therapy, where you follow a set sequence: first you do step A, then step B, then step C, and so on.

ACT's nonlinearity comes with a big upside: it gives you incredible flexibility as a therapist. If you get stuck at one point, you can move to another process; then when you think the time is right, you can head back to where you left off. The downside to this nonlinearity is that it makes ACT harder to learn initially than "follow-the-steps" models.

But despair not! In recent years, this task has gotten a whole lot easier, thanks to a simple but powerful tool called the *choice point*, which I'll introduce soon. First, though, let's quickly zip through the six core processes.

The Six Core Therapeutic Processes of ACT

The six core therapeutic processes in ACT are *contacting the present moment*, *defusion*, *acceptance*, *self-as-context*, *values*, and *committed action*. Before we go through them one by one, take a look at the diagram below, which is lightheartedly known as the ACT "hexaflex."

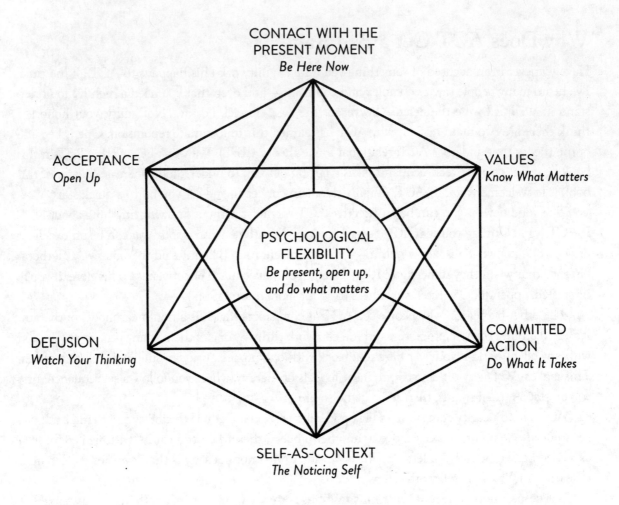

CONTACT WITH THE
PRESENT MOMENT
Be Here Now

ACCEPTANCE
Open Up

VALUES
Know What Matters

PSYCHOLOGICAL
FLEXIBILITY
*Be present, open up,
and do what matters*

DEFUSION
Watch Your Thinking

COMMITTED
ACTION
Do What It Takes

SELF-AS-CONTEXT
The Noticing Self

The ACT Hexaflex

Let's take a look now at each of the six core processes of ACT.

Contact with the present moment (be here now). *Contacting the present moment* means flexibly paying attention to our experience in this moment: narrowing, broadening, shifting, or sustaining your focus, depending upon what's most useful. This may involve consciously paying attention to the physical world around us or the psychological world within us, or both at the same time, connecting with and engaging fully in our experience.

Defusion (watch your thinking). *Defusion* means learning to "step back" and separate or detach from our thoughts, images, and memories. The full technical term is *cognitive defusion*, but usually we just call it defusion. We step back and watch our thinking instead of getting tangled up in it. We see our thoughts for what they are—nothing more or less than words or pictures. We hold them lightly instead of clutching them tightly. We allow them to guide us, but not to dominate us.

Acceptance (open up). *Acceptance* means opening up and making room for unwanted private experiences: thoughts, feelings, emotions, memories, urges, images, impulses, and sensations. Instead of fighting them, resisting them, running from them, we open up and make room for them. We allow them to freely flow through us—to come and stay and go as they choose, in their own good time (if and when this helps us to act effectively and improve our life).

Self-as-context (the noticing self). In everyday language, there are two distinct elements to the mind: a part that thinks and a part that notices. Usually when we talk about "the mind," we mean that part of us that is thinking—generating thoughts, beliefs, memories, judgments, fantasies, plans, and so on. We don't usually mean "the part that notices": that aspect of us that is aware of whatever we're thinking, feeling, sensing, or doing in any moment. In ACT, the technical term for this is *self-as-context*. We often don't explicitly label self-as-context with clients—but if and when we do, we usually call it the "noticing self" or "observing self" or simply "the part of you that notices." (Note: less commonly, self-as-context can also refer to a process called "flexible perspective taking." Don't concern yourself with this for now; we'll look at it later.)

Tricky Terminology   Defusion, acceptance, self-as-context, and contacting the present moment (also called "flexible attention") are the four core mindfulness processes of ACT. So whenever you encounter the term "mindfulness" in ACT, it could be referring to any or all of these processes, in any combination.

Values (know what matters). What do you want to stand for in life? What you want to do with your brief time on this planet? How do you want to treat yourself, others, and the world around you? *Values* are desired qualities of physical or psychological action. In other words, they describe how we want to behave on an ongoing basis. We often compare them to a compass because they give us direction and guide our life's journey.

Committed action (do what it takes). *Committed action* means taking effective action, guided by our values. This includes both physical action (what we do with our physical body) and psychological action (what we do in our inner world). It's all well and good to know our values, but it's only through putting them into action that life becomes rich, full, and meaningful.

And as we take this action, a wide range of thoughts and feelings will show up, some of them pleasurable and others very painful. So committed action means "doing what it takes" to live by our values, even when that brings up difficult thoughts and feelings. Committed action involves goal setting, action planning, problem solving, skills training, behavioral activation, and exposure. It can also include learning and applying any skill that enhances and enriches life—from negotiation, communication, and assertiveness skills to self-soothing, crisis-coping, and mindfulness skills.

Psychological Flexibility: A Six-Faceted Diamond

The six core processes of ACT aren't separate. They're like six facets of a diamond, and the diamond itself is psychological flexibility: the ability to act mindfully, guided by our values. The greater our psychological flexibility—our capacity to be fully conscious, to open to our experience, and to act guided by our values—the greater our quality of life.

How so? Because we can respond far more effectively to the problems and challenges life inevitably brings. Furthermore, when we engage fully in life and allow our values to guide us, we develop a deep sense of meaning and purpose and we experience a sense of vitality.

We use the word "vitality" a lot in ACT, and it's important to recognize that vitality is not a feeling; it is a sense of being fully alive and embracing the here and now, regardless of how we may be feeling in this moment. We can even experience vitality on our deathbed or during extreme grief because "There is as much living in a moment of pain as in a moment of joy" (Strosahl, Hayes, Wilson, & Gifford, 2004, p. 43).

The ACT Triflex

The six core processes can be lumped together into what I call the *triflex* (because it sounds more impressive than the *triangle*). The triflex comprises three functional units, as shown in the figure below.

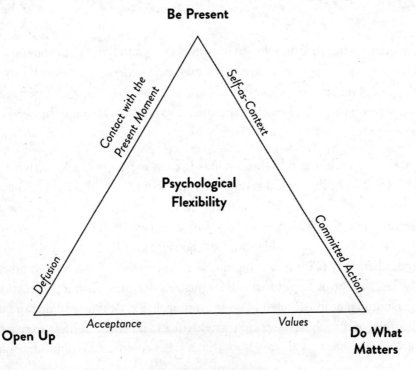

The ACT Triflex

Self-as-context (a.k.a the noticing self) and contacting the present moment both involve flexibly paying attention to and engaging in your here-and-now experience (in other words, "Be present").

Defusion and acceptance are about separating from thoughts and feelings, seeing them for what they truly are, making room for them, and allowing them to come and go of their own accord (in other words, "Open up").

Values and committed action involve initiating and sustaining life-enhancing action (in other words, "Do what matters").

So we can describe psychological flexibility as the ability to "be present, open up, and do what matters."

Now that you have a sense of the six core processes and how we can chunk them into three larger units, I want to introduce you to my all-time-favorite ACT tool, which brings them all together in an easy-to-understand and simple-to-use format.

Welcome to the Choice Point

When I wrote the first edition of *ACT Made Simple* in 2009, the choice point didn't exist. It was only in 2013 that I cocreated this tool with my colleagues Joe Ciarrochi and Ann Bailey (for the book we were writing on an ACT approach to weight loss: *The Weight Escape* [Ciarrochi, Bailey, & Harris, 2014]). Since then, I've fallen in love with the choice point and I now make it the central tool in all my training. Why? Because it gives you and your clients a simple map to follow, while retaining the great flexibility of the ACT model.

You'll see throughout this book there are many ways we can use the choice point, but for now I just want to give you a brief introduction. One of the beauties of the choice point is that it provides a clear overview of the ACT model. (Note: the choice point has similarities with but also significant differences from a popular ACT tool called the matrix [Polk & Schoendorff, 2014]; see Extra Bits for an explanation.) As I take you through it, I'm going to use the same nontechnical language that I use with clients because I want to achieve two things simultaneously: (a) simply explaining the ACT model to you and (b) demonstrating how you can explain ACT to your clients.

The choice point is a tool that rapidly maps out problems, identifies sources of suffering, and formulates an ACT approach to handling them. We can bring it in at any stage of therapy and use it for many different purposes. I often introduce it for the first time about halfway through my first session with a new client, as part of informed consent (chapter 5). Typically, it would go something like this:

Therapist: Would it be okay with you if I take a few moments to draw something? It's kind of a road map for helping us work together effectively. (*Therapist produces a pen and a sheet of paper.*) So you and I, and everyone else on the planet, we're always doing stuff. We're eating, drinking, walking, talking, sleeping, playing—always doing something. Even if we're just staring at the wall, that's still doing something, right? And some of these things we do are pretty useful; they help us move toward a better life. So I call them "towards moves." Towards moves are basically the things you want to start or do more of, if our work here is successful.

While saying this, the therapist draws an arrow and writes:

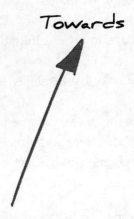

The therapist continues: So when we're doing towards moves, that means we're acting effectively, behaving like the sort of person we want to be, doing stuff that's likely to make life more meaningful and fulfilling. The problem is, that's not all we do. There are other things we do that have the opposite effect: they take us away from the life we really want to build. So I like to call these "away moves." When we do away moves, that means we're acting ineffectively, behaving unlike the sort of person we want to be, doing stuff that tends to make life worse in the long term. So basically, away moves are anything you will stop doing or do less of if our work here is successful.

While saying this, the therapist draws a second arrow and writes:

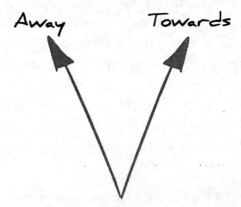

The therapist now continues: And this applies to us all, right? All day long we're all doing towards and away moves, and it changes from moment to moment. And when life isn't too hard, when things are going okay, when we're getting what we want in life, it's a lot easier to choose those towards moves. But as you know, life isn't like that a lot of the time. Life is tough, and a lot of the time we don't get what we want. So throughout the day, we're going to encounter all sorts of difficult situations, and difficult thoughts and feelings are going to show up.

At the bottom of the diagram, the therapist now writes, "Situation(s), Thoughts & Feelings." (Note: throughout this book, the term "thoughts and feelings" is used as shorthand for thoughts, feelings, emotions, memories, urges, impulses, images, and sensations. Any or all of these private experiences can be mentioned or written down on the choice point.)

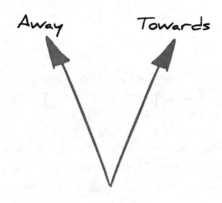

The therapist continues: The problem is, the default setting for most of us is that when these difficult thoughts and feelings show up, we tend to get "hooked" by them. They kind of hook us, and they reel us in, and they jerk us around, and they pull us all over the place. You know what I mean? They might hook us physically, so we start acting out in various ways with our arms and our legs and our mouth. Or they might hook our attention, so instead of focusing on what we're doing, we get lost in our inner world. And the more tightly we're hooked…the more we do those away moves, right?

The therapist now writes "Hooked" alongside the "Away" arrow.

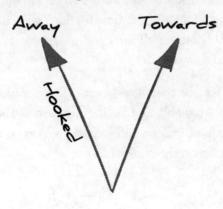

The therapist continues: So everyone does this stuff to some extent; that's normal. No one's perfect. But if this kind of thing happens a lot, it creates big problems. In fact, almost every psychological problem that we know of—anxiety, depression, addiction, you name it—boils down to this basic process: we get hooked by difficult thoughts and feelings and we start doing away moves. Does that make sense?

However, there are times when we are able to unhook ourselves from these difficult thoughts and feelings and do some towards moves instead. And the better we get at doing this…well, the better life gets.

While saying this, the therapist writes "Unhooked" alongside the "Towards" arrow.

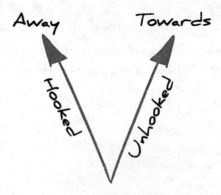

The therapist now draws a little circle at the point where the arrows converge. (If desired, she can write in the words "choice point" or the initials "CP.") While doing this, she continues: So when we're in these challenging situations, and these difficult thoughts and feelings are showing up, there's a choice for us to make: how are we going to respond to this? The more hooked we get, the more likely we are to do away moves. But the more we can unhook ourselves, the easier it is to do towards moves.

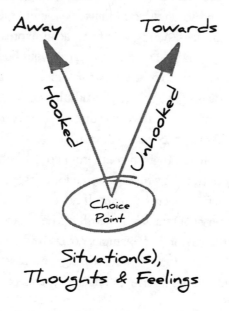

The therapist continues: So if we want to get good at doing this (*points to the towards arrow*), we need to do two things: We need to learn some unhooking skills. And we need to get clear about what towards moves we want to make. Once that's in place, we've got a lot more choice about how we're going to respond to all of this difficult stuff life is giving us. And that's basically what this type of therapy is all about: learning how to unhook from this stuff (*points to "Thoughts & Feelings"*), cut back on this stuff (*points to away moves*), and help you to get better at doing this stuff (*points to towards moves*).

Tricky Terminology   Some ACT practitioners use the term "hooked" to mean cognitive fusion only. The choice point uses the term in a broader sense to mean both cognitive fusion and experiential avoidance. We'll explore this more in chapter 2.

The "Bare Bones" Choice Point

What you've just read is a "bare bones" summary of the choice point: a generic overview with no specific details. Ideally, you'd want to put a lot of flesh on that skeleton: make it personal for the client, with specific examples of her difficult thoughts and feelings, the difficult situations she faces, her away moves, and her towards moves. As you progress through the book, I'll show you how to flesh this diagram out. For now, I just want to flag three important points:

1. **The choice point includes overt and covert behavior.** In ACT, we define behavior as "anything that a whole being does." Yes, you read that correctly: anything that a whole being does is behavior. This includes overt behaviors such as eating, drinking, walking, talking, watching *Game of Thrones*, and so on. *Overt behavior* basically means physical behavior: actions you take with your arms, legs, hands, and feet; facial expressions; everything you say, sing, shout, or whisper; how you move, eat, drink, breathe; your body posture; and so on. However, the term "behavior" also refers to *covert behavior*, which basically means psychological behavior, such as thinking, focusing, visualizing, mindfulness, imagining, and remembering. (This inner psychological behavior can never be directly observed by others, so it's often called "private behavior" rather than "covert behavior.")

    Here's a simple way to distinguish overt from covert behavior. Suppose a video camera magically appears out of thin air while the behavior is happening. Could that camera record the behavior? If yes, then it's overt behavior. If no, it's covert behavior.

    As you'll see in later chapters, when we fill in the choice point with a client, we include both overt and covert behavior. For example, covert away moves might include rumination, worrying, disengaging, losing focus, and obsessing, and covert towards moves might include defusing, accepting, refocusing attention, engaging, strategizing, and planning.

2. **The client defines what is an away move.** The choice point always maps things out from the client's perspective. In other words, it's the client who defines what behavior is "away," not the therapist. Early in therapy, a client may see self-defeating or self-destructive behavior as a towards move. For example, a client with an alcohol or gambling addiction may initially class drinking and gambling as towards moves.

    If so, we would not start debating this with the client. We would simply take a moment to clarify: "Can I just check we're using these terms the same way? Away moves are anything you want to stop or do less of if our work here is successful, and towards moves are the things you want to start or do more of if our work here is successful."

    If the client still labels the self-defeating behavior as "towards," then we acknowledge that and write it down alongside the towards arrow. Why? Because this is a snapshot of the *client's* life *as he or she currently sees it*, not as the therapist sees it. Our aim is to get a sense of the *client's* worldview, the *client's* level of self-awareness: what the client see as problems, and what he doesn't. So if we challenge the client at this point, try to get him to change his mind and see this destructive or self-defeating behavior as an away move, we're likely to get into a fruitless struggle. For now, we put it down as a towards move, and we make a note to ourselves to address this in later sessions.

Initially, we want to find therapy goals that will build the therapeutic alliance, rather than strain it. So we find out what the client *does* see as his away moves, and we use ACT to work with him on those behaviors. Then, later in therapy, once the client has a higher level of psychological flexibility, we can return to the behavior and reassess it: "When you first came to see me, you classed gambling as a towards move; do you still see it that way?" Usually, as therapy progresses and the client's psychological flexibility develops, she will change her mind and class her self-defeating behavior as away—especially when she realizes it is getting in the way of other important life goals.

3. **Any activity can be a towards move or an away move, depending on the context.** When I watch TV primarily to avoid going to the gym or to procrastinate on some other important task, or when I eat a block of chocolate mindlessly to escape boredom or anxiety, I class those as away moves. But when I watch TV as a conscious, values-guided choice that enriches my life (e.g., catching the latest episode of *The Walking Dead*) or when I eat chocolate mindfully, savoring it as part of a celebration with friends, I class those as towards moves. So it's not about the activity we're doing; it's about the effects that activity is having.

   In contexts where an activity takes us toward the life we want, behaving like the person we want to be, it's a towards move; and in contexts where that activity takes us away from the life we want, behaving unlike the person we want to be, it's an away move. If we're writing examples such as these on a choice point, we'd include information to specify when it's towards and when it's away. For example, on my away arrow I'd write "watching TV to avoid important tasks" and on my towards arrow, "watching TV as a balanced lifestyle choice."

The Choice Point, the Hexaflex, and the Triflex

Let's now look at how the hexaflex and triflex processes map onto the choice point.

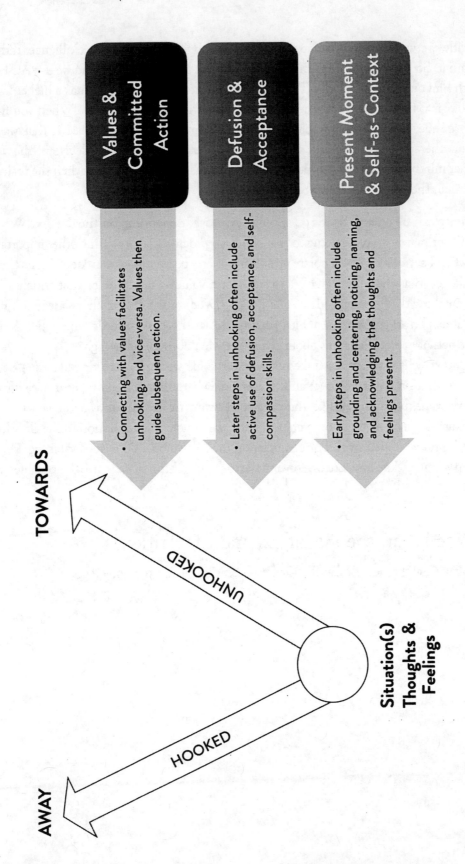

Unhooking skills refers to all four core ACT mindfulness processes: defusion, acceptance, self-as-context, and contacting the present moment. We can use any combination of these processes to "unhook" ourselves from difficult thoughts and feelings, reducing their impact and influence over overt and covert behavior.

Towards moves refer to committed action—physical and psychological—guided by our values.

Hooked refers to two core processes—*cognitive fusion* and *experiential avoidance*—that ACT sees as responsible for most of our psychological suffering. Cognitive fusion basically means we are "dominated" by our cognitions. And experiential avoidance is the ongoing struggle to avoid or get rid of unwanted thoughts and feelings. I'll explore these terms in depth in the next chapter.

Extra Bits

Please download the pdf called *ACT Made Simple: The Extra Bits* from the "Free Stuff" page at http://www.actmindfully.com.au and turn to chapter 1. There you'll find (a) printable versions of the hexaflex, the triflex, and the choice point and (b) a discussion of the main differences between the choice point and the *matrix*.

Skilling Up

Simply reading this book will not give you ACT skills, just as reading a cookbook will not give you cooking skills. If you want to learn to cook well, you gotta practice, practice, practice those skills, and the same goes for ACT. So at the end of most chapters, I'll ask you to do something to build your ACT skills. Here are a few suggestions to get you started:

- Run through the choice point with an imaginary client as if you're an actor rehearsing for a play. Act it out loud, if you're willing to; but if not, do it in your head. Ideally, draw it out as you rehearse it.

- Once you've rehearsed the choice point in private, run through it with a friend or colleague to see if you can summarize what ACT is about.

- After that, give it a go for real with some of your clients.

You may be somewhat reluctant to do this; you may be thinking it's silly, unimportant, or just not your style. However, even if you never do this with a real client, rehearsing it will help you to grasp the ACT model. (Plus it'll also help you enormously if you ever want to explain ACT to curious friends, colleagues, relatives, or guests at your next dinner party.)

Takeaway

ACT is a behavioral therapy that creatively uses values and mindfulness skills to help people build rich and meaningful lives. It is based on six core processes: values, committed action, and the four mindfulness processes of defusion, acceptance, self-as-context, and contacting the present moment. We can chunk these into three larger processes of being present, opening up, and doing what matters. In technical terms, the aim of ACT is to help people develop psychological flexibility: the ability to focus on and engage in what we are doing, to open up and make room for our thoughts and feelings, and to act effectively, guided by our values.

CHAPTER 2

Getting Hooked

What Is a "Mind"?

This is too hard. I can't do this. I wish there was a real therapist here to tell me what to do. Maybe I'm not cut out for this sort of work. I'm so dumb.

Does your mind ever say things like this to you? Mine certainly does. As does the mind of every therapist I've ever known. And what other unhelpful stuff does your mind do? Does it ever compare you harshly to others, or criticize your efforts, or tell you that you can't do the things you want to do? Does it ever dredge up unpleasant memories? Does it find fault with your life as it is today and conjure up alternative lives where you'd be so much happier? Does it ever drag you into scary scenarios about the future and warn you about all the things that might go wrong?

If so, that means your mind is normal. No, that's not a typo. In ACT, we assume that the normal psychological processes of a normal human mind readily become destructive and create psychological suffering for all of us. And ACT speculates that the root of this suffering is human language itself.

Language and the Mind

Human language is a highly complex system of symbols that includes words, images, sounds, facial expressions, and physical gestures. Humans use language in two domains: overt and covert. Overt language includes speaking, talking, miming, gesturing, writing, painting, sculpting, singing, dancing, acting, and so on. Covert language includes thinking, imagining, daydreaming, planning, visualizing, analyzing, worrying, fantasizing, and so on.

The word "mind" refers to an incredibly complex set of interactive cognitive processes, which includes analyzing, comparing, evaluating, planning, remembering, visualizing, and so on. And all of these complex processes rely on the sophisticated system of symbols we call human language. Thus, in ACT, when we use the word "mind," we're using it as a metaphor for "human language."

The Mind Is a Double-Edged Sword

The human mind is a double-edged sword. On the bright side, it helps us make maps and models of the world, predict and plan for the future, share knowledge, learn from the past, imagine and create things that have never existed, develop rules that guide our behavior effectively and help us to thrive as a community, communicate with people who are far away, and learn from people who are no longer alive.

On the dark side, we use it to lie, manipulate, and deceive; to spread libel, slander, and ignorance; to incite hatred, prejudice, and violence; to make weapons of mass destruction and industries of mass pollution; to dwell on and "relive" painful events from the past; to scare ourselves by imagining unpleasant futures; to compare, judge, criticize, and condemn both ourselves and others; and to create rules for ourselves that can often be life-constricting or destructive.

This "dark side" of the mind is completely normal and natural, and a source of suffering for just about everyone. And if we dare to explore the dark side (can you tell I'm a *Star Wars* fan?), we will soon encounter the surreptitious siblings of psychological suffering: cognitive fusion and experiential avoidance.

Cognitive Fusion

Cognitive fusion—usually shortened to *fusion*—basically means that our cognitions dominate our behavior (overt or covert) in a manner that is self-defeating or problematic. In other words, our cognitions have a negative influence on our actions and our awareness.

> **Tricky Terminology**   In ACT, the term "cognition" refers to any and all categories of thinking—including beliefs, ideas, attitudes, assumptions, fantasies, memories, images, and schemas—as well as to aspects of feelings and emotions. Many models of therapy set up an artificial distinction between cognition and emotion, as if they are separate entities. But if we explore any emotion—sadness, anger, guilt, fear, love, joy, you name it—we will find the experience "saturated" in cognition; there will be a wealth of images, thoughts, ideas, meanings, impressions, or memories "mixed in" with all the physical impulses, urges, and sensations in the body. This is why you'll often hear me talking about fusion with "thoughts and feelings."

With clients I only use the term "fusion" if they already know it prior to therapy. Mostly, I talk about "getting hooked"—a useful term that covers both fusion *and* experiential avoidance. We can talk about how our thoughts and feelings "hook" us: they hook our attention, reel us in, jerk us around, and pull us off track.

Two Main Ways That Fusion Shows Up

Cognitive fusion manifests in two main ways:

1. **Our cognitions dominate our physical *actions* in problematic ways.** In response to our cognitions, we say and do things that are ineffective for building the life we want. For example, in response to the thought *No one likes me*, I cancel going to an important social event.

2. **Our cognitions dominate our *awareness* in problematic ways.** In other words, we get "pulled into" or "lost in" our cognitions so that our awareness is reduced and we are no longer paying attention in an effective way. For example, I get so "caught up" in worrying or ruminating, I can't keep my attention on the important tasks I need to do at work, and I start making lots of mistakes.

There's a general consensus in ACT that the term "fusion" should only be used if and when the process gives rise to problematic, self-defeating behavior. In other words, if in response to our cognitions, our overt or covert behavior becomes narrow, rigid, and inflexible to an extent that is ineffective and self-defeating (e.g., makes life worse in the long term, impairs health and well-being, pulls us away from our values), then we would use the term "fusion." But if not, we wouldn't.

For example, if I'm "lost in my thoughts" in a way that is life-enhancing—such as daydreaming while lying on the beach on holiday, or mentally rehearsing an important speech at an appropriate time—we'd call that "absorption" rather than fusion.

I'll now introduce you to one of my favorite metaphors to briefly convey the concepts of fusion and defusion. I'm going to have you do the exercise part by part so you can experience it for yourself.

The Hands as Thoughts and Feelings Metaphor

[Note to readers: Read through this first paragraph, and then put this book down so you can use both your hands. Act out the exercise as if you are the client following the therapist's instructions.]

Therapist: Imagine for a moment that your hands are your thoughts and feelings. Look all around you and imagine that what you see represents everything that's important in your life. Then hold your hands together, palms open, as if they're the pages of an open book. Then slowly and steadily—take about five seconds to do this—raise your hands up toward your face. Keep going until they're covering your eyes. Then take a few seconds to look once more all around you (through the gaps in between your fingers) and notice how this affects your view of the world.

[Please do this part now, before reading on.]

* * *

Therapist: So what would it be like going around all day with your hands covering your eyes in this manner? How much would it limit you? How much would you miss out on? How would it reduce your ability to respond to the world around you? This is what I mean by "getting hooked": we get so caught up in our thoughts and feelings that we miss out on life and we can't act effectively.

[Now once again, when you reach the end of this paragraph, please do this next part of the exercise.]

Therapist: Now cover your eyes with your hands again, but this time, lower them from your face very, very slowly. And as the distance between your hands and your face increases, notice how much easier it is to connect with the world around you.

[Please do this now before reading on.]

Therapist: This is what I call "unhooking." How much easier is it now to take effective action? How much more information can you take in? How much more connected are you with the world around you?

* * *

This metaphor (Harris, 2009a) demonstrates the two main purposes of defusion: to engage fully in our experience and to facilitate effective action. (A quick note: the aim of defusion is not to get rid of unwanted thoughts and feelings or to make ourselves feel better. These things often happen as a result of defusion, but as we'll explore later, in ACT, we consider that a bonus or by-product, not the main intention.)

A Quick Summary of Fusion vs. Defusion

When we fuse with a cognition, it can seem like:

- something we have to obey, give in to, or act upon;

- a threat we need to avoid or get rid of; or

- something very important that requires all our attention.

When we defuse from that cognition, we can see it for what it is: a group of words or pictures "inside our head." We can recognize that it:

- is not something we have to obey, give in to, or act upon;

- is definitely not a threat to us; and

- may or may not be important—we have a choice as to how much attention we pay it.

Workability

The whole ACT model rests on a key concept: *workability*. Please engrave that word—workability—into your cerebral cortex, because it underpins every intervention we do. To determine workability, we ask this question: "Is what you're doing working to give you the sort of life you want, in the long term?" If the answer is yes, then we say it's "workable," so there's no need to change it. And if the answer is no, then we say it's "unworkable," in which case, we can consider alternatives that may work better.

Thus, in ACT, we don't focus on whether a thought is true or false, but whether it is workable. In other words, we want to know if a thought helps a client move toward a richer, fuller, and more meaningful life. To determine this, we may ask questions like "If you let this thought guide your behavior, will that help you create a richer, fuller, and more meaningful life?" "If you hold on to this thought tightly, does it help you to be the person you want to be and do the things you want to do?"

EXPLORING WORKABILITY IN SESSION

Here's a transcript that exemplifies this approach:

Client: But it's true. I really am fat. Look at me. (*The client grabs hold of two large rolls of fat from around his abdomen and squeezes them to emphasize the point.*)

Therapist: Okay, can I share something very important? In this room, we're never going to debate whether or not your thoughts are true or false. What we're interested in here is whether your thoughts are useful or helpful—whether they help you to live a better life. So when your mind starts telling you *I'm fat*, those thoughts really hook you, right? And once you're hooked, what happens next?

Client: I feel disgusted with myself.

Therapist: Okay. And then what?

Client: Then I get depressed.

Therapist: So it snowballs pretty rapidly. You get all these difficult thoughts and feelings showing up for you: depression, disgust, "I'm fat," and so on. And when you get hooked by that lot, what do you do then?

Client: What do you mean?

Therapist: Well, if I were watching a video of you at home, when you're hooked by all those difficult thoughts and feelings, what would I see? What would I see or hear you doing on that video that would show me "Aha! Steve's really hooked by this stuff right now"?

Client: I'd probably be sitting in front of the TV and eating chocolate or pizza.

Therapist: And that's not what you want to be doing?

Client: Of course not! I'm trying to lose weight! Look at this. (*He slaps his abdomen.*) It's disgusting.

Therapist: So when you get hooked by "I'm fat," you do things that take you away from the sort of life you want?

Client: Yes, but it's true! I am fat!

Therapist: Well, as I said, in this type of therapy, we don't get into whether a thought is true or false. What we want to know is, does it help you move toward the life you want? In other words, when you get hooked by these thoughts, does that help you to exercise, or eat well, or spend time doing the things that make life rich and rewarding?

Client: No. Of course not. But I can't help it!

Therapist: That's right. At this point in time, you can't help it. Those thoughts and feelings show up and they hook you instantly, before you even know it. So what if we could do something to change that? Would you like to learn a new skill—an "unhooking" skill—so that next time your mind starts beating you up with "I'm fat," you can unhook from it?

* * *

When we use the basic framework of workability, we never need to judge a client's behavior as "good" or "bad," "right" or "wrong"; instead we can ask, nonjudgmentally and compassionately, "Is this working to give you the life you want?" Likewise, we never need to judge thoughts as irrational, dysfunctional, or negative, or debate whether they're true or false. Instead we can simply ask questions such as:

- How does it work in the long run, if you let that belief/idea/rule run your life/dictate what you do/guide your actions?

- If you get all caught up in/hooked by those thoughts, does that help you to do the things you want?

- If you let those thoughts guide you, does that help you to be the person you want to be?

Note that in the transcript above, the therapist makes no attempt to change the content of the thoughts. In ACT, the content of a thought is rarely considered problematic; it's usually fusion with the thought that creates the problem. In many psychology textbooks, you'll discover this quote from William Shakespeare: "There is nothing either good or bad, but thinking makes it so." The ACT stance would be fundamentally different: "Thinking does not make anything good or bad, but fusion with your thinking creates problems."

On a separate note, did you notice how the therapist responded when the client said, "But I can't help it!"? Our clients will often say thing like this, especially when it comes to impulsive, addictive, or aggressive behaviors. And when they do, we want to validate it and say something like "That's right. At this point in time, you can't help it. These thoughts and feelings hook you instantly and jerk you around like a puppet on a string." We can then go on to ask, "So would you like to change that?" If the client answers yes, we can then invite her to learn some new skills, as at the end of the transcript above. ("That's all very well, Russ," I hear you say, "but what if the client answers no or says, 'That's not possible'?" We'll explore those questions in later chapters.)

WORKABILITY AND THE CHOICE POINT

As you know (unless you skipped chapter 1, in which case our specially trained sniffer dogs will track you down and then tickle you mercilessly until you promise never to skip a chapter again), I'm a big fan of the choice point, and one of the reasons for this is that it makes it easy to use the concept of workability with clients. Let's revisit the session above and see how it would go if the therapist were mapping it out on a choice point. We'll assume the therapist has already introduced the choice point as covered in chapter 1, and we'll start about halfway through the previous transcript.

Client: Then I get depressed.

Therapist: Okay. So it seems like it snowballs. Would it be okay if I jot some of this down, so we can get a better handle on it? (*The therapist can write on her hand-drawn choice point, or, if preferred, can use a fresh preprinted worksheet, as in the figures below.*) So you get all these difficult thoughts and feelings showing up for you: "I'm fat," disgust, depression, and so on. (*While saying this, the therapist writes key words at the bottom of the choice point, as shown below.*)

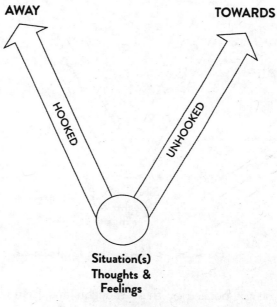

"I'm fat," self-disgust, depressed.

Therapist: And this stuff hooks you straight away, right?

Client: You bet!

Therapist: So if I were watching a video of you at home, what would I see or hear you doing that would show me "Aha! Steve's really hooked by this stuff right now"?

Client: I'd probably be sitting in front of the TV and eating chocolate or pizza.

Therapist: Okay. And would that be a towards move or an away move?

Client: Err, remind me what those words mean again?

Therapist: Sure. Towards moves mean stuff we do that helps us build the sort of life we want: doing stuff that's effective, making life better, acting like the sort of person we really want to be. Things you'll start or do more of if our work here is successful. And away moves are the opposite: all the stuff we do that takes us away from the life we want, keeps us stuck, or makes our problems worse—what you'll stop or do less of if our work here is successful.

Client: Gotcha. It's definitely an away move!

Therapist: Okay, so I'll just write that in. (*Therapist writes this on the diagram, as shown below.*)

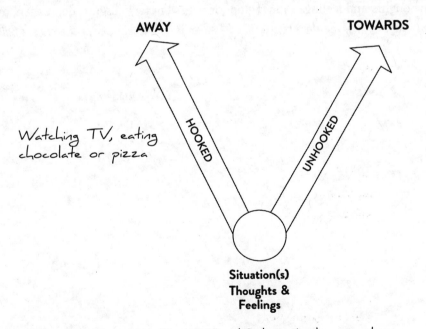

Therapist: So when you get hooked by these thoughts and feelings (*points to the bottom of the diagram*), this is the kind of stuff you tend to do (*points to the away moves*)?

The rest of the transcript would be much the same as the original, leading up to the invitation to learn unhooking skills (i.e., skills based on any of the four ACT mindfulness processes: acceptance, defusion, flexible attention, self-as-context). Note that in each of the transcripts above, the words spoken by the therapist are almost identical. The main difference between them is not the therapist's language but her use of the choice point as a visual reference, to clarify and reinforce the main points of the discussion. Note also that workability is "inbuilt" into the choice point; away moves are unworkable behaviors, and towards moves are workable.

Thoughts and Feelings Aren't the Problem

Did you notice that in the transcripts above, the therapist never describes thoughts and feelings as a problem? The ACT stance is that thoughts and feelings are not problematic in and of themselves; it's only when we respond to them in rigid, inflexible ways, such as fusion and avoidance, that they have problematic effects.

In a context of fusion and (excessive) experiential avoidance, thoughts and feelings readily become pathological or life-distorting. But if we respond to them flexibly—with defusion, acceptance, flexible attention, or self-as-context—then in this new context of mindfulness, those very same thoughts and feelings function differently. For sure, they may still be painful or unpleasant, but they no longer function in a way that impairs well-being or quality of life.

The therapist gently paves the way for the client to discover this radically new viewpoint through constructive use of the word "hooked": "So *when you get hooked by* these thoughts and feelings, you start doing XYZ." This way of speaking lays a good foundation for later work: in later sessions, the client will get to experience that he can have those difficult thoughts and feelings but respond to them mindfully, thereby reducing their impact and influence without trying to avoid or get rid of them.

Six Broad Categories of Fusion

If we really wanted to, we could create a huge range of different categories of fusion. But hey, life is short and we all have more important things to do with our time. So to keep it simple, there are six main categories of fusion to look for clinically: fusion with the past, the future, self-concept, reasons, rules, and judgments. (Keep in mind, these are not discrete categories; they all overlap and interconnect.)

Fusion with the past. This refers to all types of past-oriented cognition, including:

- rumination, regret, and dwelling on painful memories (e.g., of failure, hurt, and loss)

- blame and resentment over past events

- idealizing the past: *My life was wonderful before XYZ happened.*

Fusion with the future. This refers to all types of future-oriented cognition, including:

- worrying, catastrophizing

- predicting the worst, hopelessness

- anticipating failure, rejection, hurt, loss, etc.

Fusion with self-concept. This refers to all types of self-descriptive and self-evaluative cognition, including:

- negative self-judgment: *I am bad, unlovable, worthless, dirty, damaged, nothing, broken*

- positive self-judgment: *I am always right, I am better than you*

- overidentifying with a label: *I am borderline, I am depressive, I am alcoholic*

Fusion with reasons. Humans are great at "reason-giving": coming up with reasons for why we can't change, won't change, or shouldn't even have to change. This category includes all such reasons. *I can't do* X *(important action) because…*

- *I'm too* Y *(*Y *= depressed, tired, anxious, etc.)*

- Z *might happen (*Z *= bad outcomes such as failure, rejection, making a fool of myself)*

- *It's pointless, It's too hard, It's scary*

- *I am* B *(*B *= borderline, shy, a loser, or other self-concepts)*

- C *says I shouldn't (*C *= parents, religion, the law, cultural beliefs, workplace, etc.)*

Fusion with rules. This category includes all the "rules" I subscribe to about how I, others, or the world should be. Rules can usually be identified by words like "should," "have to," "must," "ought," "right," "wrong," "fair," or "unfair." And they often specify conditions like *can't until, shouldn't unless, mustn't because, must do this in order to, will not tolerate,* or *refuse to allow.* Here are some examples:

- I must not make mistakes.

- She needs to change before I do.

- I can't go to work when I feel this way.

Fusion with judgments. This category refers to any type of judgment or evaluation, either positive or negative, including judgments about:

- the past and future

- self and others

- our own thoughts and feelings

- our body, our behavior, our life

- the world, places, people, objects, events, and just about anything

These six categories of fusion all overlap and readily interweave into complex narratives like this one: *Because bad things have happened to me* (past), *I am damaged* (self-concept, judgment), *which means I can't do X* (reason-giving), or *so I will never be able to have Y* (future). Keep in mind, these six categories don't cover the entire spectrum of fusion, but they do account for the most common repertoires we encounter in clinical practice.

Experiential Avoidance

Let's now look at the other core process that gets people hooked: *experiential avoidance*. This term refers to our desire to avoid or get rid of unwanted "private experiences" and anything we do to try to make that happen.

Tricky Terminology   A *private experience* means any experience you have that no one else knows about (unless you tell them): thoughts, feelings, memories, images, emotions, urges, impulses, desires, and sensations.

All humans are experientially avoidant to some degree. Why should this be? Well, here's a classic ACT metaphor we can use to explain it to clients.

The Problem-Solving Machine

Therapist: If we had to pick one ability of the human mind that has enabled us to be so successful as a species, it'd have to be problem solving, which basically boils down to this:
A problem is something unwanted. And a solution means we avoid it or get rid of it. Now in the physical world, problem solving often works very well. Got a wolf outside your door? You get rid of it: you throw rocks or spears at it. Or you shoot it. Snow, rain, hail? Well, you can't get rid of those things, but you can avoid them by hiding in a cave, building a shelter, or wearing protective clothes. Dry, arid ground? You can get rid of it by irrigation and fertilization, or you can avoid it by moving to a better location.

So the human mind is like a problem-solving machine, and it's very good at its job. And given that problem solving works so well in the material world, it's only natural that our mind tries to do the same with our inner world: the world of thoughts, feelings, memories, sensations, and urges. But unfortunately, when we try to avoid or get rid of unwanted thoughts or feelings, it often doesn't work—or if it does, we end up creating a lot of new problems that make life even harder.

How Experiential Avoidance Increases Suffering

We'll return to the Problem-Solving Machine metaphor in later chapters. For now, let's consider how experiential avoidance increases suffering. Addictions provide an obvious example. Many addictions begin as an attempt to avoid or get rid of unwanted thoughts and feelings such as boredom, loneliness, anxiety, guilt, anger, and sadness. In the short run, gambling, drugs, alcohol, and cigarettes will often help people to avoid or get rid of these feelings temporarily, but over time, a huge amount of pain and suffering results.

The more time and energy we spend trying to avoid or get rid of unwanted private experiences, the more we're likely to suffer psychologically in the long run. Anxiety disorders provide another good example. It's not the presence of anxiety that creates an anxiety disorder. After all, anxiety is a normal human emotion that we all experience. At the core of any anxiety disorder lies excessive experiential avoidance: a life dominated by trying very hard to avoid or get rid of anxiety. For example, suppose I feel anxious in social situations, and in order to avoid those feelings of anxiety, I stop socializing. My anxiety gets deeper and more acute, and now I have "social phobia." There's an obvious short-term benefit of avoiding social situations—I get to avoid some anxious thoughts and feelings—but the long-term cost is huge: I become isolated, my life "gets smaller," and I find myself stuck in a vicious cycle.

Alternatively, I may try to reduce my anxiety in social situations by playing the role of "good listener." I become very empathic and caring toward others, and I discover lots of information about the thoughts, feelings, and desires of the people I talk to, but I reveal little or nothing of myself. This helps in the short run to reduce my fear of being judged or rejected, but in the long run, it means my relationships lack intimacy, openness, and authenticity.

Now suppose I take Valium, or some other mood-altering substance, to reduce my anxiety. Again, the short-term benefit is obvious: less anxiety. But long-term costs of relying on benzodiazepines, antidepressants, marijuana, or alcohol to reduce my anxiety could include (a) psychological dependence on the substance, (b) physical addiction, (c) physical and emotional side effects, (d) financial costs, and (e) failure to learn more effective responses to anxiety, which therefore maintains or exacerbates the issue.

Still another way I might respond to social anxiety would be to grit my teeth and socialize despite my anxiety—that is, to tolerate the feelings even though I'm distressed by them. From an ACT perspective, this too would be experiential avoidance. Why? Because, although I'm not avoiding the situation, I'm still struggling with my feelings and desperately hoping they'll go away. This is tolerance, not acceptance.

There's a big difference between tolerance and acceptance. Would you want the people you love to *tolerate* you while you're present, hoping you'll soon go away and frequently checking to see if you've gone yet? Or would you prefer them to completely and totally *accept* you as you are with all your flaws and foibles, and to be willing to have you around for as long as you choose to stay?

The cost of tolerating my social anxiety (that is, gritting my teeth and putting up with it) is that it takes a huge amount of effort and energy, which makes it hard to fully engage in social interaction. As a consequence, I miss out on much of the pleasure and fulfillment that commonly accompanies socializing. And this in turn increases my anxiety about future social events because "I won't enjoy it" or "I'll feel awful" or "It's too much effort."

Sadly, the more importance we place on avoiding anxiety, the more we develop anxiety about our anxiety. It's a vicious cycle, found at the center of any anxiety disorder. (After all, what is at the core of a panic attack, if not anxiety about anxiety?) Indeed, attempts to avoid unwanted thoughts and feelings can often paradoxically increase them. For example, research shows that suppression of unwanted thoughts can lead to a rebound effect: an increase in both intensity and frequency of the unwanted thoughts (Wenzlaff & Wegner, 2000). Other studies show that trying to suppress a mood can actually intensify it in a self-amplifying loop (Feldner, Zvolensky, Eifert, & Spira, 2003; Wegner, Erber, & Zanakos, 1993).

A large and growing body of research shows that higher experiential avoidance is associated with anxiety disorders, excessive worrying, depression, poorer work performance, higher levels of substance abuse, lower quality of life, high-risk sexual behavior, borderline personality disorder, greater severity of posttraumatic stress disorder (PTSD), long-term disability, and higher degrees of overall psychopathology (Hayes, Masuda, Bissett, Luoma, & Guerrero, 2004).

It's hardly surprising then that a core component of most ACT protocols involves getting the client in touch with the costs and futility of experiential avoidance. This is often an essential first step to pave the way for a radically different agenda: *experiential acceptance*. Of course, although we want to facilitate mindful, values-based living, we don't want to turn into…

Mindfulness Fascists

We are not "mindfulness fascists" in ACT; we don't insist that people must always be in the present moment, always defused, always accepting. That would be ridiculous. Experiential avoidance is not inherently "bad" or "pathological"; it's normal. We only target it when it's excessive, rigid, or inappropriate, to such an extent that it's getting in the way of a rich and meaningful life.

So in ACT textbooks when we talk about experiential avoidance as problematic or pathological, we don't mean *all* experiential avoidance; we mean excessive, rigid, inappropriate experiential avoidance. In other words, it's all about workability. If we take aspirin from time to time in order to get rid of a headache, that's experiential avoidance, but it's workable—that is, it improves our quality of life in the long run.

If we drink one glass of red wine at night primarily to get rid of tension and stress, that too is experiential avoidance—but unless we have certain medical conditions, it's not likely to be harmful, toxic, or life-distorting. However, if we drink two entire bottles of red wine each night, that's a different story.

A Very Important Point About Acceptance vs. Avoidance

In ACT, we do not advocate acceptance of *all* thoughts and feelings under *all* circumstances. That would be not only very rigid but also quite unnecessary. ACT advocates experiential acceptance under two circumstances:

1. when avoidance of thoughts and feelings is limited or impossible

2. when avoidance of thoughts and feelings *is* possible, but the methods used make life worse in the long term

If experiential avoidance is possible and assists you in living your values, then go for it. *Please remember this point.* Many ACT newbies get the impression that all experiential avoidance is bad, or experiential avoidance is the opposite of living by your values. Not so!

How Fusion Gives Rise to Experiential Avoidance

When experiential avoidance becomes excessive, it's largely due to fusion with two categories of thinking: *judgments* and *rules*. Our mind judges our difficult thoughts and feelings as "bad" and formulates the rule "I have to get rid of them!" Often this happens faster than the speed of conscious thought; as soon as difficult thoughts and feelings arise, we instantly start trying to avoid or get rid of them. (So it might help you to think of excessive experiential avoidance as a by-product of fusion with this rule: "These thoughts and feelings are bad, so I have to get rid of them.")

In summary, then, fusion is the overarching pathological process in ACT, and experiential avoidance is one of the many problems that fusion can cause. So if you're ever doing a case formulation and trying to figure out "Is this fusion or avoidance?" the answer is usually: it's both! For example, a client may drink alcohol motivated by both the desire to avoid anxiety (experiential avoidance) and fusion with "I need a beer."

This overlap between processes is why I use the term "hooked" to refer to *both* fusion *and* avoidance. To flesh this out, I often refer to two different modes of being hooked: automatic mode and avoidance mode.

Automatic mode means that in a state of fusion, we automatically obey our thoughts and feelings; we do whatever our cognitions tell us to do. We fuse with our angry cognitions, and we act aggressively. We fuse with our anxious cognitions, and we act fearfully. We fuse with the cognitive elements of our urges and cravings, and we do whatever it is they urge us to do—take drugs, smoke cigarettes, overeat, and so on.

Avoidance mode means that in a state of fusion, we do whatever we can to avoid or get rid of unwanted thoughts and feelings. What dominates our behavior are efforts to avoid or get rid these difficult inner experiences: in other words, experiential avoidance.

When we are hooked by thoughts and feelings, we may go into automatic mode, avoidance mode, or, commonly, both at once.

The Six Core Pathological Processes of Psychological Rigidity

The core pathological processes of ACT, as shown in the figure below, are fusion, experiential avoidance, inflexible attention, remoteness from values, unworkable action, and fusion with self-concept. Any or all of these processes can give rise to psychological rigidity. You can think of these as the "flip sides" of the core therapeutic processes of psychological flexibility. As we go through them, I'll provide examples of clients with clinical depression to illustrate each process.

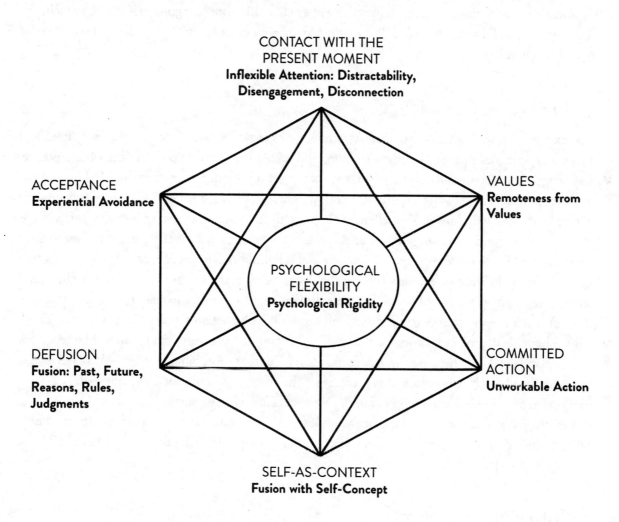

An ACT Model of Psychopathology

Fusion

As you know, fusion means our thoughts dominate our physical actions and our awareness to a problematic extent. In a state of depression, for example, clients may fuse with all sorts of unhelpful thoughts: *I'm bad, I don't deserve any better, I can't change, I've always been this way, Life sucks, It's all too hard, Therapy won't work, It'll never get any better, I can't get out of bed when I feel this way*, or *I'm too tired to do anything*. They also often fuse with painful memories of rejection, disappointment, failure, or abuse. (Extreme fusion with a memory—to such an extent that it seems to be reality, happening right here and now—is commonly called a "flashback.") In clinical depression, fusion often manifests as worrying, ruminating, trying to figure out "why I'm like this," or an ongoing negative commentary: *This party sucks. I'd rather be in bed. What's the point of even being here? They're all having such a good time. No one really wants me here.*

Experiential Avoidance

Experiential avoidance—the ongoing attempt to get rid of, avoid, or escape from unwanted private experiences such as thoughts, feelings, and memories—is the very opposite of acceptance. Depressed clients commonly try very hard to avoid or get rid of painful emotions and feelings such as anxiety, sadness, fatigue, anger, guilt, loneliness, lethargy, and so on. Let's take the commonplace example of social withdrawal. Your client is planning to go to her best friend's birthday party, but as the time draws near, she fuses with thoughts such as *I'm boring, I'm a burden, I've got nothing to say, I won't enjoy it, I'm too tired*, or *I can't be bothered*, plus painful memories of recent social events that haven't gone well. She has feelings of anxiety, which grow ever stronger as the hour approaches, until she is consumed by a sense of dread. So she calls her friend and says she's feeling too sick to come. And in that moment, there's instant relief: all those difficult thoughts and feelings instantly disappear. The relief doesn't last for long, of course. A short while later she's fused with self-hatred: *Look what a loser I am! Can't even go to my best friend's party*. But that short burst of relief—that brief escape from her dread—is highly reinforcing; it increases the chance of future social withdrawal.

Fusion and avoidance go hand in hand. Our clients fuse with all sorts of painful cognitions (e.g., ruminating, worrying, self-criticism, or memories of failure and disappointment) while simultaneously trying to avoid or get rid of them (e.g., through drugs, alcohol, cigarettes, watching TV, or sleeping excessively).

Inflexible Attention

Contacting the present moment, or flexible attention, means the ability to make full conscious contact with both your inner and outer worlds and to narrow, broaden, shift, or sustain your focus, depending upon what's most useful. Its inverse, *inflexible attention*, refers to a wide range of deficits in this ability, especially the "three Ds": distractibility, disengagement, and disconnection.

DISTRACTIBILITY

Distractibility refers to difficulty sustaining one's attention on the task or activity at hand; attention easily shifts to other stimuli that aren't relevant. The more distracted we are during any task or activity, the more poorly we will perform and the less satisfying it will be.

DISENGAGEMENT

Disengagement refers to the many different ways we lose conscious interest or involvement in our experience: going through the motions; doing things mindlessly, on autopilot, or in a bored, disinterested, or absentminded manner.

DISCONNECTION

Disconnection is a term I use to describe a lack of conscious contact with our own thoughts and feelings. If we aren't able to notice how we are thinking or what we are feeling, then we lack self-awareness, so it's much harder to change our behavior in adaptive ways. We are prone to emotional dysregulation and impulsive, reactive, or mindless behavior.

We commonly see all of the three Ds—distractibility, disengagement, and disconnection from thoughts and feelings—not just in clients with depression, but across the entire spectrum of clinical issues.

Remoteness from Values

As our behavior becomes increasingly driven by fusion and experiential avoidance, our values often get lost, neglected, or forgotten. And if we're not clear about our values, or not able to contact them, we can't use them as an effective guide for our actions. As an example, clients who are depressed often lose touch with their values around caring, connection, and contribution; being productive and helpful; self-care; playfulness; intimacy; reliability; and so on.

Our aim in ACT is to bring behavior increasingly under the influence of values rather than of fusion or avoidance. Consider the differences between going to work under these three conditions:

- motivated by fusion with beliefs such as *I have to do this job. It's all I'm capable of.*

- motivated by experiential avoidance: to avoid "feeling like a loser" or to escape unpleasant feelings due to marital tension at home

- motivated by values such as caring, connection, and contribution

Which form of motivation is likely to bring the greatest sense of vitality, meaning, and purpose?

Unworkable Action

The term "unworkable action" (or "away moves") describes patterns of behavior that pull us away from mindful, values-based living. This includes action that's impulsive, reactive, or automatic (as opposed to mindful, considered, or purposeful); action persistently motivated by fusion or experiential avoidance (rather than by values); or inaction or procrastination where effective action is required. Common examples of unworkable action in cases of depression (and many other disorders) include using drugs or alcohol excessively; withdrawing socially; ceasing previously enjoyable activities; sleeping, watching TV, or gaming excessively; and attempting suicide.

Fusion with Self-Concept

We all have a story about who we are. This story is complex and multilayered. It includes objective facts (e.g., name, age, sex, marital status, occupation), descriptions and evaluations of the roles we play, our strengths and weaknesses, our likes and dislikes, and our hopes, dreams, and aspirations. If we hold this story lightly, it can help us to define who we are and what we want in life.

But when we fuse with our self-concept, it seems as if all those self-descriptive thoughts are the very essence of who we are. We lose the ability to step back and see this self-concept as nothing more or less than a complex cognitive construction, a rich tapestry of words and images. (Many ACT textbooks refer to such fusion with the somewhat confusing term "self-as-content.")

In depression, clients generally fuse with a very negative self-concept: *I am bad/worthless/ hopeless/ unlovable* and so on. However, you may also get "positive" elements in there—for example, *I'm a strong person; I shouldn't be reacting like this* or *I'm a good person; why is this happening to me?*

Who Is ACT Suitable For?

Therapists often ask me, "Who is ACT suitable for?" My reply is "Can you think of anyone it's not suitable for?" Who wouldn't benefit from being more psychologically present; more in touch with their values; more able to make room for the inevitable pain of life; more able to defuse from unhelpful thoughts, beliefs, and memories; more able to take effective action in the face of emotional discomfort; more able to engage fully in what they're doing; and more able to appreciate each moment of their life, no matter how they're feeling? Psychological flexibility brings all these benefits, and more. ACT therefore seems relevant to just about everyone.

Of course, if people have significant deficits in their ability to use language, such as some people with severe autism, acquired brain injury, or other disabilities, then ACT may be of limited use. However, RFT (relational frame theory) has all sorts of useful applications for these populations.

ACT has been scientifically studied and shown to be effective with a wide range of conditions including anxiety, depression, obsessive-compulsive disorder, social phobia, generalized anxiety disorder, schizophrenia, borderline personality disorder, workplace stress, chronic pain, drug use, psychological adjustment to cancer, epilepsy, weight control, smoking cessation, and self-management of diabetes (Bach & Hayes, 2002; Bond & Bunce, 2000; Branstetter, Wilson, Hildebrandt, & Mutch, 2004; Brown et al., 2008; Dahl, Wilson, & Nilsson, 2004; Dalrymple & Herbert, 2007; Gaudiano & Herbert, 2006; Gifford et al., 2004; Gratz & Gunderson, 2006; Gregg, Callaghan, Hayes, & Glenn-Lawson, 2007; Hayes, Bissett, et al., 2004; Hayes, Masuda, et al., 2004; Lundgren, Dahl, Yardi, & Melin, 2008; Ossman, Wilson, Storaasli, & McNeill, 2006; Tapper et al., 2009; Twohig, Hayes, & Masuda, 2006; Zettle, 2003).

Extra Bits

See chapter 2 in *ACT Made Simple: The Extra Bits* (downloadable from the "Free Stuff" page at http://www.actmindfully.com.au) for the Six Core Pathological Processes worksheet, which you can use in the Skilling Up section, below.

Skilling Up

To help you start thinking in terms of this model, let's do an exercise in case conceptualization:

- Pick one of your clients and find examples of the six core pathological processes outlined in this chapter, which you'll notice all overlap with each other. Use the worksheet from Extra Bits.

- If you get stuck on any heading, don't fret about it, just move on to the next one. And keep in mind there's a lot of overlap between these processes, so if you're wondering, *Is this fusion or avoidance?* then it's probably both, so write it down under both headings. This exercise is purely to get you started. Later on in the book, we'll focus on case conceptualization in more detail. For now, just give it a shot, and see how you do.

- Better still, run through this exercise for two or three clients because (like pretty much everything) with practice, it gets easier.

- And even better still: if you really want to get your head around this approach to human psychopathology, pick two or three disorders in the DSM-5 (*Diagnostic and Statistical Manual of Mental Disorders*, 5th ed.; American Psychiatric Association, 2013) and identify the fusion, avoidance, and unworkable action going on: What kind of cognitive content do people with these disorders fuse with (in terms of past, future, self-concept, reasons, rules, and judgments)? What feelings, urges, sensations, thoughts, and memories are they unwilling to have or actively trying to avoid? What unworkable actions do they typically take? What core values do they lose touch with? What kind of distractibility, disengagement, and disconnection is common?

- Last but not least: run through this exercise on yourself. If you want to learn ACT, the best person to practice on is you. So take some time to do this seriously: identify your own areas of fusion, avoidance, inflexible attention, remoteness from values, and unworkable action. (You may be surprised at what you discover.) The great thing is, the more we apply ACT to our own issues, the better we'll be able to do it with our clients. And when we see that it works in our own life, it gives us not only confidence in the model, but a sense of authenticity in the therapy room.

Takeaway

The ACT model rests on the core concept of workability: is what you are doing working to make your life richer and fuller? The overarching pathological process in ACT is cognitive fusion, of which there are six broad categories: past, future, self-concept, reasons, rules, and judgments. Fusion can give rise to many problems, and one of the most common is experiential avoidance; so when we use the term "hooked" in the choice point, it refers to both fusion and experiential avoidance.

The core pathological processes of cognitive fusion, experiential avoidance, inflexible attention, remoteness from values, unworkable action, and fusion with self-concept can be found to some extent in all humans, which is why ACT sees itself as a model for the human condition.

CHAPTER 3

"Mindfulness" and Other Dodgy Words

ACT and Mindfulness

ACT has been described as an existential, humanistic, transpersonal, client-centered, mindfulness-based, cognitive behavioral therapy. And I think that's a fair description because most of the core ACT processes can be found, to at least some extent, in many other models of therapy. However, there are some big differences between ACT and most other mindfulness-based approaches. So let's consider for a moment...

Where Does "Mindfulness" Come From?

Mindfulness is an ancient concept, found in a wide range of ancient spiritual and religious traditions, including Buddhism, Taoism, Hinduism, Judaism, Islam, and Christianity, as well as in practices such as tai chi and martial arts such as kung fu and aikido. Many books and articles attribute mindfulness to Buddhism, but this is not accurate; Buddhism is 2,600 years old, whereas mindfulness practices go back at least 4,000 years in Yogic, Taoist, and Judaic traditions. (Indeed, Buddhist scriptures clearly state that Buddha learned his mindfulness skills from a Yogi.) Having said that, there's no doubt that the majority of Western mindfulness-based approaches are based on, derived from, or borrow heavily from Buddhism; ACT is a notable exception.

So What IS Mindfulness?

If you read a few books on the subject, you'll find a variety of definitions of mindfulness; there is not one agreed-upon overarching definition. But if you put them all together, they all boil down to this:

Mindfulness is a set of psychological skills for effective living that involves paying attention with openness, curiosity, kindness, and flexibility.

This simple definition tells us five important things.

- First, mindfulness refers to a set of diverse skills. These include everything from accepting painful feelings to savoring pleasurable experiences, from gently observing your thoughts to grounding yourself amid overwhelming emotions. (As you know from reading chapter 1, in ACT, the term "mindfulness" refers to any combination of defusion, acceptance, contacting the present moment, and self-as-context—and to any or all of the skills, methods, practices, tools, and techniques used to instigate and reinforce any or all of these processes.)

- Second, mindfulness is an attention process, not a thinking process. It involves paying attention to your experience, as opposed to being "caught up" in your thoughts.

- Third, mindfulness involves a particular attitude: one of *openness and curiosity*. Even if your experience in this moment is difficult, painful, or unpleasant, you can be open to it and curious about it instead of running from it or fighting with it.

- Fourth, mindfulness involves *flexibility* of attention: the ability to consciously broaden, narrow, sustain, or redirect your focus so you can attend to different aspects of your here-and-now experience, as desired.

- Fifth, mindful attention includes the quality of kindness. It's not like the cold, clinical, detached attention of a scientist dissecting a rat; it's like the warm, caring attention that a loving parent gives to a child.

We can use mindfulness to "wake up," connect with ourselves, and appreciate the fullness of each moment of life. We can use it to improve our self-knowledge—to learn more about how we feel, think, and react. We can use it to connect deeply and intimately with the people we care about, including ourselves. And we can use it to consciously influence our own behavior and increase our range of responses to the world we live in. It is the art of living consciously—a profound way to enhance psychological resilience and increase life satisfaction.

Of course, there's a lot more to ACT than just mindfulness. It's also about values-based living: taking action, on an ongoing basis, that is guided by and aligned with core values. Indeed, we teach mindfulness skills in ACT for the primary purpose of helping people to live by their values.

THE BASIC MINDFULNESS INSTRUCTION: "NOTICE X"

There is one basic instruction that you'll find at the core of every single mindfulness exercise—from a ten-second ACT technique to a ten-day silent meditation retreat. It's "notice X."

Common alternatives to the word "notice" include "observe," "pay attention to," "focus on," "be aware of," or "bring awareness to." The "X" that we're noticing can be anything that's here in this moment: a thought or a feeling; a sensation, urge, or memory; our body posture; our actions; and anything that we can see, hear, touch, taste, or smell. X might be the view from a window, the expression on the face of a loved one, the sensations of a hot shower, the taste of a piece of chocolate, the action of tying our shoelaces, the movement of our lungs, or the sounds we can hear in the room around us.

At times, we may want to broaden our focus, for example, if we're walking in the countryside and we want to take in all the sights and sounds and smells. At other times, we may want to narrow our attention: if we're driving in pouring rain, we want to be absolutely focused on the road, not chatting with the passengers or looking around to take in the scenery. At times, we may want to direct our attention inward to the world of thoughts, feelings, and sensations; at other times, outward to the world around us; and much of the time, to both worlds at once—freely shifting attention from one thing to another, as required by the demands of the situation. A useful term for this ability is *flexible attention*.

The "notice X" technique is without a doubt the single most flexible technique in the whole of ACT, and as you go through the book, you'll see how we can use it to instigate and reinforce every core process.

MINDFULNESS ISN'T MEDITATION

A psychologist told me that he'd just had a first session with a new client, and early on in the session, he told the client that he liked to use "mindfulness" in his work. The client screwed up his face and said in a grumpy voice, "I know what mindfulness is, mate. You can take your mindful raisin and stick it up your arse!" Have you ever had similar negative reactions from clients? Mindfulness is, at least in some quarters, getting a bad name.

Part of the problem is that many people—clients and therapists alike—conflate the words "meditation" and "mindfulness." So let's be clear: they are not one and the same. First off, mindfulness doesn't necessarily refer to formal meditative practice, such as observing your breath or scanning your body. It does sometimes, for sure, but it also refers to a wide array of skills, tools, and practices that bear little or no resemblance to formal meditation.

Also keep in mind that there are many different types of meditation styles and practices, some of which are extremely different from formal mindfulness meditation. For example, in some types of meditation the aim is to "clear the mind of all thoughts." This is the very opposite of mindfulness meditation, where you have no expectation the "mind will clear," and you are open to and interested in the many thoughts that continually appear. (More about this distinction in a minute.)

In some ACT protocols, such as Eifert and Forsyth's (2005) *Acceptance and Commitment Therapy for Anxiety Disorders*, formal mindfulness meditation practice does play a big role. In later weeks of this protocol, clients meditate for up to forty minutes a day (in two sittings of twenty minutes each). However, this is an outlier in ACT. Most protocols place much less emphasis on formal meditation and instead emphasize informal, quick mindfulness skills that can be incorporated easily into everyday life, any time, any place, and any activity.

Why do ACT protocols tend to do this? It's purely pragmatic. If we wanted to get as many people as possible doing more exercise, we wouldn't insist, "You have to go the gym for forty minutes a day!" If we did, we'd get a lot of resistance and high drop-out rates. Instead, we might suggest things like "Take the stairs instead of the elevator," "Park a block away from the supermarket," "Go for a ten-minute walk at lunchtime," and so on. In ACT, we take a similar approach to developing mindfulness skills; we aim to make it simple for people to slot these new mindfulness practices into their everyday life, and easy enough that people are willing to do them.

"MINDFULNESS" IS BECOMING A DODGY WORD

When I wrote my first book, *The Happiness Trap*, back in 2006, the word "mindfulness" was so little known that I didn't even mention it until halfway through the book. Now, twelve years later, it seems that almost everyone knows the word. Unfortunately, there are now so many different connotations that go with this word, you're often better off not using it. I've already mentioned that many people conflate mindfulness with Buddhism or meditation. Others confuse it with positive thinking, relaxation, or distraction, or think of it as a way to get rid of unwanted thoughts and feelings. As we've already explored, it doesn't mean any of these things (at least as we use the term in ACT). So throughout this book, I will encourage you to use other words instead: "unhooking," "engaging," "dropping anchor," "task-focused attention," "expansion," and so on. And I will encourage you to be very clear with your clients about which specific skill you are teaching (i.e., don't just vaguely call it "mindfulness") and how it is likely to help them with their issues.

For example, if clients are hooked by difficult thoughts or worrying or rumination, we could talk about helping them to "unhook" or learn some "unhooking skills." Or if making room for difficult feelings will help clients live their values and pursue their goals, we can talk about helping them "expand around" or "open up and make room for" those feelings and then refer to "expansion skills" or "opening-up skills." And if they're having difficulty focusing on important tasks, engaging in life, or being present with their kids, then we can help them "focus," "refocus," "engage," "train their attention," or "be present." Basically, as a term, "mindfulness" is often just too abstract, too heady, too generic, and too far removed from clients' issues.

One thing to watch for is the enormous difference between "practicing mindfulness" and "practicing mindfulness *meditation*." Again, they aren't the same thing. There are zillions of ways to practice mindfulness in everyday life, without ever meditating. The simple fact is most clients won't get into meditation in a big way, if at all. And for many, even the thought of meditation will be a turnoff. If you're running a mindfulness meditation program and that's what people are coming along for, great. But in a therapy context, if you start trying to push "meditation," you'll often find it a hard sell.

The bottom line is that we need to link each of the four specific mindfulness skills covered in ACT—defusion, acceptance, contacting the present moment, and self-as-context—to clients' specific issues and their goals for therapy. We need to make sure that they not only see why this is relevant but also get to experience the benefits during the actual session.

But if you do use the word "mindfulness" with a client and it does elicit a negative reaction, then you want to respectfully explore that response. Does the client see it as a religious practice? Has he heard bad things about it? What are his past experiences with mindfulness? What mindfulness practices has he already tried? What was he hoping would happen, and what actually did happen?

If you explore such questions, you'll often find your clients have not experienced the kind of flexible, nonmeditative, practical approach to mindfulness that ACT offers. Instead, they have probably experienced formal mindfulness meditation practices—which, let's face it, are hard and boring for many people. In such cases, we could reassure them: "That's a very different approach to mindfulness than we have in this model. But given that the word has negative connotations for you, let's not use it again. Let's just talk about unhooking skills."

In addition, you'll often find clients don't really understand how mindfulness is supposed to help with everyday life. Very commonly, they have misunderstood it to be a relaxation technique and expected it to get rid of their anxiety or other difficult feelings, and are disappointed that it didn't do so. In such cases, we need to provide some psychoeducation about the purpose of mindfulness in ACT.

Takeaway

"Mindfulness" is only one dodgy word in ACT. There are quite a few others, including "values," "commitment," "acceptance," and "self-compassion." These words have many negative connotations; they're fine to use with some clients, but with others they can elicit negative responses. So when we get to these topics, I'm going to give you a variety of other words you can use instead. Remember, as I said in chapter 1 (and I'll say again later), adapt and modify everything in ACT to suit your own style and the clients you work with. If you suspect a certain word, metaphor, tool, or technique will not go down well with your client, then change, modify, or adapt it. Don't stick to the script; be creative and improvise around it.

Now, enough about dodgy words! It's time to…

CHAPTER 4

Get Your Geek On

Please—Do Not Skip This Chapter!

This chapter, unlike the rest of the book, is a bit geeky. In fact, it contains more technical jargon than the entire rest of the book put together. So if geeking out is your thing, you're in for fun. If, however, geeking out is *not* your thing, please don't skip this chapter. Please stick with it for three good reasons: (a) it will enrich your understanding of ACT in valuable ways that will make you a better ACT therapist; (b) later in the book we'll often refer back to the concepts in this chapter, so if you skip it you'll be wondering what the hell we are talking about; and (c) after you get to the end of this chapter, everything else in the book will seem so much simpler in comparison. Are you game? Good. Your first mission is to understand functional contextualism.

Functional What??!!

Functional contextualism. It's a mouthful, isn't it? Functional contextualism is the philosophy of science that underpins the ACT model. It gets its name because it looks at how behavior *functions* in different *contexts*. The word "function" is a technical term (not one that you'd use with clients) that you'll find in most ACT textbooks. When we ask, "What is the function of this behavior?" we mean "What effect does this behavior have in this situation? What is it achieving?" To clarify this, imagine five different people, in five different situations, each making cuts across their forearm with a sharp knife. Now see if you can come up with five possible functions for such behavior.

* * *

Here are some possibilities:

- Getting attention

- Self-punishment

- Release of tension

- Distraction from painful emotions

- Creating body art

- Feeling something if you are "totally numb"

- Attempting suicide

Notice that in all these scenarios, the form of the behavior is the same—cutting one's arm with a knife—but the function of the behavior, or the effect it is having in this situation, is different. Now let's suppose your friend is lost in thought and you wish to gain his attention. Think of five different forms of behavior that might have this effect.

* * *

Here are a few ideas:

- Wave at him.

- Shout "Hello, is there anybody in there?"

- Pour a cup of water over his head.

- Bang loudly on some furniture.

- Say, "Can I have your attention for a moment, please?"

In this example, you can see that many different forms of behavior all have the same function: they all have the effect of getting attention in this situation. In functional contextualism, we're much more interested in the function of a behavior—the effect it has—than the form of it. When we use the choice point, for example, we're continually analyzing the function of client behavior *in the context of the client's life* (more on what "context" means in a minute). We ask whether it functions as a towards move or as an away move. This enables us to take a nonjudgmental view of client behavior; instead of evaluating whether it's good or bad or right or wrong or positive or negative, we can simply look at in terms of workability. Remember: if your behavior functions in such a way as to help you effectively build the life you want, it's workable; if it functions in the opposite way, it's unworkable.

Tricky Terminology   A quick reminder that the word "behavior" means anything a whole being does. Overt behavior is physical behavior: actions you take with your body, facial expressions, what you say, how you move, your body posture, and so on. Covert behavior means psychological action, such as thinking, focusing, defusing, accepting, and remembering; behavior that goes on in your inner world; behavior a video camera, if present, could never record.

Okay, so now that we're clear on what "function" means, let's take a look at…

Context!

All behavior happens within a context. And the technical term "context" means everything that influences the behavior we are analyzing.

This may include:

- Emotions, feelings, moods

- Cognitive events (thoughts, beliefs, attitudes, assumptions, schemas)

- Cognitive processes (attention, memory)

- Interpersonal factors (who else is present, your past relationship history with them)

- Social and cultural events (public holidays, traditional celebrations and rituals)

- The physical environment (location, furnishings, weather, time of day, temperature, smell)

- Genetic and epigenetic factors

- Physiological states such as thirst, hunger, fatigue

- Consumption of drugs, alcohol, food

- Physical health or illness

- Social and cultural status (social class, position and rank, peer groups)

- Developmental and learning history, including attachment style

Our behavior occurs amid a vast and ever-changing nonstop stream of influences. So vast and complex is this stream, it's impossible for us to ever know everything that's influencing our behavior in this moment. Collectively these influences are referred to as the "context" in which the behavior happens. And we can conveniently divide any context into two broad categories of influence: antecedents and consequences.

Antecedents are factors that trigger the behavior in question—that is, they immediately precede it and cue its occurrence. Clinically, the main antecedents we focus on are situations, thoughts, and feelings. When using the choice point, antecedents always go at the bottom, as illustrated in the figure below. In this example, the away moves are all forms of social withdrawal. As the diagram illustrates, there are many possible antecedents for such behaviors.

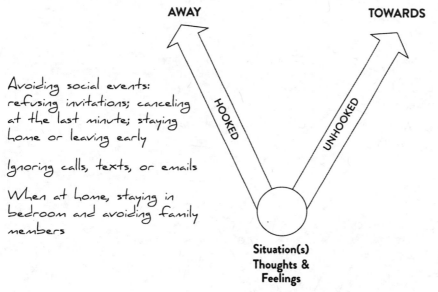

AWAY

TOWARDS

HOOKED

UNHOOKED

Avoiding social events: refusing invitations; canceling at the last minute; staying home or leaving early

Ignoring calls, texts, or emails

When at home, staying in bedroom and avoiding family members

Situation(s)
Thoughts &
Feelings

Social events, social interactions, social invitations

"I'm boring," "No one likes me," "I'll have a bad time"

Anxiety, fear of rejection, racing heart, sweaty hands

In lay terms, we can say that every behavior we do has both payoffs (outcomes that convey some sort of benefit or gain) and costs (outcomes that are in some way detrimental).

If the costs of a behavior lead to it reducing or stopping over time, then in technical terms, we call them *punishing consequences*. For example, if the client cancels a social event but then feels intensely lonely and miserable for the rest of the evening, and as a result, she starts to cancel social events less often, then technically we'd call that a punishing consequence.

If the payoffs of a behavior lead to it maintaining or increasing over time, then technically we call them *reinforcing consequences*. For instance, if the client cancels a social event and gets a huge sense of relief from doing so, and this leads to her canceling even more in future, then this is a reinforcing consequence.

It's often useful to include costs and payoffs in the choice point. For example, in the next figure, to help the client understand why she keeps doing her problematic behavior (i.e., what is reinforcing it), the therapist adds in payoffs at the top of the diagram.

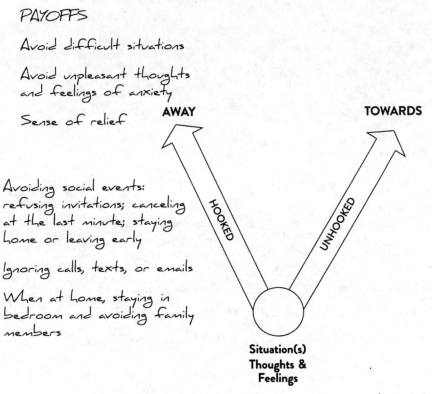

PAYOFFS

Avoid difficult situations

Avoid unpleasant thoughts and feelings of anxiety

Sense of relief

AWAY   TOWARDS

HOOKED   UNHOOKED

Avoiding social events: refusing invitations; canceling at the last minute; staying home or leaving early

Ignoring calls, texts, or emails

When at home, staying in bedroom and avoiding family members

Situation(s)
Thoughts &
Feelings

Social events, social interactions, social invitations

"I'm boring," "No one likes me," "I'll have a bad time"

Anxiety, fear of rejection, racing heart, sweaty hands

It's often very useful to map out the antecedents and consequences of a behavior in this manner, especially when a client says, "I don't understand why I keep doing this." The technical term for such mapping is *functional analysis*, more playfully called *function spotting*. When we run through this process with a client, it can rapidly raise his awareness and give him valuable insight into his behavior: what triggers it (antecedents) and what keeps it going (reinforcing consequences).

At the same time, it provides a great springboard for clinical interventions. For example, in the figure above, we can readily identify thoughts to target with defusion, feelings to target with acceptance, and challenging situations to target with values-guided problem solving, goal setting, and action planning (which would include training in social skills, if the client has deficits in this area).

Of course, there's a whole lot more to functional contextualism than this, but we've covered enough to get us started.

Takeaway

In ACT, we continually make use of all the concepts covered in this chapter. For example, we use mindfulness both to raise awareness of the antecedents (i.e., to notice the thoughts, feelings, and situations that trigger the behavior in question) and to track the consequences of behavior (what effects it has, both short term and long term). We also use mindfulness and values to help people change the way they respond to antecedents so that those very same situations, thoughts, and feelings that once triggered away moves now become antecedents for towards moves. In later chapters, as we explore the core ACT processes in depth, I'll link what we're doing again and again to these basic behavioral concepts. But for now, geek time is over. (You can now mindfully breathe a sigh of relief.)

PART 2

Getting Started

CHAPTER 5

Setting Up for Success

First Things First

About half the problems I encounter in supervision happen because therapists launch into ACT without effectively setting up their sessions. If we take the time to set our sessions up well, right from the word go, we're likely to get much better results. So in this chapter and the next, I'll give you a bunch of suggestions for doing this. (And of course, like everything else you read in this book, adapt and modify everything to suit your own way of working.)

The First Session

Therapists come to ACT from a vast array of backgrounds and therefore often have widely differing ideas about the first session. For example, many therapists like to do an "intake session" or "pretreatment session" before the first session of "active" therapy. This typically involves taking a history, filling in assessment forms, conducting specialized assessments such as a mental status examination, and agreeing to a therapeutic contract. However, practitioners with a brief therapy orientation prefer not to do a pretreatment session; instead they jump into active therapy on the very first encounter with the client. There are pros and cons to both approaches, and this isn't the place to discuss them; so if the way you currently work is giving you the results you want, then stick with it. Throughout this book, I will treat session one as the very first client-therapist encounter (that is, I will assume there's no pretreatment session). So if you don't work this way, modify all the suggestions that follow to include a pretreatment session or to "stretch out" the first session into two.

Ideally, in session one we aim to:

- establish rapport

- obtain informed consent

- take a history

- establish behavioral goals

If we have enough time, we can also:

- do a brief experiential exercise

- give some simple "homework"

With high-functioning clients or those who have a very specific problem, we can often accomplish all of the above tasks in one session. However, for low-functioning clients or those with multiple problems and complex histories, this could easily spill over into two sessions or more.

Also keep in mind that if your client has a long history of trauma or repeated experiences of abuse and betrayal in intimate relationships, there may be significant trust issues. If so, you may want to spend two or three sessions primarily taking a history and building rapport—going slowly and taking your time to establish a trusting relationship.

In chapter 6 we'll look at taking a history and establishing behavioral goals, and in chapter 7 we'll explore brief experiential exercises and simple homework tasks you can bring into any session, including the first. In this chapter, we're going to focus on building rapport and obtaining informed consent.

Building Rapport and Seeing the Rainbow

The therapeutic relationship is of central importance in ACT. And one of the best ways we can strengthen it is to embody ACT in the therapy room. When we're fully present with our clients, open to whatever emotional content arises, defused from our own judgments, and acting in line with our core therapeutic values of connection, compassion, caring, and helping, then we naturally facilitate a warm, kind, open, and authentic relationship. Indeed, when we give our full attention to another human being with openness, compassion, and curiosity, that is therapeutic in itself.

For any given client, it's useful to ask ourselves, *Do I see this person as a rainbow or as a roadblock?* A rainbow is a unique and beautiful work of nature. We don't look at it as a problem or an obstacle; rather, we feel grateful and awed to be in its presence. So can we bring a similar attitude to our clients? Can we truly appreciate their uniqueness and the gift we have been granted of working at such a deep level with our fellow human beings?

When clients are deeply stuck—that is, extremely fused and avoidant—therapy often becomes extremely difficult, or stalls. Not surprisingly, therapists find this challenging. When we're working with very stuck clients, and we're not making progress, our minds are usually quick to start judging. And if we get hooked by those judgments, we start to see our clients as roadblocks: getting in our way, stopping us from doing our jobs, becoming a nuisance.

So it's essential to apply ACT to ourselves in these situations—to unhook from our judgments, and instead, pay attention to our clients with openness, curiosity, and appreciation.

A compassionate and respectful relationship with our clients is essential for doing ACT well; without it, our interventions are almost guaranteed to fail, backfire, or invalidate. To develop and maintain the therapeutic relationship is a huge topic, so in chapter 30 we'll explore it in more depth. For now, I just have one more point to emphasize: ACT's stance of radical equality between clients and therapists—the idea that we are all "in the same boat." Just like our clients, we therapists readily get entangled in our minds, lose touch with the present, and engage in futile battles with our own thoughts and feelings. Just like our clients, we repeatedly lose touch with our core values and act in self-defeating ways. And just like our clients, we struggle with many aspects of a full human life: disappointment, rejection, failure, betrayal, loss, loneliness, conflict, sickness, injury, grief, resentment, anxiety, insecurity, and death. So given that clients and therapists are fellow travelers on the same inspiring and painful human journey, we can both learn a lot from each other.

The Two Mountains metaphor (Hayes, Strosahl, & Wilson, 1999) is a good way to convey this stance of equality. Many therapists share this on the first session.

THE TWO MOUNTAINS METAPHOR

Therapist: You know, a lot of people come to therapy believing that the therapist is some sort of enlightened being, that he's resolved all his issues, he's got it all together—but that's not the way it is. It's more like you're climbing your mountain over there, and I'm climbing my mountain over here. And from where I am on my mountain, I can see things on your mountain that you can't see—like there's an avalanche about to happen, or there's an alternative pathway you could take, or you're not using your pickaxe effectively.

But I'd hate for you to think that I've reached the top of my mountain, and I'm sitting back, taking it easy. Fact is, I'm still climbing, still making mistakes, and still learning from them. And basically, we're all the same. We're all climbing our mountain until the day we die. But here's the thing: you can get better and better at climbing, and better and better at learning to appreciate the journey. And that's what the work we do here is all about.

Obtaining Informed Consent in ACT

At some point in the first session, we need to get the client's informed consent to do ACT. My personal preference is to do this before we are halfway through the session. We might say something like "There's a lot more I want to know about what's going on for you, what you're struggling with, and so on, and we'll come back to that shortly, but can we just take a couple of minutes to talk about the sort of therapy I do—what it involves, how long it takes—and just make sure it's the right approach for you. Is that okay?"

EXPLAINING WHAT ACT IS AND WHAT IT INVOLVES

At the bare minimum, I recommend you include the following points when obtaining consent to do ACT. (And please remember to modify the language to suit your way of speaking and your clientele):

- ACT is a very active form of therapy/coaching. It's not just talking about your problems and feelings.

- The idea is that we work together as a team, to help you build the sort of life you want to live.

- One big part of this approach involves learning skills to unhook yourself from difficult thoughts and feelings—learning how to reduce their impact and take away their power, so they can't jerk you around or hold you back or bring you down.

- It also involves clarifying your values: finding out what matters to you, what you want to stand for in life, what strengths and qualities you want to develop and how you want to treat yourself and others. And taking action to solve your problems, face your challenges, and do things that make life better.

- I want you to leave here after each session with an action plan: something practical to take away and use to actively make a difference in your life.

- I will ask you at times to try new things that may pull you out of your comfort zone—like learning new skills to handle difficult thoughts and feelings—but you never have to do them. You are always free to say no to anything I suggest.

Once you've covered these points, the following two metaphors can come in extremely handy.

The "Press Pause" Metaphor

The "Press Pause" metaphor is not essential, but I highly recommend it, for reasons I'll explain shortly. Ideally, introduce it immediately after informed consent. It goes like this:

Therapist: Can I have permission to "press pause" from time to time, so if I see you doing something that looks like it might be really helpful or useful, in terms of dealing with your problems and improving your life, I can just slow the session down and get you to really notice what you are doing?

For example, I may ask you to pause or slow down, take a couple of breaths, notice what you're thinking or feeling or saying or doing. That way, you'll be able to see more clearly what you're doing, and we can look at ways you can use it outside of this room. Is that okay?

And can I also "press pause" if I see you doing something that looks like it may be contributing to your problems or making them worse, so we can address it?

And of course, this goes both ways—you can also "press pause" on me, any time you like.

With this mutual agreement to "press pause," you now have a really simple mindfulness intervention you can bring in at any point in session, either to interrupt problematic behavior or to reinforce psychologically flexible behavior as it arises during the session.

For example, suppose the client is raising his voice and becoming aggressive with his words and intimidating with his body language. The therapist could say, "Um, do you remember you said I could 'press pause' at times? I think this is one of those times it would be useful. Could I ask you just to pause for a moment; just take a breath, take a moment to notice how you're speaking, your tone of voice, the things you're saying…the way your fists are clenched…? Can I get you just to check in, notice what you're feeling right now? I'm doing this myself, and I notice that I'm feeling quite intimidated." The therapist has interrupted the client's behavior and can now intervene in numerous ways: work on grounding and centering, or defusion from angry thoughts, or exploring the feelings of anger, or practicing assertiveness skills, and so on.

The therapist may also take an interpersonal tack: "Right now, it doesn't feel to me like we are a team. Feels like there's a lot of tension between us. Is it okay if we take a look at what's going on here? See if we can get back to working as a team again?"

Now suppose your client is usually distracted and disinterested, but all of a sudden, you notice she's really engaged: she's sitting up straight instead of slouching, she's looking at you instead of the floor, and she looks interested instead of bored. This is psychologically flexible behavior that you want to reinforce. If you ignore it, take it for granted, or fail to comment on it, you are missing an opportunity. So you could say something like "Can I press pause for a moment? I can't help but notice that you're doing something very different right now. A few minutes ago you were slouched down and staring at the floor…and now, do you notice how you're sitting differently and looking interested? I have to say, it makes a huge difference to me. I feel much more connected with you; I feel like we're really a team now."

Practical Tip   We can never know for sure in advance what will reinforce a client's behavior, but we can make a good guess. When we help the client to notice her behavior and the positive effect it is having, this will usually be a reinforcing consequence; that is, we'll see the behavior increase. But suppose we see the behavior in question reduce—for example, if the client feels embarrassed or self-conscious and stops doing it. If so, then what we said was actually a punishing consequence, in which case, we would stop doing it and try a different strategy.

After the spiel about pressing pause (above), you could go on to try the guitar metaphor, which goes like this:

The Guitar Metaphor

Therapist: Doing ACT is a bit like playing guitar. We can't learn to play guitar by thinking about it, reading about it, or talking about it; the only way we can learn is to actually pick it up and start strumming. So these new skills—I'm going to take you through them in session, here with me, and that will be helpful. But what makes all the difference is how much you practice them at home. Again, it's like learning guitar; if you want to get any good, you have to practice. So I'll be asking you to take these new skills home and practice between sessions.

DEFUSION FROM DOUBT

Suppose your client now expresses some doubt or uncertainty: "I don't think this will work for me." Such thoughts are perfectly natural, and they're only problematic if the client fuses with them. So here we have a perfect opportunity to establish a context of acceptance and defusion. For example, we might say, "That's a perfectly natural thought. Many people feel doubtful at first. And the truth is, there's no known treatment that's guaranteed to work for everyone. So I can't promise that this will work for you. I could tell you it's worked for lots of other people, and I could pull out all the published studies and the research papers, and so on, but that still wouldn't guarantee it will work for you. In fact, if you ever go and see any health professional—doctor, dentist, psychologist, therapist, whatever—and they guarantee you, one hundred percent, 'This will work'—I recommend you don't go back and see them, because they're either lying or deluded."

The client will often smile or chuckle at this point. We may then go on to introduce some simple defusion as follows:

Therapist: Of course, I'm expecting this will help you—otherwise I wouldn't keep working with you. But here's what I predict. Your mind is going to be doubtful, at least for the first couple of sessions. It will keep saying things like *This won't work.* And each time those kinds of thoughts pop up, there's a choice to make: we can give up and stop the session because your mind says it won't work—or we can let your mind say that and carry on working and give it our best shot.

Client: I get that.

Therapist: So, even though your mind is saying *This won't work*, we can keep going?

Client: Sure.

Notice in the transcript above, we're not challenging the client's thought. Rather, we're validating it as natural and normal. And we're establishing a context where (a) it's okay for the client to have that thought (acceptance) and (b) the thought is present but doesn't control the client's actions (defusion). In chapter 12, we'll look at how to take this simple intervention a step further, when clients are fused with hopelessness.

REDUCING RISK OF DROPOUT

If you know or suspect that your client is likely to drop out of therapy, then it's useful to say something like this: "Sometimes therapy can be bit of a roller-coaster ride. But you and I are a team here, and I will be there in the roller-coaster car with you. And sometimes you might feel an urge to drop out of therapy. And that's completely normal, especially if you're facing up to some very important issue or problem or challenge. So if you ever do start feeling that way, would you be willing to share it with me please, so we can work with those feelings during our sessions? Because I'd hate for you drop out when you're just about to make a breakthrough."

AGREEING ON THE NUMBER OF SESSIONS

How many sessions of ACT does a client need? Well, how long is a piece of string? I've seen amazing things happen from a single session of ACT, and I've also had clients I worked with on a regular basis for three or four years! As a general rule, the greater your clients' problems in number, duration, severity, and impact on their quality of life, the longer the duration of therapy. However, this is not necessarily so.

ACT can be delivered in many different formats, including these:

- Long-term therapy: for example, one protocol for ACT for clients with borderline personality disorder goes for forty group sessions, each two hours long (Brann, Gopold, Guymer, Morton, & Snowdon, 2007).

- Brief therapy: for example, a popular protocol for ACT for clients with anxiety disorders is based on twelve one-hour sessions (Eifert & Forsyth, 2005), and one published study for ACT with chronic stress and pain is based on an eight-hour protocol (Dahl et al., 2004).

- Very brief therapy: for example, one published study on ACT for clients with chronic schizophrenia consisted of only three or four one-hour sessions. That very brief intervention led to an almost 50 percent reduction in hospital readmission rates (Bach & Hayes, 2002). (Obviously with these very brief ACT interventions, it's not as if the client fully and completely embraces mindful, values-based living and never has any issues ever again. It's more the case that we can deliver the core elements of ACT—be present, open up, do what matters—quite quickly and with significant benefits. The client then becomes his own ACT therapist, and life throws up all sorts of problems and challenges, which provide opportunities to further develop his skills.)

Quite a few ACT textbooks suggest you agree to twelve sessions initially, but there is nothing magical about this number, so you can adjust it to suit your clientele. For example, in Australia, the country where I live and practice, there's not the same degree of openness to therapy as there is in the US; therefore, I typically contract for only six sessions initially.

At this juncture, we tell the client that therapy isn't a smooth journey but involves ups and downs. For example, you might say, "One thing I should mention is that therapy doesn't always progress smoothly. Sometimes you make a huge leap forward, and sometimes you take a step backward. So I usually recommend six sessions initially—and after that we can assess how it's going and see if you need more. And you'll be the one who makes the call on that, not me. You'll judge whether we're making progress or not. The truth is, some people don't need the full six sessions, and others end up needing more than that. It really varies. So would you be willing to initially commit to six?"

How Directive Is ACT?

When doing ACT, we can be as directive or nondirective as we wish. It depends on the capabilities of the client and the demands of the situation. For low-functioning clients, with many problems and significant deficits in coping skills, we will usually need to be fairly directive: we'll need to set a clear agenda at the start of each session, and steer the client back to it as often as needed in order to ensure she actively learns new skills, clarifies values, sets goals, and creates action plans during the session. But with higher-functioning, self-motivated clients, we can be much less directive. So we can titrate how directive we are in any given session to suit the needs of the unique client in front of us. It's impossible, however, to be completely nondirective when teaching people mindfulness skills; we do need to give instructions, suggestions, and feedback to people to ensure they learn and apply their new skills.

Skilling Up

If you're anything like me, you have a tendency to read textbooks and hope everything "sinks in" so you can readily trot it out in the therapy room. If only! There's no two ways about it: you won't learn ACT simply by reading a book. So I really hope you've been doing these Skilling Up sections. For this chapter, your challenge is simply to do the following:

- Read through all the therapist spiels above. Read them aloud, as if you're an actor rehearsing lines for a play; or if you're not willing to do this, at least run through them in your head.

- As you read each script, modify it: put it into your own words.

Ideally, do this quite a few times, until the spiel rolls off the tip of your tongue, so that you could, if you wanted to, quickly summarize all the key points to colleagues, allied health professionals, or people you meet at the grand finale of the World Chess Championship. I can't overstate the importance of this: if you don't practice this out of session, you likely won't remember it when you're in session.

Takeaway

The main takeaway from this chapter is this: set your sessions up effectively. It's like laying a foundation for the house you're going to build. If the foundation isn't laid properly, expect lots of problems with the building process. Informed consent is an essential part of this foundation; you can't afford to skip it. And so is building a strong alliance—so see your clients as rainbows, not as roadblocks!

CHAPTER 6

What's the Problem?

Looking with ACT Eyes

One of the things ACT newbies often find hard is to see a client's issues through the lens of the six core processes. To help you do this, let's take another quick look at the choice point, shown below. This summarizes the essence of most clinical issues from an ACT perspective.

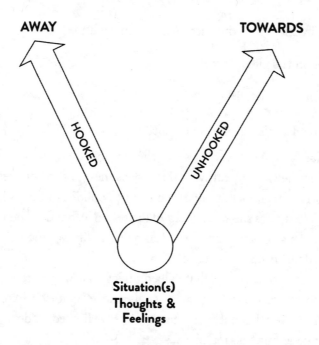

The bottom and left side of the diagram summarize the main features of almost all clinical issues and psychiatric disorders:

A. The client is dealing with difficult situations (which could include all manner of health, relationship, financial, legal, medical, domestic, lifestyle, and occupational problems) and experiencing a variety of difficult thoughts and feelings. (Remember: "thoughts and feelings" is short for all private experiences, including emotions, memories, urges, impulses, and physical sensations.)

B.   When the client responds inflexibly to his thoughts and feelings, with fusion and/or avoidance (getting "hooked"), she behaves in values-incongruent, self-defeating ways that make her life worse in the long term ("away moves").

The right side of the diagram reminds us that the outcome we want from ACT is mindful ("unhooked"), values-based living ("towards moves"). In other words, we want to develop "unhooking skills" (defusion, acceptance, self-as-context, flexible attention) and take values-guided committed action (towards moves) to create as rich, full, and meaningful a life as possible.

When we take a history, our clients generally find it far easier to describe their suffering and their struggles (bottom and left arrow) than to describe what they want to do to build a rich and meaningful life (right arrow). However, in order for us to be effective as therapists, we need to know both sets of information. Fortunately, there are all sorts of tools and techniques to help people clarify their values and goals, as we shall see in chapter 19.

There are two key questions that allow us to quickly conceptualize any issue or problem from an ACT perspective:

1.   What valued direction does the client want to move in?

2.   What is getting in the client's way?

Let's look at these in more detail.

What valued direction does the client want to move in?

Here we seek to clarify values: How does the client want to grow and develop? What personal strengths or qualities does he want to cultivate? How does she want to behave? How does he want to treat himself? What sorts of relationships does she want to build? How does he want to treat others in those relationships? What does she want to stand for in life? What does he want to stand for in the face of this crisis or challenging situation? What domains of life are most important to her? What values-congruent goals does he currently have?

Once we can answer the question "What valued direction does the client want to move in?" we can use that knowledge to set values-congruent goals and to guide, inspire, and sustain ongoing action. And if we can't answer this question, that tells us we'll need to do some work on clarifying values, setting goals, or generating action plans.

What is getting in the client's way?

This question refers to psychological barriers: what prevents the client from acting effectively in the face of life's challenges? Psychological barriers can include any or all of the six processes of psychological rigidity that we covered in chapter 2: cognitive fusion, experiential avoidance, inflexible attention, remoteness from values, unworkable action, and fusion with self-concept. Not all of these processes will be relevant for every client, but most will be relevant, at least to some extent, in most clients.

When we take a client's history, much of it will involve gathering answers to the two key questions above.

Taking a History

Taking a history is rarely a neat, orderly, linear process; usually, we gather bits and pieces as we go, jumping backward, forward, and sideways to progressively fill in the picture of the client's current life, the issues she's struggling with, and relevant past history. Luckily, we don't need to gather all our information in one session; we can always gather more history later, as needed. To make history-taking quicker and easier, I ask clients to fill out a couple of worksheets before the first session. (I either mail or email the worksheets or ask the client to arrive twenty minutes early and complete them in the waiting room.) Two worksheets that I've found especially useful for this purpose are Dissecting the Problem and the Bull's Eye. You'll find these at the end of the chapter (and for printable versions, see Extra Bits). Please take a quick look at them now, then come back to this point.

If we want to rapidly get a sense of values in different domains of life, the quickest and easiest worksheet I know of is the Bull's Eye. This divides life into four domains: work/education, personal growth/health, relationships, and leisure. When clients fill this in for the first time, you are likely to get quite a mixture of values, desires, wants, needs, and goals: a great starting point for further exploration.

The Dissecting the Problem worksheet breaks down the client's suffering into four key components: fusion with thoughts, fusion with feelings, experiential avoidance, and unworkable action. I ask my clients to complete these worksheets to the best of their ability and bring them along to the first session. I explain that even if they only write a few words, that's a good start. Alternatively, you can fill these worksheets in during the session or give them as "homework" to complete after the session.

How Much History Do We Take?

Gathering a client history can take anywhere from a few minutes to an hour, depending upon the situation. For example, the textbook *ACT in Practice* (Bach & Moran, 2008) recommends an entire session to take a detailed history and carefully conceptualize your client's issues. On the other hand, in primary care settings, where the therapist may have only two or three sessions of fifteen to thirty minutes each, the history needs to be very brief (Robinson, 2008).

So once again, the message is: adapt ACT to your own way of working, your own style, and your own clientele. And when you take the history, feel free to use whatever standardized assessment tools you like. A word of caution though: many popular assessment tools measure changes in the number, frequency, or severity of symptoms (that is, changes in symptom *form*) but fail to measure changes in the impact or influence of symptoms (that is, changes in symptom *function*). However, in ACT, our interest is in changing symptom function rather than form. So while there's no absolute necessity for you to use ACT-specific assessment tools, such as the AAQ-II (Acceptance and Action Questionnaire—II; Bond et al., 2011), they can be very helpful. I won't discuss such tools in this book, but you can download a wide variety from https://www.contextualscience.org.

Now, I'm assuming you already have a procedure for history taking, so what follows are some tips to help you adapt what you already do to ACT.

Eight Key Areas of History

When taking a history in preparation for doing ACT, there are eight key areas to explore:

1. the presenting complaint(s)

2. initial values assessment

3. current life context

4. relevant past history

5. psychological rigidity

6. motivational factors

7. psychological flexibility

8. client resources

I just want to briefly touch on each of these.

1. *The Presenting Complaint(s)*

    Basically here, you want to gather the information that's bottom and left on the choice point: the difficult situation(s) the client is facing, the thoughts and feelings hooking him, and his self-defeating behaviors when hooked. (And remember: you never have to use the choice point; it's a tool for your convenience, to use only if you like it.)

2. *Initial Values Assessment*

    As part of our history, we want to get a sense of the client's values. Sometimes, it's almost impossible to get this information up front, so we'll look at how to do this in chapters 19 and 20. However, a good starting point is the Bull's Eye.

3. *Current Life Context*

   The current life context includes health, medications, work, finances, relationships, social situation, family, culture, lifestyle (including diet, exercise, smoking, drugs, and alcohol), legal or financial issues, and so on. When we explore the current life context, we uncover external barriers (as opposed to psychological barriers) to building a rich and full life such as unemployment, medical illness, and poverty. These will require values-based problem solving and action planning.

4. *Relevant Past History*

   ACT is very focused on the present, but it's important to gather past history where it's directly relevant to current issues. In particular, we want to know about significant relationships (past and present) and how clients have been impacted by them. Such history can be especially helpful for developing self-acceptance and self-compassion.

5. *Psychological Rigidity*

   Look for the six core processes of psychological rigidity we outlined in chapter 2. Again, these are fusion (with reasons, rules, judgments, past, and future), experiential avoidance, remoteness from values, unworkable action, inflexible attention, and fusion with self-concept. Don't rely solely on clients' reports; be on the lookout for such behavior as it arises spontaneously during the session.

6. *Motivational Factors*

   Start identifying positive motivational factors, for example, goals, dreams, desires, visions, and values. And also identify negative motivational factors, for example, fusion with helplessness or the reinforcing consequences for problematic behaviors.

7. *Psychological Flexibility*

   Look for evidence of the six core processes of psychological flexibility: values, committed action, defusion, acceptance, flexible attention (contacting the present moment), and self-as-context. Again, don't rely solely on clients' reports; be on the lookout for such behavior as it arises spontaneously during the session.

8. *Client Resources*

   What strengths, skills, and other personal resources does the client have that could be utilized? What external resources could the client access? Who can the client turn to for help, support, encouragement?

In later chapters, you'll discover many useful questions you can ask to flesh out these key areas of history, but for now, I want to turn to an extremely important issue.

Establishing Behavioral Goals for Therapy

Whatever you do, don't skip or skim over this part of the chapter. It's so important. Numerous issues I encounter in supervision are due to one main error: the coach or therapist has failed to establish *behavioral* goals for therapy. Behavioral goals are "doing" goals: they describe what you want to *do*. (Quick reminder: covert behavior is psychological action: what we do in our inner, private world. Overt behavior is physical action: all the things we do with our physical body.)

To establish behavioral goals, we can ask:

If the work we do here is successful, then…

- What will you do differently?

- What will you start doing/stop doing?

- What will you do more of or less of?

- How will you treat yourself, others, the world differently?

- What people, places, events, activities, challenges will you approach, start, resume, or contact (rather than avoid, withdraw, quit, or stay away from)?

The questions above often tend to elicit *overt* behavioral goals. To establish *covert* behavioral goals, we can ask questions such as:

- Are there any tasks or activities you'll be better able to focus on or engage in?

- Are there any people you'll be more attentive to or more present with?

- Is there anyone or anything you'll be able to appreciate more?

Emotional Goals vs. Behavioral Goals

When we set therapeutic goals in ACT, we must keep sight of this crucial distinction:

Emotional goals = how I want to *feel*

Behavioral goals = what I want to *do*

Guess which type of goals our clients almost always present with? Yes! They bring their *emotional* goals into the room: how I want to *feel* ("I want to feel Y"—e.g., happy, relaxed) or *not feel* ("I want to stop feeling X"—e.g., depressed, anxious).

Common emotional goals include "recover from depression (or other mental health disorder)," "stop feeling so anxious," "increase self-worth," "build self-esteem," "get over what happened," "get my old self back," "feel happy," "feel good," "stop feeling like shit," "have more confidence," "stop doubting myself," "feel calmer," "reduce anxiety," "stop getting so angry."

These goals basically all boil down to the same agenda:

Get rid of my unwanted thoughts and feelings; I want to feel good!!!

And of course, it's completely natural and fully expected that clients will present with emotional goals. We all want to feel good; no one likes feeling bad. Unfortunately, however, if we agree to such goals, it will not be possible to do ACT. Why not? Because emotional goals reinforce the agenda of experiential avoidance: the ongoing attempt to avoid and get rid of unwanted thoughts and feelings. In ACT, we aim to actively undermine experiential avoidance and open the client to a radically different agenda: experiential acceptance (which is also known as "willingness"). So if we agree to emotional goals, we will not be able to do ACT.

However, we don't want to actively confront such emotional goals (unless we are doing a specific intervention called "creative hopelessness," which we cover in chapter 8). What we want to do is gently reframe them as behavioral goals; these we can work with.

Reframing Emotional Goals as Behavioral Goals

Are you fully awake? Hope so, because the next sentence is very important to remember.

"To learn a new skill" is a behavioral goal.

Yes, that's right. And this of course includes learning psychological skills as well as physical skills. So for many clients, one of the first behavioral goals we agree to is "learning new skills to handle these difficult thoughts and feelings more effectively." (I'm sure you'll recall this in part of the informed consent process we looked at in chapter 5.) So let's have a look at a few examples of how we can use this idea of skill building to reframe emotional goals as behavioral ones.

Emotional Goal #1

Client: I don't want to do anything differently. I just want to stop feeling like this. I just want to get rid of these thoughts/feelings/emotions/memories.

Behavioral Goal Reframe

Therapist: So it seems like a big part of our work here will need to be about *learning new skills to handle these difficult thoughts/feelings/emotions/memories more effectively.*

Emotional Goal #2

Client: I just want to feel good (or happy, confident, calm, in love, etc.).

Behavioral Goal Reframe

Therapist: So you don't feel the way you want to. Can you tell me what kind of difficult thoughts and feelings are showing up for you? (*Therapist gathers this information.*) So it seems like a big part of our work here will need to be about *learning new skills to handle these difficult thoughts and feelings more effectively.*

Emotional Goal #3

Client: (*In reply to previous reframe*) I don't want to *handle* them. I just want to get rid of them!!!

Behavioral Goal Reframe

Therapist: Of course you do. Who wouldn't? They're really painful and difficult and they're having a huge negative impact on your life. So we'll *do something to improve that situation* as fast as possible. Is there anything else you want to get out of our work together?

Practical Tip   If this is all the client wants—to feel good and get rid of unwanted feelings—and he is not interested in anything else, the therapist will need to move to creative hopelessness, as covered in chapter 8. If the therapist skips creative hopelessness with such clients, she won't be able to get any further with ACT.

Emotional Goals Disguised as Behavioral Goals

Sometimes clients will present with what appear to be behavioral goals, but they're really just emotional goals in disguise. This is common with addictive and impulsive behaviors, and it usually takes the form "I want to stop doing this." If we dig beneath the surface, the hidden agenda is something like "Get rid of the thoughts and feelings (or urges, sensations, impulses, compulsions, withdrawal symptoms) that trigger this behavior, because until they are eliminated, I can't stop doing it." Here's how this might sound.

Emotional Goal In Disguise

Client: I want to stop… (drinking, smoking, gambling, overeating, yelling at my kids, etc.).

Behavioral Goal Reframe

Therapist: Sure. So part of our work here is to identify the thoughts and feelings (or memories, urges, impulses, obsessions, compulsions, and so on) that trigger this behavior, and *learn new skills to handle them more effectively* so they stop jerking you around and pulling you back into doing these things. And another part of the work is to explore what *you want to do instead*, so if you're ever in a similar situation again, you can choose *to do something different that will hopefully work better.*

Watch Out For "Dead Person's" Goals

As we've been discussing, often your client's goals will be to stop feeling or acting a certain way—for example, "I want to stop using drugs," "I want to stop procrastinating on my study," "I don't want to have any more panic attacks," or "I don't want to feel depressed." In ACT, these are called a "dead person's goals" (Lindsley, 1968). A dead person's goal is anything that a corpse can do better than a living human being. For example, a corpse will never use drugs, never procrastinate, never have a panic attack, and never feel depressed.

In ACT, we want to set "living person's" goals—things that a living human being can do better than a corpse. To move from a dead person's goal to a living person's goal, you can ask simple questions like these:

- So if that happens, what would you do differently? What would you start or do more of? How would you behave differently with friends or family?

- If you weren't using drugs, what would you be doing instead?

- If you weren't yelling at your kids, how would you be interacting with them?

- If you weren't feeling depressed or having panic attacks, what would you be doing differently with your life?

Two useful questions to turn emotional goals and dead person's goals into behavioral goals are the magic wand question and the seven-day documentary question. Let's take a quick look at each of these now.

THE MAGIC WAND QUESTION

This is a great question for cutting through experiential avoidance. (Note the phrase "are no longer a problem for you"; this is very different from saying "have all disappeared.")

Therapist: Suppose I had a magic wand here. I wave this wand, and all the thoughts and feelings you've been struggling with are no longer a problem for you; they're like water off a duck's back. What would you then do differently? What sort of things would you start doing or perhaps do more of? How would you behave differently toward others? What would you do differently at work, at home, on weekends?

THE SEVEN-DAY DOCUMENTARY QUESTION

This is a good question for helping the client become more specific about the changes she wants to make in her life.

Therapist: Suppose we followed you around with a camera crew for a week, filmed everything you did, and edited it into a documentary. And then suppose we did the same at some point in the future, after our work together has finished. What would we see or hear on the new video that would show that therapy had been helpful? What would we see you doing or hear you saying? What would we notice differently about the way you treat other people, the way you treat yourself, the way you treat your body, the way you spend your time?

In addition to emotional goals and dead person's goals, there is another category of goals we want to gently reframe: *outcome goals*.

Outcome Goals vs. Behavioral Goals

Here's the formula for outcome goals:

Outcome goals = what I want to *get* or *have*

Many clients come to therapy with outcome goals: what they want to get or have. For example, a client may want to find a partner, have a baby, get a job, lose ten pounds, cure an illness, recover from an injury, get a promotion, buy a house, or "get my kids to obey me." We want to validate these outcome goals; they are often useful for motivational purposes and are a good starting point for values and committed action. At the same time, we want to empower our clients through helping them to focus on what is within their control. We all have a lot of control over our own behavior, especially our overt behavior (what we say and do). And we all have zero control over what the *outcome* of our behavior will be; there's never a guarantee that we will get the outcome we are hoping for. So as soon as possible, let's convert these outcome goals into behavioral goals. Here are a few examples:

Outcome Goal #1

Client: I want to find a partner/get a better job.

Behavioral Goal Reframe

Therapist: So part of our work here is to get you doing things differently, saying and doing things that are likely to increase your chances of finding a partner/getting a better job.

Outcome Goal #2

Client: I want my kids to obey me/my husband to stop drinking.

Behavioral Goal Reframe

Therapist: So part of our work here is to get you doing things differently, saying and doing things that are likely to be more effective in influencing your children's/husband's behavior.

Outcome Goal #3

Client: I want to cure this illness/recover from this injury.

Behavioral Goal Reframe

Therapist: So there are two important parts to our work here: one part of it is to get you doing everything possible to improve your health—from cooperating with your medical team to looking after your diet and exercise. And the other part is to get you doing everything possible to make your life as good as it possibly can be right now, given all the difficulties imposed by your illness/injury.

   Insight goals are a subset of outcome goals. In this case, what the client wants to get or have (her desired outcome) is insight or self-understanding. Clients may express this as "I want to understand why I'm like this," "I need to figure out why I keep doing this," or "I want to discover who I really am." Therapy goals like these—primarily aimed at developing insight into one's own behavior—can easily lead to "analysis paralysis": session after session of intellectual/theoretical/conceptual discussions and endless reflections on the past instead of the development of new skills for mindful, valued living.

   As it happens, during ACT, clients will develop a lot of understanding and insight into their own behavior, thoughts, feelings, habits, personality, and identity. They will generally have powerful realizations around who they are, how their mind works, what they really want in life, how the past has influenced them, and why they do the things they do. But they will develop this insight via experiential work, not through lengthy analytical discussions. Furthermore, this insight is not an end in itself: it's simply something that happens on the journey toward the desired outcome of mindful, valued living.

   Thus, to move to a more useful therapy goal, I say, "Here's the thing. As we do this work together, you'll get a lot more understanding of who you are, how your mind works, why you do the things you do, and what you really want in life. That's already a given; it's all part of the process. What I'm curious to know is once you have that understanding, what do you want to do differently? If you had that knowledge, what would you do that you're not doing now? How would you behave differently? What would others notice that was different about you, in terms of what you say or do or how you interact with them?"

   So to recap, there are three kinds of goals:

Behavioral goals = what I want to *do*

Emotional goals = how I want to *feel*

Outcome goals = what I want to *get* or *have*

Overt and Covert Behavioral Goals

When we use a choice point to plot out the client's problems and therapy goals, the towards and away arrows can include both overt and covert behaviors. For example, *covert* towards moves could involve focusing, engaging, self-compassion, accepting, forgiving, appreciating, effective planning and strategizing, reflecting on values, being mindful, and so on. Covert away moves might involve disengaging, paying attention to thoughts and feelings instead of the current activity (often described as "distractedness" or "lack of focus"), and cognitive activities such as worrying, ruminating, and obsessing.

At times, you'll encounter clients who are quite content with their overt behavior; they're going through life doing all the things they want to be doing (or at least, this is what they say). The problem they complain about is they aren't able to enjoy or appreciate what they are doing because they are consumed by worrying (or other cognitive processes, such as ruminating, fantasizing, obsessing, or dwelling on the past). In this next example, the client—who has recently had cancer—is consumed by worry that she or someone she loves will become ill. She also worries about social situations, both before and during the event (whether people will like her, whether she's boring them).

Her anxiety doesn't stop her from doing the things she would like to do—she will still see friends, spend time with her kids, go to work, and so on—but it makes it hard for her to enjoy these things. She came to therapy with a number of emotional goals: stop worrying, stop thinking about illness, feel happier, and feel less anxious.

The therapist elicits that if therapy is successful, the client's overt behavior (i.e., her physical actions) will not change, but her covert behavior (i.e., her inner psychological behavior) will. For example, although this client currently attends social events, she gets hooked by her worries, and that leads to away moves that are mainly covert behaviors such as disengaging and focusing on her thoughts and feelings instead of being fully present with her loved ones (with clients, we would call this "getting distracted"). In the transcript below, the therapist articulates what a successful outcome (i.e., a change in covert behavior) would look like.

Therapist: So part of our work here is to help you develop some new skills to handle all these anxious thoughts and feelings more effectively, and especially to help you focus better when you're in those social situations so you can truly engage in what you're doing and be fully present with your loved ones—so you can actually appreciate these events.

Client: But what about the worrying? I really want to stop all this worrying; it's not good for me.

Therapist: Sure. So what "worrying" basically means is "getting hooked by anxious thoughts." Now I don't know how to stop your mind from coming up with thoughts about bad things that might happen; everyone's mind does that to some extent. But when we get hooked by those thoughts—all caught up in them, completely lost in them—that's what we mean by "worrying." So another part of our work here is to learn how to unhook from those anxious thoughts and refocus your attention on what you're doing; that's the antidote to worrying.

* * *

Did you notice how the therapist reframed the dead person's goal of "stop worrying" to the living person's goal of "unhook from anxious thoughts and refocus attention on the activity at hand"? We can use a similar reframe for other cognitive processes: rumination, dwelling on the past, revenge fantasies, blaming, obsessing, and so on. We can reframe these covert behaviors as "getting hooked by" the cognitive content in question (e.g., thoughts about "why I'm like this," painful memories, fantasies about revenge). The antidote, then, is learning how to unhook from such cognitive content and refocus attention on the activity at hand.

On a choice point, we could plot the above therapist summary as follows. (Note how both the towards and away moves are covert behaviors.).

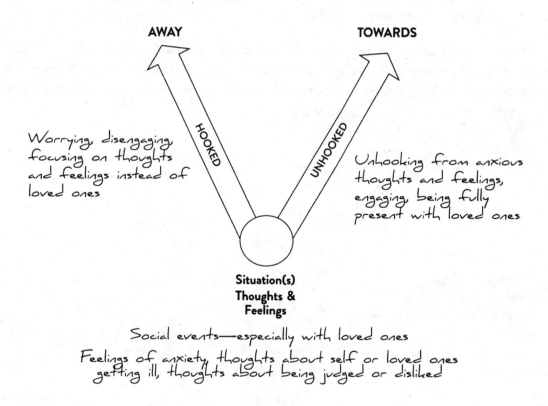

AWAY

TOWARDS

HOOKED

UNHOOKED

Worrying, disengaging, focusing on thoughts and feelings instead of loved ones

Unhooking from anxious thoughts and feelings, engaging, being fully present with loved ones

Situation(s)
Thoughts &
Feelings

Social events—especially with loved ones

Feelings of anxiety, thoughts about self or loved ones getting ill, thoughts about being judged or disliked

Therapy Goals: Two Examples

There's a lot to take in in this chapter, so to help you bring it all together, I'm going to give you a couple of examples of behavioral goals for therapy, as they would be summarized by the therapist.

BEHAVIORAL GOALS FOR DEPRESSION

In response to the magic wand question, this client replied that what she'd do differently is get back to work, start exercising again, and spend more time with her friends and family.

Therapist: So can we say it like this? It seems that what you mean by depression is that you're getting hooked by a lot of unpleasant thoughts—negative self-judgments, a sense of hopelessness, memories about painful events from the past, and worries about the future. And you're also getting hooked by some really painful feelings including guilt, sadness, anxiety, and physical tiredness. Does that sound right? And when you get hooked by these thoughts and feelings, your away moves include spending a lot of time in bed, socially isolating yourself, staying indoors, avoiding the gym, avoiding going to work, watching a lot of TV, and so on. Am I getting this right? So what we're aiming for here is (a) to learn some new skills to handle all those difficult thoughts and feelings—to unhook from them so they no longer bring you down or hold you back—and (b) to get you back into doing things that used to matter to you, such as socializing, working, exercising, and generally doing things that fulfill you. Is that about right?

Notice how the therapist breaks the issue down into two elements that correlate well with the choice point: (1) getting hooked by (fusion with and avoidance of) thoughts and feelings, and (2) unworkable actions. If desired, the therapist could map this out on a choice point while she is running through the spiel above. It would look like this:

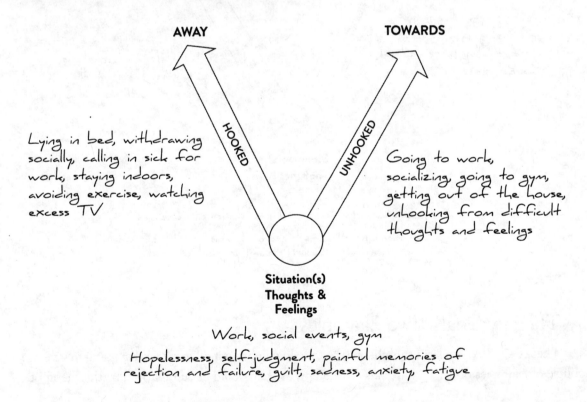

AWAY   **TOWARDS**

HOOKED   UNHOOKED

Lying in bed, withdrawing socially, calling in sick for work, staying indoors, avoiding exercise, watching excess TV

Going to work, socializing, going to gym, getting out of the house, unhooking from difficult thoughts and feelings

Situation(s)
Thoughts &
Feelings

Work, social events, gym
Hopelessness, self-judgment, painful memories of rejection and failure, guilt, sadness, anxiety, fatigue

Note that right from the word go, we can subtly lay the groundwork for two key insights:

1. Our thoughts and feelings are not the main problem; it's getting hooked by them (fusion and avoidance) that creates our problems.

2. Our thoughts and feelings do not have to control our behavior.

This second key insight often takes therapists by surprise, so let's take a moment to explore it. Our thoughts and feelings *influence* our behavior, but they don't necessarily *control* our behavior. As we explored in chapter 4, our behavior in any moment is under the influence of multiple streams of stimuli, coming both from the world inside our skin and from the world outside us.

So when do thoughts and feelings have the most influence over behavior? You guessed it: in a context of fusion and avoidance. However, in a context of defusion and acceptance (that is, mindfulness), those same thoughts and feelings have much less influence over our behavior (i.e., we unhook from them), which makes it easier for us to act on our values.

What this means is the greater our psychological flexibility, the greater our capacity to choose our behavior, regardless of the thoughts and feelings we're having. With this in mind, we want to repeatedly draw a distinction between (a) the client's thoughts and feelings (antecedents) and (b) what the client does when those thoughts and feelings show up (behavior). Ultimately, we want to shatter the illusion that the former controls the latter.

Now let's look at another example of good behavioral goal setting.

BEHAVIORAL GOALS FOR ADDICTION

This client wanted to quit drinking for two reasons: one, his wife was threatening to leave him, and two, at a recent medical checkup, his liver was in bad shape. In response to the magic wand question, he said he wanted to be a "better husband" and "fix up" his liver.

Therapist: So to summarize, when you've tried to quit drinking in the past, it would never last long because you'd get strong cravings or feelings of anxiety showing up, and when you get hooked by those feelings, you start drinking. So our aims here are to (a) learn some new skills so you can handle these cravings and feelings more effectively—unhook from them so they don't keep jerking you around and pulling you back into drinking, (b) start saying and doing things differently, to help build a better relationship your wife, and (c) start looking after your liver, to help make it as healthy as possible. Is that about right?

Again, if desired, the therapist could map these goals out on a choice point:

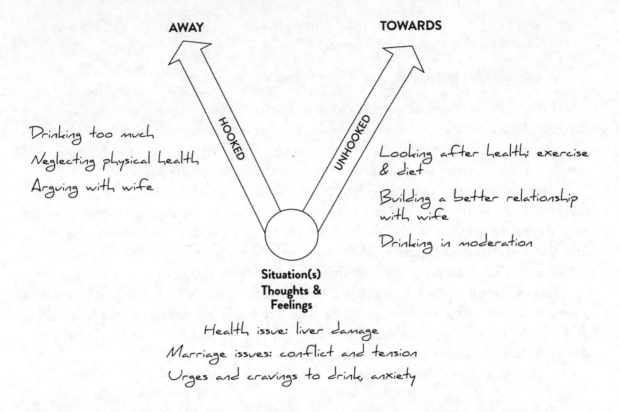

AWAY

TOWARDS

HOOKED

UNHOOKED

Drinking too much
Neglecting physical health
Arguing with wife

Looking after health: exercise
& diet

Building a better relationship
with wife

Drinking in moderation

Situation(s)
Thoughts &
Feelings

Health issue: liver damage
Marriage issues: conflict and tension
Urges and cravings to drink, anxiety

> **Practical Tip**   The choice point diagrams in this chapter are all "minimalist": just a few notes to highlight key themes. If you wish, either you or the client can write in a lot more detail. You can also do a separate choice point for each issue you focus on. For example, suppose in a later session with the client above, you focus primarily on improving his relationship with his wife; you might then do a fresh choice point purely on the relationship problems.

"Catch-All" Behavioral Goals

Sometimes, despite all your best efforts, your client will be unable or unwilling to give you any specific behavioral goals. She may just keep answering, "I don't know," "Nothing matters," "I just want to stop feeling like this," or "I just want to feel happy." In such cases, don't try to force the point. For now, just stick to the nonspecific catch-all generic behavioral goals you introduced in the informed consent process:

Therapist: So how does this sound to you? Part of our work here will involve learning some new
          skills to unhook from your thoughts and feelings so they don't jerk you around or hold

you back from living the life you want. And another part of it, even though right now you have no idea what you want and you feel like nothing matters, is to make this a place where that can change. We can work on finding out what matters to you, and experiment with doing things differently to make your life better.

Extra Bits

See chapter 6 in *ACT Made Simple: The Extra Bits* (downloadable from the "Free Stuff" page at http://www.actmindfully.com.au). There you'll find (a) printable versions of two worksheets, Dissecting the Problem and the Bull's Eye, and (b) more tips for establishing behavioral goals in tricky cases.

Skilling Up

Here are some steps you can take to practice the skills we've just covered:

- Read out loud and paraphrase the therapist's spiels in the transcripts above to get yourself used to ACT-speak and find your own style of doing it.

- Pick two clients and write brief answers to these key questions: What valued direction does the client want to move in? What is getting in her way?

- Practice thinking in terms of behavioral goals. Pick two clients and imagine how you would summarize the therapy goals.

- If you like the choice point, fill in a diagram for one of the issues you picked in the second and third tasks above.

As you do these exercises (and all the other ones in this book), please give yourself permission to do them poorly. You're learning a new model of therapy, so allow yourself to be a beginner, a novice, a learner. Beginners make mistakes (as do experts). It's an essential part of the learning process. And if your mind starts beating you up, make a note of what it says so you can work with those thoughts in chapter 12.

Takeaway

The overarching takeaway in this chapter is to establish behavioral goals as soon as possible, even if they're just the vague generic goals covered in informed consent. It's especially important to do this when clients present with a stack of emotional goals. It may take a while, but it makes the whole rest of your therapy so much easier.

Thoughts That Hook You	Life-Draining Actions:
What memories, worries, fears, self-criticisms, or other unhelpful thoughts do you dwell on or get "caught up" in that are related to this issue? What thoughts tend to hook you, jerk you around, pull you out of your life?	What are you currently doing that makes your life worse in the long run: keeps you stuck; wastes your time or money; drains your energy; restricts your life; impacts negatively on your health, work, or relationships; maintains or worsens the problems you are dealing with?
Feelings That Hook You	Avoiding Challenging Situations:
What emotions, feelings, urges, impulses, or sensations tend to hook you and jerk you around or pull you into self-defeating actions?	What situations, activities, people, or places are you avoiding or staying away from? What have you quit, withdrawn from, dropped out of? What do you keep "putting off" until later?

The Dissecting the Problem Worksheet

YOUR VALUES: *What do you want to do with your time on this planet? What sort of person do you want to be? What personal strengths or qualities do you want to develop? Please write a few words under each heading below.*

Work/Education: includes workplace, career, education, and skills development.

Relationships: includes your partner, children, parents, relatives, friends, and co-workers.

Personal Growth/Health: may include religion, spirituality, creativity, life skills, meditation, yoga, nature; exercise, nutrition, and/or addressing health-risk factors.

Leisure: how you play, relax, or enjoy yourself; activities for rest, recreation, fun, and creativity.

THE BULL'S EYE: make an X in each area of the dart board to represent where you stand today.

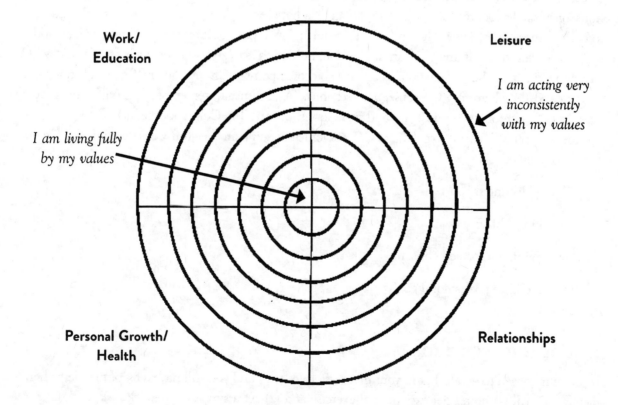

Adapted from *Living Beyond Your Pain* by J. Dahl and T. Lundgren by permission of New Harbinger Publications (Oakland, CA), www.newharbinger.com.

The Bull's Eye Worksheet

CHAPTER 7

Where Do I Start?

Beginning Well

One of the most common questions I get asked in ACT workshops is "Russ, where do you get your amazing shirts from?" To which I reply, "I'm sorry, but that's a trade secret." However, two other questions I get asked a lot are "Where do I start?" and "What process do I focus on first?" And my answer to both of those questions is "It depends." Remember, ACT is a nonlinear model, and you can work with any core process at any point in any session. So there's no fixed sequence; where you start will vary from client to client. However, I can give you some pointers around (a) the first steps in active therapy and (b) where to go in subsequent sessions. (And as usual, remember to modify and adapt everything; what follows are just tips and suggestions, not the Ten Commandments.)

Ideally, you will start off your first ACT session(s) by doing all the stuff we covered in the previous two chapters:

- establishing rapport

- taking a history

- obtaining informed consent

- establishing behavioral goals

Initial Interventions

If you've managed to do all that in your first session (or two) and you still have a bit of time left, then ideally you will (1) do a brief experiential exercise and (2) set a simple homework task. Let's take a quick look at these two interventions.

A Brief Experiential Exercise

Throughout this book, you'll find a wide range of brief experiential exercises, many of which take less than five minutes to do. One of the simplest is dropping anchor, which we cover in chapter 10. Another is the defusion technique "I'm having the thought that," described in chapter 12. There are many others covered in other chapters, and you can pare back any mindfulness technique (e.g., observing the breath or a body scan) to a simple three- or four-minute version.

Keep in mind, however, if you're going to introduce an experiential exercise, you need to ensure that you have time not only to complete the exercise, but also to debrief it afterward, to make sure the client understands the purpose and sees how it's relevant to her therapy goals.

Also keep in mind what we discussed in the last chapter: if your client is only interested in feeling good and getting rid of pain, and resists your efforts to establish behavioral goals, your first experiential work will need to be creative hopelessness (chapter 8).

A Simple Homework Task

It's a good idea to ask your clients to do a bit of homework between sessions. For example, if you took your client through a mindfulness exercise in session, then for homework, you could ask her to practice it. Alternatively, you might ask her to keep a diary or fill in a worksheet, such as those mentioned at the end of this chapter.

Practical Tip   Many clients dislike the word "homework," so I recommend you use alternative words. You might ask, for example, "Would you be willing to play around with this [or try it out, test it out, experiment with it, practice this, fill this in, give it a go, work on this, apply this, spend some time on this]?"

If you've introduced the choice point, it readily lends itself to simple homework tasks. Here's my favorite:

Noticing Towards and Away Moves

Therapist: Between now and next session, can I ask you to do a couple of things? First, notice your towards moves. When and where do you do them? What difference do they make? See if you can really appreciate them as you're doing them.

Second, notice your away moves. When and where do you do them? And especially see if you can notice: what are the thoughts and feelings that hook you, and pull you into doing them?

* * *

There are many ways to modify this homework. For example, you might ask the client to write his observations down in a diary. Or you might give the client a blank choice point to put in a prominent place as a reminder. Or you might ask him to fill in a choice point between sessions, focused on a specific issue (e.g., a "bad habit" he is trying to break, such as smoking or drinking too much, or a recurring situation he struggles with, such as looking after his three young children) and bring it back completed to the next session. This deceptively simple choice point homework serves a number of different purposes:

- It increases client self-awareness.

- It provides useful information for the next session, which helps with setting an agenda and deciding what to target first.

- It's a good first step in getting the client to notice his thoughts and feelings and become more aware of his behavior.

- The information gathered on towards moves is usually very useful for exploring values, goals, and committed action.

Practical Tip   If you aren't keen on the choice point, you can set exactly the same homework task as above without drawing it or referring to it. The language and concepts (hooking, unhooking, towards and away moves) are more powerful for most people when you visually illustrate them, but you certainly don't need to.

Client Worksheets

Worksheets are often helpful because they act as a reminder of the session, increase the chance that your client will follow through, and provide good material for the next session. However, if clients are not keen on filling in forms (or if you as a therapist dislike them), then you don't have to use them. They are simply aids to ACT, not essentials.

At the end of the first session, if you didn't get much information about values, and you didn't get the client to fill out a Bull's Eye worksheet (chapter 6), you could now ask her to do so for homework. For example, you might say, "We've talked quite a lot about your problems today—the thoughts and feelings you struggle with, and the things you do that make your life worse—but we haven't talked much about what sort of life you want to live, what really matters to you in the big picture. So I'm wondering, between now and next session, would you be willing to fill in this worksheet, which asks you to think about these things?"

Other worksheets you might give out are the Vitality vs. Suffering Diary or the Problems and Values worksheet (see Extra Bits). You can explain that these worksheets help gather more information to guide therapy.

After the First Session, What's Next?

Hopefully this chapter and the previous one have given you a reasonably clear idea about what to do in your first session (or two). And the burning question now is "What next?" And again the answer is "It depends." That's right: there is no "correct" answer to this question, no such thing as the "right" or "wrong" next step. All six core processes are interconnected and overlapping, and you can use any of them at any point during therapy. What follows are some ideas as to where you *could* go next, but this will vary depending on your assessment of the client's needs. So make sure to hold these pointers loosely—and feel free to make different choices, tailored to suit your unique client.

- *When clients are overwhelmed by their feelings, extremely fused, dissociated, emotionally dysregulated, or highly impulsive:* begin with mindful grounding exercises such as dropping anchor (chapter 10).

- *When clients are experiencing major grief or loss:* begin with self-compassion (chapter 18) and/ or dropping anchor (chapter 10).

- *For the poorly motivated or those fused with hopelessness:* begin with values (chapter 19) and defusion from hopelessness (chapter 14).

- *For clients fixated on feeling good and getting rid of painful feelings:* begin with creative hopelessness (chapter 8).

(Clients who are mandated or coerced to get counseling are beyond the scope of this book, but I cover this in my advanced level textbook, *Getting Unstuck in ACT* [Harris, 2013].)

Choosing Which Path to Follow

Broadly speaking, after the first session, ACT protocols tend to follow one of two paths, which flow from these two questions:

A. *What valued direction does the client want to move in?*

    If this is the path chosen, the steps followed (not necessarily in this order) are typically:

- Values clarification

- Goal setting

- Action planning

- Problem solving

- Skills training

- Exposure

Speaking in terms of the choice point, when we take this path, we focus on clarifying and planning *towards moves*.

B. *What's getting in the client's way?*

If this is the path chosen, the steps followed (often in this order, but not necessarily) are typically:

- Target inflexible attention with contacting the present moment.

- Target fusion with defusion.

- Target experiential avoidance with acceptance.

- Target self-criticism, self-hatred, and self-neglect with self-compassion.

In the language of the choice point, all of the above are *unhooking skills*, chosen to match the client's specific *away moves*.

Whichever path you start on, sooner or later it's going to cross over with the other path. Remember, all core processes are interconnected. But don't concern yourself about this for now; as you progress through the book, we'll look at how to jump from path to path.

Determining What to Do in Each Session

Recall that the aim of ACT is to cultivate psychological flexibility: the ability to be fully conscious and open to your experience while acting on your values—or, said more simply, the ability to "be present, open up, and do what matters." The outcome we're looking for is mindful, values-based living: doing what is meaningful while embracing each moment of life.

ACT practitioners need to learn how to do three things really well:

1. develop a client's openness to her own thoughts and feelings;

2. help the client be fully present—engaging in life and focusing on what's important; and

3. help the client do what matters, acting effectively, guided by her values.

The ACT triflex, which we first saw in chapter 1, shows how these tasks relate to each other and to the core processes:

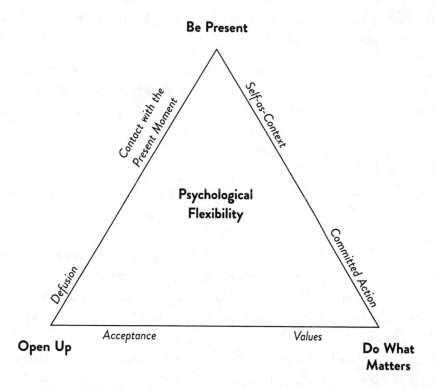

The ACT Triflex: Be Present, Open Up, Do What Matters

In any session, if we do any intervention—no matter how brief or long, how simple or complex—that helps the client with being present, opening up, or doing what matters, it's useful; it helps develop psychological flexibility.

Tricky Terminology   In many ACT textbooks, the terms "being present," "opening up," and "doing what matters" are referred to respectively as "aware," "open," and "engaged."

The triflex serves as a useful visual map of what we tend to do in each session, based on our assessment of what the client needs at the time:

- If the client is overwhelmed, dissociated, or extremely fused, we start up top with *being present*: grounding and dropping anchor.

- If we want to help the client get moving, we shift to the right side of the triflex: *doing what matters* (values and committed action). We clarify values, set goals, create action plans, and teach skills.

- If the client is deeply stuck, going nowhere, paralyzed by fusion and experiential avoidance, we shift to the left side: *opening up* (defusion and acceptance).

- If we run into barriers at either the left or right side (or both), we come back to center: *being present* (grounding, dropping anchor).

- If the client is successfully doing what matters, we return to being present: we help the client to engage fully in her experience and focus on what she's doing. And if she's doing something potentially enjoyable, we help her learn how to appreciate and savor it.

Setting an Agenda

The more stuck, directionless, or overwhelmed your client is, the more important it is to establish an agenda for the session. This is doubly so when your client keeps "problem-hopping": rapidly moving from problem to problem without focusing on any one of them long enough to come up with an effective action plan or strategy to address it. You could ask, "Can we pick one important problem or area of life that we can make the main focus of the session, in order to improve it?"

It's often good to give a rationale for this, such as "The reason for this is it makes our work much more efficient. If we are trying to deal with several different problems at once, it's very hard to deal effectively with any of them."

Alternatively, you could ask the client to nominate a single problem, goal, relationship, or other aspect of life to focus on for today's session. Then agree to work on a specific unhooking skill or an action plan to deal with the chosen issue.

You can of course use the choice point to set an agenda. You could present it to the client and say, "So we have two main options for today's session. We can focus on the towards moves—have a look at what you want to do differently to take your life in the direction you want. Or we can focus more on building those unhooking skills, to help you handle those difficult thoughts and feelings. Which would you prefer?"

If your client is fixated on feeling good or getting rid of her pain, and that's all she wants from therapy, then go to creative hopelessness.

If the client chooses towards moves, then start with either clarifying values or setting goals:

- If she already knows her values, set goals.

- If she doesn't know her values, clarify them. Then use those values to set goals.

- Once the client has values-based goals, turn them into action plans.

If the client chooses unhooking skills, start with the easiest ones first: dropping anchor and simple defusion.

A Rough Sequence for Teaching Unhooking Skills

When we teach unhooking skills, there is no particular sequence we have to follow. However, when I created my own ACT protocol for the general public ("The Happiness Trap Online Program"; to find out more about it, go to https://thehappinesstrap.com), this is the sequence I used:

1. Dropping anchor/mindful grounding (chapter 10)

2. Simple defusion (e.g., noticing and naming) (chapter 11)

3. Meditative defusion (e.g., Leaves on a Stream) (chapter 15)

4. Attention-training and focusing skills (e.g., mindful breathing) (chapter 17)

5. Engaging and savoring skills (e.g., mindful eating, drinking, walking, listening) (chapter 17)

6. Self-compassion (chapter 18)

7. Acceptance of pain (chapter 22)

8. The noticing self (chapter 25)

You can use this sequence as a general guideline, likely to work well with most of your clients. However, please don't regard it as something you have to follow. Vary it as needed. We always want to be flexible in how we work and adapt what we do to the unique client in front of us.

Structuring Your Sessions

Here's a good general structure (again, hold it loosely and adapt it as needed) for your sessions:

1. Mindfulness exercise

2. Review of previous session

3. Agenda

4. Main interventions

5. Homework

Let's take a quick look at each of these now.

Mindfulness exercise. It's often helpful to start each session with a brief mindfulness exercise such as dropping anchor or mindful breathing. This is not essential, but it gets both client and therapist into a mindful state and sets an expectation for experiential work.

Review of previous session. Review the previous session, including key content covered, exercises practiced, and any thoughts or reactions the client has had since. If your client followed through on his homework, what happened, and what difference did it make? And if not, what got in the way?

Agenda. Agree on an agenda for the session, as outlined above.

Main interventions. If you're following a protocol, you'll have a good idea in advance of what you wish to cover in session. It's important, though, to be flexible—to respond to what's happening in session. Be willing to let go of everything you had planned, if need be. (You can always come back to it later.) If you're not following a protocol, you will either pick up from wherever you left off in the previous session or you will address a new issue based on the agenda you have just set.

Homework. It's important to repeatedly emphasize to clients that what they do in between sessions is what will really make all the difference in their lives. New skills require practice. Valued action requires effort. Before the end of each session, you need to collaboratively agree on what the client is going to practice, do, or experiment with between sessions. (But be careful—don't get too pushy or use values coercively.)

Extra Bits

See chapter 7 in *ACT Made Simple: The Extra Bits* (downloadable from the "Free Stuff" page at http://www.actmindfully.com.au). There you'll find the Vitality vs. Suffering Diary and the Problems and Values worksheet.

Takeaway

After we've taken a history, built rapport, obtained informed consent, and established behavioral goals for therapy, which is the main work of the first session (or two), we move into active intervention, with an emphasis on experiential work in session and homework between sessions.

When you get into the experiential work, dance around the three overarching processes depicted in the ACT triflex: being present, opening up, doing what matters.

- To get the client moving: work on values and committed action (towards moves).

- When the client is stuck: work on defusion and acceptance (unhooking skills).

- And if you're blocked at either side: work on getting back to being present and dropping anchor (more unhooking skills).

PART 3

The Nitty Gritty Stuff

CHAPTER 8

Creative What?!

I Just Want to Be Happy!

Have you ever had a client who just wanted to be happy? And that's all she wanted from therapy? Of course you have. And I'm sure you remember well how challenging that was! Luckily, from now on, you will have something to help you with these clients: *creative hopelessness*. (Please don't let the name put you off.)

Creative Hopelessness in a Nutshell

In Plain Language: *Creative hopelessness* is a process in which one becomes aware that trying hard to avoid or get rid of unwanted thoughts and feelings tends to makes life worse rather than better. This leads to a sense of hopelessness in the agenda of avoiding one's difficult thoughts and feelings, out of which can emerge a creative attitude toward finding new and different ways of dealing with them.

Aim: To increase the client's awareness of the emotional control agenda (see below) and the costs of excessive experiential avoidance; to consciously recognize and acknowledge that clinging tightly to this agenda is unworkable.

Synonym: Confronting the agenda.

Method: We look at what the client has done to avoid or get rid of unwanted thoughts and feelings, examine how they work in the short term and the long term, uncover all the costs of these strategies, and explore whether they are making life better or worse.

When to Use: When we know or suspect that the client is excessively experientially avoidant, strongly attached to an agenda of emotional control: *I must feel good; I must get rid of these unwanted thoughts and feelings.*

The Emotional Control Agenda

Creative hopelessness is a part of the ACT model that we bring in if we know for a fact or are pretty sure that the client is clinging tightly to the agenda of emotional control: *I've got to control how I feel. I have to get rid of the unwanted, unpleasant, and difficult thoughts, feelings, emotions, and memories—and replace them with good, pleasant, and desirable ones.*

Now we've all got this agenda to some extent; you'll recall that in chapter 2, we looked at how this is normal and how experiential avoidance in moderation is not problematic. But when the client is clinging desperately to this agenda, experiential avoidance is high and almost always very problematic. (Remember: high levels of experiential avoidance directly correlate with risk of depression, anxiety disorders, long-term disability, poor work performance, PTSD, addiction, and many other psychiatric disorders.)

Creative hopelessness gets its name because what we aim to do is create a sense of hopelessness *in this agenda of controlling your feelings.* (It's not about hopelessness in your future, yourself, or your life). We aim to undermine this agenda so we can open our clients up to a new one: the agenda of acceptance. (ACT textbooks often refer to this new agenda as "willingness": that is, the willingness to have your difficult thoughts and feelings, as opposed to fighting with or avoiding them.)

Creative hopelessness (CH) is rarely a once-off intervention. It's usually something you need to revisit session after session. But usually each time you revisit it, it gets quicker and easier to do. Now before we get into the nitty gritty of CH, let's get clear on the concept of…

Emotional Control Strategies

Emotional control strategies (ECS) are anything we do primarily to try to get rid of unwanted thoughts and feelings: overt or covert behavior that's predominantly motivated by experiential avoidance. ECS can include everything from exercise, prayer, and meditation to alcohol, heroin, and suicide attempts. (Note: if exercise, prayer, and meditation are predominantly motivated by values, we wouldn't call them ECS. We'd call them ECS only if the main intention of such activities is to avoid or get rid of unwanted feelings.) In CH work, we ask the client to look openly and nonjudgmentally at all the emotional control strategies she's using. But we never judge these ECS as good or bad, right or wrong, positive or negative; our aim is purely and simply to see how these strategies are working (or not) in terms of creating a better life.

Do We Target All Emotional Control Strategies?

In a word: nooooooo! Recall that the whole ACT model rests on the concept of workability: is this behavior working to help you build a rich and meaningful life? So if your emotional control strategies are working to enrich and enhance your life, keep doing them! However, the reality is that most human beings overrely on ECS, and when we use them excessively, rigidly, or inappropriately, our quality of life suffers.

Take eating chocolate, for example. When we mindfully eat a piece of good-quality chocolate, appreciating and savoring it, we feel good (assuming we like chocolate). So if we use this as an ECS, flexibly and moderately, it enriches our life: it's workable. But if we do it excessively, it may start to have costs to our health, such as weight gain. Plus, if we are in intense emotional pain and we eat chocolate to try to distract ourselves from it, that's unlikely to work.

Exercise is another example. When we exercise, we often feel better (at least afterward, if not at the time). And exercise also improves our quality of life. Therefore, if we use exercise as an ECS, and we do so flexibly and moderately, that's generally workable. But if it becomes excessive—like the client with anorexia who spends three hours in the gym each day to keep her body in a state of wasted thinness—then even something as positive as exercise will have costs.

Furthermore, ACT postulates that even life-enhancing activities (such as exercise, meditation, and healthy eating) will be more satisfying and rewarding when they're motivated by values (such as self-care) rather than by experiential avoidance (trying to escape unwanted feelings).

For example, have you ever eaten yummy food primarily to push away unwanted feelings such as boredom, stress, or anxiety? Was it a deeply satisfying experience? Contrast that with occasions when your eating was motivated by values around savoring and appreciating your food, or connecting and sharing with loved ones. Which was more rewarding? Similarly, if you do charity work motivated by values around sharing, caring, giving, and helping, you'll likely find that far more rewarding than if you're mainly motivated by trying to avoid feelings of guilt or worthlessness.

Therefore, we aim to help clients take action guided by their values rather than by experiential avoidance: we want to get them consciously moving toward what is meaningful rather than simply running from what is unwanted.

To really hammer this point home, suppose you exercise primarily motivated by values such as self-care, or you pray motivated by values around connecting with God. We wouldn't class those as ECS because your *primary aim* isn't to control how you feel. But we *would* class them as ECS if your main purpose in doing them is to get rid of unwanted thoughts and feelings.

CH is an intervention based on workability. We ask the client to take a good, long, honest, and mindful look at all his ECS and see what they are costing him. We want him to connect with the reality that his ECS often work in the short run to make him feel better, but do not work in the long run to make his life rich, full, and meaningful.

Is CH Necessary for Everyone?

Again, the answer is nooooooooooo. (I like that word!) If a client is motivated to change and not deeply attached to an agenda of emotional control, or if she's already familiar with mindfulness or ACT and open to the approach, then there's no need for CH, and we can skip it.

How Long Does It Take?

CH interventions vary enormously in length. In Zettle's (2007) sample protocol for depression, the initial CH intervention lasts for twenty minutes. But we can also do CH more quickly, in the space of a few minutes (Strosahl, 2005). At the other extreme, some therapists spend an entire session on CH. So ideally we'll "titrate" the intervention to suit our client's issues. Take for example a high-functioning client with plenty of self-awareness and openness to new ideas compared with a client with a lifelong history of substance abuse who clings desperately to the emotional control agenda. The latter will need a far more extensive CH intervention than the former.

How Do We Ease the Client Into It?

Whatever the length of the CH intervention, we want to gently lead the client into the shallow waters of creative hopelessness, then gradually wade in deeper; we do not want to push him head first into the deep end. This may go something like this:

Therapist: Okay, so it seems like the main thing you're wanting from our work together is to get rid of these difficult thoughts and feelings, such as… (*therapist recaps the main thoughts, feelings, emotions, memories, urges, and so on that the client wishes to avoid*).

Client: Yeah. That's about right. I hate feeling like this. I just want to be happy.

Therapist: Of course you do. Who wouldn't? These feelings are really painful and difficult and they are having a huge negative impact on your life. So we want to change that situation as fast as possible. But before we try something new, we first need to get clear about everything you've already tried in the past—find out what's worked and what hasn't. So is it okay if we just take a few minutes to zip through what you've tried in the past?

You're now set up to confront the agenda, by taking the client through five basic questions.

Five Basic Questions

There are many different ways of doing CH, but they all boil down to these questions:

1.   What have you tried?

2.   How has it worked?

3.   What has it cost?

4.   What's showing up?

5.   Are you open to something new?

We're now going to explore these questions in depth. There's a lot to take in, but don't worry, you can download my Join the DOTS worksheet, which summarizes all the key points (see Extra Bits). You can also use Join the DOTS (or another worksheet or tool, or just your notepad) to record the valuable information you and your client will glean from these five questions.

Question 1: What Have You Tried?

The first question in CH is "What have you tried doing so far to avoid and get rid of these unwanted thoughts and feelings?" We'll usually need to prompt our clients' memories, so I have a little acronym—DOTS—that helps me remember the prompts:

D = *Distraction*

O = *Opting out*

T = *Thinking strategies*

S = *Substances and other strategies*

Let's go through these one by one.

D = DISTRACTION

I'll say to clients, "Have you ever tried distracting yourself from these feelings? What have you tried? Watching television? Listening to music? Getting out of the house? Getting busy? Playing computer games? Any other ways you've tried to distract yourself?"

O = OPTING OUT

This is a layperson's term for overt avoidance, that is, avoiding stuff outside my skin—people places, situations, activities, events. So we can ask the client, "Have you ever tried opting out, withdrawing, or staying away from situations and people and activities that tend to trigger these uncomfortable thoughts and feelings? What kind of things have you quit or opted out of?"

The easiest place to begin is usually with procrastination, so I ask clients:

Are there important things you are procrastinating on?

Are there important tasks you are avoiding?

Are there people or places you're staying away from?

Are there important activities you're putting off?

T = THINKING STRATEGIES

The question we ask here is, "How have you tried to think your pain away?" Run through some common thinking strategies with your clients: "Have you tried thinking of people who are worse off than you? Positive thinking? Challenging your thoughts or debating with yourself? Pushing the thoughts out of your head? Minimizing it? Criticizing yourself? Telling yourself to just *snap out of it* or *get on with it*?"

S = SUBSTANCES AND OTHER STRATEGIES

Here we first ask, "What kinds of substances have you tried putting into your body to get rid of pain? Drugs? Alcohol? Prescription medications? Aspirin? Paracetamol? Coffee? Tea? Cigarettes? Pepsi? Pizza? Ice cream? Double-coated chocolate Tim Tams? (Tim Tams are the greatest invention in the history of Australia—a truly amazing chocolate-coated cookie that forms a staple food source for most Australians.)

And after that we explore, "Are there any other strategies you ever use to try to escape these feelings? Have you seen doctors or therapists? Read self-help books? Tried things like exercise, yoga, meditation, diet change? Self-harming? Suicide? Taking risks or doing dangerous things? Picking fights or quarrels? Keeping busy? Planning holidays? Doing house work? Prayer? Beating yourself up? Giving up? Gritting your teeth and forcing yourself to get on with it? Asking yourself, *Why am I like this?*"

Here's an example of how this process sounds in a session:

Therapist: By the time most folks get to therapy, they've already tried doing a lot of different things to feel better or not feel so bad, and some of them work, and some of them don't. And I'm guessing it's the same for you. And one of the things I want to ensure here is that we don't do more of what doesn't work. So could we spend a bit of time recapping all the things you've tried to avoid or get rid of these painful thoughts and feelings?

Client: To be honest, I can't really think of anything.

Therapist: Well, let me help you out here. One of the most common things people do is try to distract themselves, to take their mind off how they feel. Do you ever do that?

Client: Of course!

Therapist: Me too. So what sort of things do you do to distract yourself?

Client: I watch TV. Listen to music. Read. Smoke dope.

Therapist: Computers?

Client: Yeah—computer games, surfing the Net, a lot of time on YouTube, just watching crap.

Therapist: Anything else?

Client: (*pauses, shakes his head*)

Therapist: Well, another thing people often do is they start opting out of things that bring up painful feelings. Are there any important people, places, activities that you've withdrawn from? Anything important you're putting off or staying away from?

* * *

In this way, the therapist works through DOTS, taking anywhere from five to fifteen minutes. You might just evoke two or three strategies for each category of DOTS, or you might go through all the different strategies the client has ever used. It really depends on (a) how attached the client is to the agenda of emotional control and (b) how much time you have in session.

Question 2: How Has It Worked?

The second question we explore in CH is "How has it worked *in the long term?*" We want to validate that most of these ECS work in the short term to relieve the client's pain, and then we want to ask compassionately and respectfully, "How do they work in the long term? Do these thoughts and feelings permanently go away, or do they come back?"

The purpose of this question is to help the client join the dots: she's been trying and trying and trying to get rid of this pain, and she's found a zillion and one ways of achieving this *in the short term*—but in the long term it keeps coming back!

There are two ways to run through question 2. Some people bring in question 2 as a discrete second phase of CH. In phase one, you list all the client's ECS, and in phase two you say something like this:

Therapist: So most of these strategies give you some relief in the short term, right? (*Client agrees.*) And did any of these permanently eliminate those feelings, so they never came back?

Client: I don't know. Maybe some of them.

Therapist: Okay, but mostly they keep coming back, right? Otherwise you wouldn't be here, right?

Client: Yeah.

Other people prefer to interweave question 1 and question 2, rather than address them in separate phases. So after the client identifies an ECS (or a category of ECS), the therapist asks, "So did that work in the short term? Did it give you a bit of relief?" The client will usually answer "yes" or "at first" or "a bit" or "It helped a bit to begin with." The therapist then replies, "And what about in the long term?" or "And how long did that last?" or "And how long before the feelings came back?"

Either way, the therapist brings question 2 to an end with something like this: "So you've tried lots of different strategies. And in the short term, most of these strategies work; they give you some relief; but in the long term, these difficult thoughts and feelings keep coming back."

It's also worth asking, "And would you say, from year to year, your pain/anxiety/depression is staying the same, getting better, or getting worse?" Almost all of these clients will report that it's getting worse.

Question 3: What Has It Cost?

A little bit of experiential avoidance is rarely a problem for most of us, but high levels usually come with significant costs. So we now ask the client, "Can we take a few moments to explore the costs of using all these strategies to avoid discomfort?" Again, we'll usually need to prompt our clients to help them contact the costs. Fortunately, we can once again use the DOTS acronym to help us with this process; we can look at each type of emotional control strategy (distraction, opting out, thinking strategies, substances, and other strategies) to discover the costs when the client relies on it excessively.

> **Practical Tip**   Remember, we aren't "mindfulness fascists" in ACT; we aren't opposed to all ECS. So be crystal clear about this with your clients, saying something like "If any of these strategies are working long term to help build the life you want to live, then please keep doing them! I'm not asking you to stop. What I would like to do, please, if it's okay with you, is look at the costs of these strategies when you use them excessively."

COSTS OF DISTRACTION

Distraction, in moderation, used flexibly, is rarely a problem and sometimes very helpful. But what are some of the costs of excessive distraction? We want to ask the client, "How much time do you spend on distracting yourself?" "How much of that seems time well spent, and how much feels like time wasted?" "How much money do you spend on it?" "Do these things have any costs to your health, work, or relationships?"

COSTS OF OPTING OUT

Next, we want to explore the costs of excessive opting out (overt avoidance). For most people, the biggest cost is missed opportunities. The more we start avoiding important and meaningful people, places, situations, activities, and events, the smaller our lives get and the more we miss out on. If your client is avoiding asking the boss for a pay raise, what's the financial cost of that? If she's avoiding having a difficult heart-to-heart conversation with her partner, what are the intimacy costs to the relationship? If he's avoiding going to the doctor or the dentist or going to the gym, what are the health costs?

COSTS OF THINKING STRATEGIES

One of the biggest costs of thinking strategies is spending your day caught up in your thoughts, thereby missing out on life, disengaging, doing things on autopilot, or getting lost in "analysis paralysis." Of course, when emotional pain is mild—when there's only a little bit of anxiety or sadness or guilt—it's often possible to reduce the pain through thinking strategies; but the more challenging the situation and the greater the emotional pain, the more ineffective thinking strategies are.

Another cost for most clients is wasted time: all that time spent in one's head rather than engaging in life. Usually, the therapist will need to ask leading questions here: "How much time have you spent in your head, trying to think away your pain? How much did you miss out on?"

COSTS OF SUBSTANCES AND OTHER STRATEGIES

The costs of excessive substance use—on health, work, well-being, finances, and relationships—are often the easiest for clients to identify. The costs of "gritting your teeth, sucking it up, and forcing yourself to get on with it" are dissatisfaction and exhaustion. If any other strategies have been mentioned, we should explore the costs of these, too.

CLOSING QUESTION 3

We want to round off question 3 by validating that the client has worked hard and is not stupid. For example, we might say, "You've really worked hard at this. You have tried and tried and tried for a long, long time to get rid of these painful thoughts and feelings. No one can call you lazy. You've put a lot of effort into this. And no one can call you stupid, either, because everyone does these things; we all try to distract ourselves, or avoid difficult tasks and situations, or try to think our pain away, or put substances into our bodies to feel better. We all do it, and our culture promotes it; these kinds of strategies are widely recommended by friends, family, health professionals, women's magazines, self-help books, and so on. And of course, these things *do* work in the short term: they give you those sweet moments of relief. But in the long term, those feelings keep returning, right? And what I'm wondering is, are these strategies really giving you the life you want, and helping you to be the sort of person you want to be?"

Practical Tip   For this work to be effective, we need to come from a space of compassion, equality, and respect. We aim to validate the client's experience—that she's trying very hard, and in the long term it isn't working. Obviously, if we come across as critical or judgmental, then our client will feel invalidated. This is why it's so important to highlight that these are strategies we all use to some extent, and short term, they do often work to make us feel better.

Question 4: What's Showing Up?

At this point we inquire, with great compassion, about how the client is feeling. We might say, for example, "You know, a lot of people at this point experience some quite intense feelings…like sadness, or anger, or anxiety…and I'm wondering, what's showing up for you right now?"

Many clients will have an emotional reaction—often some combination of sadness, anger, anxiety, or guilt—and we want to normalize and validate whatever it may be. At the same time, they often have a sense of relief, because we are validating their experience: they've been using all these ECS and getting a bit of short-term relief, but in the long term, it's not working.

Sometimes at this point the client fuses with negative self-judgment (e.g., "I'm such a loser!"). If so, we want to reiterate that these are common strategies that everyone uses, and our culture encourages us to do these things. Then we can segue into some quick basic defusion, as in this example:

Therapist: So notice what your mind's doing here. Notice how quick it is to jump in and start beating you up. And believe it or not, what your mind's trying to do here is help you. It's got a strategy here: "If I can beat myself up and give myself a hard enough time, that'll help me get on with my life and stop screwing up." So it's completely natural and normal that your mind would be doing this; it's just not particularly helpful. So how about we let your mind have its say, but let's not get sidetracked by it; and can we come back to what we're dealing with here?

This response will enable many clients to unhook, but if not we may need to spend more time on defusion, using strategies from chapters 12 to 16. Similarly, if the client at this point becomes overwhelmed by intense emotion, we could segue into grounding and dropping anchor (chapter 10). The point is, whatever the client's reaction, let's validate it, normalize it, and respond with great compassion and understanding.

Question 5: Are You Open to Something New?

Once we sense that the client is in contact with the futility of trying very hard to control his emotions, we can ask, "Are you open to something new?"

This may sound a bit like this:

Therapist: So, can I just quickly recap? You've been trying hard for a long, long time to get rid of your unwanted feelings. You've found a whole bunch of strategies that give you relief in the short term, but they either don't work or make life worse in the long term. And there have been some big costs for you. Living your life this way has taken a toll. So given all that, I'm wondering…are you up for something new? A new way of responding to difficult thoughts and feelings that's radically different from everything else you've ever tried?

As long as we run through this process with openness, curiosity, and compassion, clients will find it validating; it nonjudgmentally confirms their experience: that they've been trying hard to control their feelings, but it's not working in the long term, and life is getting worse, not better.

What Next?

Clients' reactions vary enormously at this point. They may be nonchalant ("Okay"), excited ("Let's do it!"), or anxious ("I don't know. What does it involve?"). Whatever their emotional reaction, we want to acknowledge it, validate it, and also make a judgment call: has the client truly contacted the unworkability of the emotional control agenda? If not, we'll need to persist with CH a bit longer. But if so, most therapists would now segue into a group of interventions called "dropping the struggle" (chapter 9).

Extra Bits

See chapter 8 in *ACT Made Simple: The Extra Bits* (downloadable from the "Free Stuff" page at http://www.actmindfully.com.au). There you'll find the Join the DOTS worksheet (which I created to help myself remember all the various steps in CH). You can fill in this worksheet with the client or draw it up on a whiteboard. You'll also find two other useful forms: the Vitality vs. Suffering Diary and the Problems and Values worksheet.

Skilling Up

There are quite a few steps to CH, so it takes practice. I recommend you do the following:

- Download the Join The DOTS worksheet and print out two copies. Fill one in *on yourself* (after all, the best person to practice ACT on is you) and the other based on a current client.

- After that, rehearse the various steps aloud (or at least inside your head) with an imaginary client, changing the words to fit your own way of speaking.

- Once you've rehearsed it, try it out in session with a real client.

Takeaway

Creative hopelessness is an optional part of the ACT model; you don't have to do it with every client. However, if your client is high in experiential avoidance and only interested in feeling good or getting rid of her difficult thoughts and feelings, then you absolutely must do creative hopelessness; if you skip it with such clients, you will get stuck. As long as it's done with compassion and curiosity—not with judgment, condescension, or lecturing—clients will find that it powerfully validates their own experience.

CHAPTER 9

Drop the Struggle

If Not Avoiding, Then What?

If we're not avoiding our unwanted thoughts and feelings, what's the alternative? In traditional ACT terminology, the alternative is *willingness*: that is, the willingness to have our thoughts and feelings instead of running away from them or fighting with them. Willingness can involve any one or any combination of the four core mindfulness skills: defusion, acceptance, flexible attention (contacting the present moment), and self-as-context.

> **Tricky Terminology** . The term "willingness" has two different meanings in ACT: (a) it's a synonym for acceptance: to willingly have or make room for your thoughts and feelings (as opposed to doing so grudgingly or halfheartedly, which we'd call "tolerance") and (b) it's a quality of action: you do something willingly, as opposed to resentfully or reluctantly.

The default setting for most of us is that when difficult thoughts and feelings show up, we struggle with them: we fight against them, try to suppress or conquer them, or run away and hide from them. So the very first step in willingness is simply to drop the struggle: stop fighting and fleeing our own thoughts and feelings.

Two main types of intervention come into this phase of therapy:

A. naming struggle as the problem

B. shattering the illusion of emotional control

If, following creative hopelessness, your client impatiently asks, "So what should I do?" you could reply, "Good question. You already know we're going to be learning some new skills here for handling difficult thoughts and feelings. But this approach is so different from everything else you've tried, it would probably backfire if we just leaped straight into it. So if you're willing to bear with me a little longer, what I'd like to do is lay a bit of groundwork for what comes next. Perhaps you could think about it this way…"

The therapist now uses her metaphor of choice to convey that struggle is the problem (we'll get to this shortly).

Struggle Is the Problem, Not the Solution

The above phrase means that as long as a client is hooked by the agenda of trying to control how she feels, she will remain in a vicious cycle of increasing suffering. In most ACT textbooks, you'll find an alternative phrase: "Control is the problem, not the solution"; I don't like that version because it easily creates confusion around the issue of control. Let me explain.

If we aim to empower people, we need to help them focus on what's in their control. That's why in ACT, we help people to

A. tell the difference between what is and isn't within their control,

B. relinquish trying to control what they can't control, and

C. actively exert control over what they can control (if doing so is useful).

Below is a table that clarifies these differences:

Outside My Control	Within My Control (Potentially)
Vast majority of my emotions and feelings	How I respond to my emotions and feelings
Vast majority of my thoughts	How I respond to my thoughts
Vast majority of my sensations	How I respond to my sensations
Memories	How I respond to my memories
Whether or not I achieve the outcomes I want	What I say and do to increase the chances of achieving what I want
How good I feel when I'm doing what I do	How much I focus on or engage in what I do
What other people say and do	What I say and do to influence other people
How others judge or perceive me	Whether or not I act like the sort of person I want to be
What happens in the future	What I say and do to influence the future

What happened in the past	How I respond to thoughts about the past
Painful losses	Being self-compassionate when facing loss
Whether or not life gives me what I want	The values I live by and act on, whether or not life gives me what I want
Most of life's difficult events (e.g., work issues, illness, injury, suffering of loved ones, natural disasters, economic crisis, global warming)	The values I live by and act on in the face of life's difficult events, and my degree of self-compassion

Note the word "potentially" at the top of the right-hand column; if you're highly fused, operating on autopilot, or dissociative, you obviously don't have much control in these areas, but as psychological flexibility develops and increases, your degree of control increases with it.

Hopefully you can see then that we actually *encourage* a lot of control in ACT. Indeed, I've often said to clients, "I want to help you have a lot more *control over what you say and do* when life gets tough and these difficult feelings show up."

So given this potential confusion with terminology, rather than talk about "control" as the problem, I prefer to use the term "struggle" or the longer phrase "fighting with and running from our difficult thoughts and feelings."

Intervention: Recognizing Struggle as the Problem

The first type of intervention for dropping the struggle is helping the client recognize that struggle against difficult thoughts and feelings, not the thoughts or feelings themselves, is the problem. There are many metaphors we can use to convey how struggle is the problem. In this chapter, we'll first look at my favorite—the Pushing Away Paper exercise—and then two popular alternatives, Struggling in Quicksand and Tug of War with a Monster (both from Hayes et al., 1999).

PUSHING AWAY PAPER

This exercise, which has evolved from my earlier Pushing the Clipboard exercise (Harris, 2009a), is a metaphor for acceptance and experiential avoidance. The script that follows is a generic version, suitable for just about anyone. It's much more powerful if we make it specific to each unique client, so instead of saying things like "all the people you care about," we'd say, for example, "your husband, Michael, and your teenage daughter, Sarah."

When I do this, I usually carry my chair over to the client, and we sit side by side, each with a sheet of paper. Our chairs back up to the wall, we both face toward the room, and we both do all the actions simultaneously. You don't have to do it this way, of course; you can modify and adapt it freely to suit yourself. The exercise is more powerful if we first write down on the paper the specific thoughts, feelings, emotions, memories, urges, cravings, and sensations that the client is trying to avoid or escape.

As you read through the script below, please act it out: grab a sheet of paper and push it away from you as instructed and imagine actually doing this with your client.

A *few words of warning*: this is a very physical metaphor, so if you or your client has neck and shoulder problems or other issues that would make this painful, you wouldn't do this; you'd use a purely verbal metaphor such as those we'll look at shortly: Struggling in Quicksand or Tug of War with a Monster.

* * *

Therapist: (*sitting side by side with the client, both facing the room*) Imagine that out there in front of you (*gesturing to the contents of the room and the far wall*) is everything that really matters to you, deep in your heart; everything that makes your life meaningful (*or used to, in the past*); all the people, places, and activities you love; all your favorite foods and drinks and music and books and movies; all the things you like to do; and all the people you care about and want to spend time with.

But that's not all. Also over there are all the problems and challenges you need to deal with in your life today, such as…(*therapist gives some examples based on the client's history, such as "your conflict with your son," "your financial issues," "your health problems," "your court case," "your search for a job," "your chemotherapy for your cancer"*).

And also over there are all the tasks you need to do on a regular basis to make your life work: shopping, cooking, cleaning, driving, doing your tax return, and so on.

Now, please copy me as we do this exercise. Let's imagine that this sheet of paper is all those difficult thoughts, feelings, emotions, and memories that you'd like to get rid of. Now hold it tightly at the edges like this, and push it as far away from you as you possibly can. (*Therapist holds the paper tightly at the edges with both hands, and stretches his arms out, pushing the paper as far away as possible. The client copies him.*) This is what your culture tells you to do—get these thoughts and feelings away from you. Friends tell you to do this, doctors, therapists, counselors, women's magazines; everyone. Right? But hey (*therapist says this next part humorously*), it looks like we aren't really trying very hard here; let's push harder. Push as hard as you possibly can. Straighten those elbows, dislocate those shoulders; let's get these thoughts and feelings as far away as possible. (*The therapist and client maintain this posture for the next section of the exercise: holding the paper tightly by the edges, arms straight, holding it as far from the chest as possible.*)

Now notice three things. First, how tiring is this? We've only been going for less than a minute, and already it's tiring. Imagine doing this all day; how much energy would it consume?

Second, notice how distracting it is. If the person you love were right there in front of you, how hard would it be to give her your full attention? If your favorite movie were playing on a screen over there, how much would you miss out on? If there's an important task in front of you right now or a problem you need to address or a challenge you need to tackle, how hard is it to focus on it?

Third, notice, while all your effort and energy is going into doing this, how hard it is to take action, to do the things that make your life work, such as (*therapist gives some examples based on the client's history, such as "to cook dinner," "to drive your car," "to cuddle your baby," "to type on your computer"*). So notice how difficult life is when we're struggling with our thoughts and feelings like this. We're distracted, we're missing out on life, it's hard to focus, we're exhausted, and it's so hard to do the things that make life work.

Now, let's see what happens when we drop the struggle with our thoughts and feelings. (*Therapist now relaxes his arms, drops the paper into his lap. The client copies him. Typically the client will express a sigh of relief: "Ahh—that's better."*) Big difference, huh? How much less tiring is this? How much more energy do you have now? How much easier is it to engage with and focus on what's in front of you? If your favorite person were in front of you right now, how much more connected would you be? If there were a task you needed to do or a problem you needed to address, how much easier would it be to focus on it? Now move your arms and hands about (*therapist gently shakes his arms and hands around; client copies*). How much easier is it now to take action: to drive a car, cuddle a baby, cook dinner?

Now notice these things (*therapist indicates the paper in his lap*) haven't disappeared. We haven't gotten rid of them. They're still here. But we've got a new way of responding to them. We're handling them differently.

They're no longer holding us back, or bringing us down, or jerking us around. And if there's something useful we can do with them, we can use them. You see, even really painful thoughts and feelings often have useful information that can help us, even if it's just pointing us toward problems we need to address or things we need to do differently, or simply reminding us to be kinder to ourselves. And if there's nothing useful we can do with them, we just let them sit there.

* * *

Please note well the final paragraph of the above exercise; we don't dismiss or ignore painful feelings in ACT. We look at them with openness and curiosity. Our emotions are a great source of wisdom, and we don't stop at accepting them; we actively turn them into allies, as we'll see in chapter 23.

Practical Tip   Sometimes a client will say, "Can't I do this?" and throw the paper onto the floor. The therapist would reply by summarizing some of the main avoidance strategies identified in the creative hopelessness work, as follows: "Yes, we've already established you know many ways to do that for a short period of time—take some drugs, avoid a challenging situation, distract yourself with a computer game—but how long before it comes back again? Not long, right? So this (mimes *throwing the paper away*) is basically the same thing as this (mimes *pushing the paper away*). We're talking about doing something radically different, like this (mimes *dropping the paper on his lap*).

Next, we'll look at two more popular metaphors for dropping the struggle.

Struggling in Quicksand Metaphor

Therapist: Remember those old movies where the bad guy falls into a pool of quicksand, and the more he struggles, the faster it sucks him under? In quicksand, the worst thing you can possibly do is struggle. The way to survive is to lie back, spread out your arms and legs, and float on the surface. This is very tricky, because every instinct in your body tells you to struggle. But if you do what comes naturally and instinctively, you'll drown. And notice, lying back and floating is psychologically tricky—it doesn't come naturally—but it's a lot less physical effort than struggling.

Tug of War with a Monster Metaphor

Therapist: Imagine you're in a tug-of-war with some huge anxiety monster. (Alter the name of the monster to suit the issue, for example, the depression monster.) You've got one end of the rope, and the monster has the other end. And in between you, there's a huge bottomless pit. And you're pulling backward as hard as you can, but the monster keeps on pulling you ever closer to the pit. What's the best thing to do in that situation?

Client: Pull harder.

Therapist: Well, that's what comes naturally, but the harder you pull, the harder the monster pulls. You're stuck. What do you need to do?

Client: Drop the rope?

Therapist: That's it. When you drop the rope, the monster's still there, but now you're no longer tied up in a struggle with it. Now you can do something more useful.

There are numerous other metaphors you could use to illustrate that the struggle itself is the problem. Basically, you can use anything that conveys this message: the more you do what comes naturally and instinctively in this problematic situation, the worse the situation gets. Well-known examples include slamming on the brakes when your car skids, swimming against a rip tide, trying to dig your way out of a hole, scratching an itchy rash, and leaning backward on your skis when you're going too fast. Yet another option is the Struggle Switch metaphor (Harris, 2007), which we cover in chapter 22.

Practical Tip   You can come back to these metaphors in later sessions when a client relapses into self-defeating emotional control strategies. For example, if your client reports he went on a three-day drinking binge, you may compassionately and respectfully reply, "Struggling in the quicksand again. It's so common. It's so hard for us to break old habits," or "Three days of doing this (*therapist mimes pushing away paper*); you must be exhausted."

Intervention: Shattering the Illusion of Emotional and Cognitive Control

In this type of intervention, we shatter the myth or illusion that humans can control their thoughts and feelings. You might say, "So we're all walking around, trying to control how we feel, and it just doesn't work. It's not that we've got no control at all, but we've got a lot less than we'd like. And what I'd like to do, if you're okay with it, is just take you through a few little exercises so you can check this out for yourself." You could then take the client through any or all of the following exercises, in any combination or order. (The first two are from Harris, 2007, and the others are from Hayes et al., 1999.)

Delete a Memory

Therapist: Just take a moment to remember how you got here today. Done that? Okay, now delete that memory. Just get rid of it. (*pause*) How'd you do?

Numb Your Leg

Therapist: Now make your left leg go completely numb. So numb that I could cut it off with a hacksaw and you wouldn't feel a thing. (*pause*) How'd you do?

Don't Think About...

Therapist: For the next exercise, you must not think about what I say. Not even for one microsecond. Don't think about...ice cream. Don't think about your favorite flavor. Don't think about how it melts in your mouth on a hot summer's day. (*pause*) How're you doing?

The Polygraph Metaphor

Therapist: Imagine I'm a mad scientist and I've kidnapped you for an experiment. And I've wired you up to a supersensitive polygraph, or lie detector. This machine will detect the tiniest bit of anxiety in your body. You can't kid it. Even the tiniest hint of anxiety and all the alarm bells will ring. And in this experiment I'm about to do on you, you must not feel any anxiety at all—because if you do, then I'll pull this lever, which will electrocute you with one million volts. (*pause*) What would happen?

Client: I'd be fried.

Therapist: Right. Even though your life depends on it, you can't stop the anxiety.

Falling in Love

Therapist: Now suppose I were to offer you one billion dollars—one billion—if you can do what I ask. I'm going to bring someone into this room—someone you've never met before—and if you can instantly fall head-over-heels in love with that person, then I'll give you the money. Could you do it?

Client: If it were Brad Pitt, I could.

Therapist: It's a sexist, racist, homophobic truck driver, who keeps shouting deeply offensive things, and he hasn't had a bath or brushed his teeth for a year.

Client: In that case, no!

Therapist: Not even for one billion dollars?

Client: I suppose I could try.

Therapist: Sure. You could put on an act. Hug him and kiss him and say, "I love you, I love you!" because you've got a lot of control over your actions; but could you control your feelings?

Client: No.

So What's Next?

At this point, your client is hopefully ready to start learning some new skills. If you have enough time left in this session, you can start on this straight away. The easiest skills to begin with, for most clients, are dropping anchor or simple (nonmeditative) defusion; more challenging skills to begin with are acceptance, self-compassion, and self-as-context.

If, however, you don't have enough time to start on active skill building, explain this to the client and say something like this: "Next session, if you're up for it, our main focus will be on learning some new ways of handling these difficult thoughts and feelings. How does that sound to you?" In such cases, it's useful to set a simple homework task that builds on the struggle metaphor you've used: ask your client to notice when she's "pushing hard" or "tugging on the rope" or "struggling in the quicksand" and also to notice when, if ever, she stops pushing, tugging, or struggling, and what difference that makes.

Better still, if she's willing, encourage her to keep a daily journal: When and where does the struggle happen? What triggers it? What are the consequences? When, if ever, does she drop the struggle? What difference does that make? These homework tasks can be alternatives or additions to the CH homework tasks from the previous chapter.

Extra Bits

See chapter 9 in *ACT Made Simple: The Extra Bits* (downloadable from the "Free Stuff" page at http://www.actmindfully.com.au). There you'll find (a) the Daily Struggle worksheet, (b) how to normalize and validate clients' struggles with their emotions and help them understand why they do it, (c) how to handle uncommon but tricky reactions to Pushing Away Paper, and (d) links to my YouTube animation of the Polygraph metaphor.

Skilling Up

You can probably guess what I'm going to say next. Reading this stuff ain't enough; you gotta actually practice it. Soooo:

- Read through all the exercises and metaphors aloud, as if taking a client through them. (Or at least rehearse them mentally.)

- Notice your own tendencies to struggle with your thoughts and feelings. Keep a daily journal: When and where does the struggle happen? What triggers it? What are the consequences? When, if ever, do you drop the struggle? What difference does that make?

Takeaway

Dropping the struggle metaphors provide a good segue into formal explicit work on acceptance. They also provide a useful bridge between creative hopelessness and willingness.

CHAPTER 10

Dropping Anchor

A Multipurpose Mindfulness Tool

Dropping anchor is a simple yet powerful technique for contacting the present moment. The aim of it is to help clients become "fully present," engage in what they are doing, regain control over their actions, and focus their attention on what's most important here and now. It's so effective for most people, and so easy to teach relative to other mindfulness techniques, that I hope we will see it much more widely utilized in ACT protocols than it currently is.

Personally, I recommend dropping anchor as the first mindfulness skill you formally teach clients who are struggling with:

- Emotional dysregulation

- Hypoarousal

- Hyperarousal

- Dissociation

- Overwhelming emotions

- Impulsive behavior

- Compulsive behavior

- Extreme fusion

- Flashbacks

- Panic attacks

In addition, it's a good first skill to teach any client who's interested in mindfulness or who wants to get better at unhooking from difficult thoughts and feelings. It's also an excellent choice as your first step in actively developing willingness, after creative hopelessness and dropping the struggle. (Can you tell I like this technique?)

Introducing Dropping Anchor

The Emotional Storm metaphor (Harris, 2007) is a good way to introduce dropping anchor to your clients.

The Emotional Storm Metaphor

In the transcript that follows, the client is overwhelmed by anxiety. The therapist has just asked, "Where are you feeling this most?"

Client: Everywhere! It's all churning around in here (*pointing to his chest and abdomen*).

Therapist: So it's more intense in your chest and tummy. And what's it like inside your head?

Client: Terrible. It's all just spinning around. (*He spins his finger around by the side of his head.*)

Therapist: So you've got all these thoughts spinning around your head; all these feelings whirling around your body. It's like an emotional storm blowing up inside you. And while you're being swept away by that storm, there's nothing effective you can do. You're at the mercy of the elements, right?

Client: Too right!

Therapist: So suppose your boat sails into harbor just as a huge storm is blowing up; what's your top priority?

Client: Tie it up, I guess.

Therapist: Yup. Tie it up or drop an anchor as fast as possible. And it's the same with us. When emotional storms blow up, the first thing we need to do is drop anchor. And obviously that won't make the storm go away; anchors don't control the weather; but it will hold us steady until the storm passes.

Practical Tip   It's important to mention that the boat is approaching or already in the harbor. A boat out at sea wouldn't drop anchor during a storm; it would attempt to ride the waves.

In ACT, we want to be flexible with our metaphors and always adapt or change them to fit our clients. In 2016, I was privileged to author (helped by many others) an ACT protocol for the World Health Organization for use in refugee camps around the world (Epping-Jordan et al., 2016). Assuming there'd be a lot of trauma-related disorders and emotional dysregulation among the refugees, I made dropping anchor the first mindfulness exercise in the protocol. However, the first two countries targeted were Syria and Uganda, neither of which have strong cultural ties to boats and sailing. So I changed the metaphor to "grounding," as follows:

Imagine you are high in a tree, in the topmost branches, when suddenly a storm appears. A mighty wind tosses you around, and you cling desperately to a branch to stop yourself from falling. Now what do you need to do? Obviously, you don't want to stay in the branches. You want to get down to the ground as quickly as possible. And getting down to the ground won't make the storm stop; but it's the safest place for you to be. Plus, if you stay up high in that tree, you can't really do anything useful. For example, if you have a young child at the bottom of the tree, you can't do anything to protect her or comfort her while you are high in the branches. But as soon as you are on the ground, you can hold her and comfort her until the storm passes. Our aim here is to learn how to "ground" ourselves in this way, when emotional storms blow up inside us. Whatever the emotional storm is made of—anger or sadness or fear or guilt or hopelessness—the sooner we can ground ourselves, the better.

Three Steps to Dropping Anchor

Dropping anchor exercises all follow a repeating three-step structure, which you can remember with the acronym ACE:

A—Acknowledge your inner experience

C—Come back into your body

E—Engage with the world

Let's look at these one by one.

A—Acknowledge your inner experience. The aim here is simply to acknowledge whatever thoughts, feelings, emotions, memories, sensations, and urges are present. It's often useful to put this into words (silently or aloud), for example, "Here's sadness," "I'm noticing painful memories," "I'm having a feeling of anger."

C—Come back into your body. The aim here is to regain a sense of self-control by focusing on what you have most control over when difficult thoughts and feelings are present: your physical actions. Move, stretch, change posture, sit upright, stand up, walk, alter your breathing, straighten your spine, push your feet into the floor, and so on. These things help people to rapidly regain control over their physical body: a great first step toward any type of effective physical action.

E—Engage with the world. The aim now is to expand your awareness: notice where you are, what you're doing, and what you can see, hear, touch, taste, and smell. This is not to distract from thoughts and feelings, but to notice what else is here in addition to them.

What Are the Indications for Dropping Anchor?

There are three main indications for dropping anchor:

1. The client wants to learn a simple mindfulness skill (that can serve as the foundation for defusion, acceptance, contacting the present moment, or self-as-context).

2. The client is so fused that he is unable to engage or participate in the session.

3. The client is emotionally overwhelmed, acting impulsively or compulsively, or dissociating.

Dropping Anchor: Why Shouldn't You Stick to the Script?

When you do these exercises on yourself or with your clients, please *don't stick to the script*. There are gazillions and bazillions (and maybe even trazillions) of possible variations on the script below, so please be flexible and creative. For example, if your client has chronic pain that worsens if he pushes his feet into the floor, then don't ask him to push his feet into the floor! Instead, ask him to gently nod his head, wriggle his toes, tap his fingers, or shrug his shoulders.

The Dropping Anchor Exercise

Ideally, before you start this exercise, the client has told you the elements of her emotional storm: the thoughts, feelings, emotions, and memories she's struggling with. If so, you can refer to them specifically, for example, "There's a very painful memory showing up right now, and a lot of sadness and a lot of anger." But if the client is too distressed to speak, or unable or unwilling to say what thoughts and feelings are present, then you can refer to them with nonspecific terms such as "pain," "discomfort," "hurt," "something difficult," "difficult thoughts and feelings," or even "emotional storm." (I've *italicized in bold* such phrases throughout the script because we're going to discuss them later.)

Allow a good ten seconds between instructions, and give your voice a kind and calming quality. You should model all the actions for the client (e.g., pressing feet down, pressing fingertips together) to help reduce the client's self-consciousness and build a sense of rapport: *we're in this together; we're a team.* I strongly recommend you read this script aloud in advance and act it out, as if rehearsing your lines and actions for a role in a play. But if you can't or won't do that, at least actively rehearse it in your mind.

> ***There's a lot of emotional pain showing up for you right now.*** I can see how much you're struggling with it, how difficult it is for you. And I really want to help you handle it. So please would you follow my instructions? You don't need to say anything if you don't want to, and you can speak if you feel like it.

Okay. First, take a moment to *acknowledge that there are difficult thoughts and feelings showing up* for you right now.

And at the same time, see if you can push your feet hard into the floor. Push them down (*therapist pushes his own feet down hard*) ... That's it. Feel the ground beneath you.

Now sit forward in your chair and straighten your back (*therapist does these actions himself while talking*) ... Feel the chair beneath you; notice your back supporting you.

Now slowly press your fingertips together, and as you do that, gently move your elbows and your shoulders (*therapist does these actions himself while talking*).

Feel your arms moving, all the way from your fingers to your shoulder blades.

Take a moment to *acknowledge there's a lot of pain here* that you're struggling with ... You didn't ask for it ... but here it is ... and it's challenging and it's difficult and you want it to go away, and yet it's not going ...

Silently *acknowledge to yourself what type of pain it is* ... For example, say to yourself, *Here's sadness* or *Here's anxiety* or *Here's a painful memory.* (*If the therapist knows what the pain is, he can specifically mention it.*)

Now *notice that there are painful thoughts and feelings here,* and there's also a body around all that pain—holding it, containing it. And it's a body that you can move and control. Straighten your back again, and notice your whole body now—your hands, feet, arms, legs. (*therapist straightens his back*) Gently move them, and feel them moving ... Have a good stretch (*therapist stretches his arms out*) ... Notice your muscles stretching ... Press your feet down and feel the floor (*therapist presses his feet down*).

Now also look around the room—up, down, and side to side—(*therapist looks around the room*) and notice five things that you can see.

And also notice three or four things you can hear—sounds coming from me or you or the room around you.

And also notice you and me (*therapist gestures to both himself and the client*), working here together, as a team.

So *notice, there are some difficult thoughts and feelings here* that you're struggling with, and at the same time, see if you can also notice your body in the chair ... and gently move that body, have a stretch (*therapist moves, stretches*) ... That's it, take control of your arms and legs.

And also notice the room around you (*therapist looks around the room*).

And also notice you and me here (*therapist gestures to both himself and the client*) working together as a team.

The therapist continues to cycle through the exercise—acknowledging inner experience, coming back into the body, engaging with the world—until the client is grounded, which might be indicated by nonverbal responses (e.g., facial expressions, body posture, eye contact) or verbal responses (e.g., speaking readily, asking or answering questions, verbalizing thoughts and feelings) that convey engagement. The therapist ends the exercise with simple debriefing questions such as:

Do you notice any difference now? Are you less hooked by these difficult thoughts and feelings? Are you less "swept away" or "jerked around" by them?

Is it any easier for you to engage with me, to be present, to focus on what I'm saying and what we are doing here?

Do you have more control over your actions now—over your arms and legs and mouth? Check it out, move your arms and legs, have a stretch (*therapist moves and stretches, encouraging client to copy him*). Do you have more control over what you're doing now?

Practical Tip   Note that in all these debriefing questions, the therapist never asks if the pain has reduced or the client is "feeling better." To ask such questions would send the wrong message: that the aim of the exercise is to reduce or get rid of emotional pain. Of course, this often happens; but in ACT that's a bonus, not the main aim.

Did you notice all the bold, italicized phrases in the script above? These are all variants on the instruction "Notice your painful thoughts and feelings." This is the big (and very important) difference between grounding exercises in ACT and almost all other models. In virtually all other models of therapy, you will not find these repeated instructions to notice and acknowledge painful private experiences. And why is this a problem? Because if you fail to repeatedly acknowledge the presence of the pain, these exercises are highly likely to function as distraction techniques rather than mindfulness techniques; clients will almost always use them to escape from or avoid their painful thoughts and feelings, in order to feel less distressed or anxious. (Indeed, in some models, this is the primary aim of such grounding techniques.) Remember: distraction is the very opposite of mindfulness. If you've forgotten the difference, revisit chapter 3.

How Long Does Dropping Anchor Go For?

The aim of this technique is to help the client become "fully present," engage in what he is doing, regain control over his actions, and refocus his attention on what's most important here and now. So the exercise goes for as long as is necessary to achieve this. Usually one to three minutes is enough, but I've had clients who were so emotionally overwhelmed or dissociated that we needed to do this for ten to fifteen minutes. At the other extreme, when clients only "drift off" slightly, a ten-second version might be enough.

A word of warning: Using this technique to stop the client from crying, to distract the client from her feelings, or to change the topic because you are feeling uncomfortable would all be serious misuses of the method.

We can of course repeat these exercises as often as we think it will be useful. For example, when working with clients who keep dissociating or having flashbacks, we may drop anchor many times in one session. Typically, from session to session, we can make these exercises shorter and shorter because the client responds more quickly and more dramatically. On the other hand, we can progressively build upon these simple exercises, extending them and bringing in other core processes. For example, we can easily extend them into self-compassion exercises (see chapter 18).

How Do We Help Clients Identify the Benefits?

After ending the exercise, it's good to help clients contact the benefits of doing it. Here are some useful questions to ask:

- How could this be useful outside this room?

- When and where do you experience emotional storms? How might this help you in those situations?

- When and where could you apply this? With whom, doing what?

- How might this help you with XYZ (*where XYZ = client issues or behavioral goals*)?

Once the client sees how dropping anchor can be useful outside the therapy room and relevant to her behavioral goals (see chapter 6), we can then ask, "Would you be willing to practice this between sessions?" If the answer is yes, we can then segue into "When and where will you practice?" "For how long?" "How often?" and so on.

> **Practical Tip**   Suppose you ask the client how this might be helpful, and she answers something like "It relaxes me," "It makes me less anxious," or "It distracts me from my feelings." If so, we could say, "Well, that's a nice bonus when it happens—so enjoy it when it does—but that's not actually the aim of the exercise. Can we take a moment to get clear about the real aim of this?" Then repeat the Pushing Away Paper exercise (chapter 9).

When and How Do We Apply This?

Dropping anchor is one of the most versatile skills in ACT. And have you noticed how the ACE formula maps neatly onto the triflex? Acknowledging your inner experience is a useful first step in learning how to **Open Up**. Coming back into your body is a useful first step in preparing to **Do What Matters**. Engaging with the world is learning how to **Be Present**. So with this one simple exercise, you're laying foundations for all the core ACT processes. This makes dropping anchor a great intervention with many types of problems. Let's take a quick look at some of its many applications.

Dropping Anchor When the Weather Is Fine

You can practice dropping anchor any time, any place, any activity—even when the emotional weather is wonderful. After all, even on a warm and sunny day, a boat will drift out of the harbor if you don't anchor it. And all of us, throughout the day, repeatedly "drift off": as we get caught up in our thoughts, our attention wanders away from what we are doing. So for homework, encourage your clients to practice dropping anchor throughout the day. You might phrase it something like this:

Therapist: Throughout the day, any time you realize you've "drifted off"—you know, you've gotten all caught up in your thoughts and feelings so you're not really focused or engaged in what you're doing—drop an anchor. Do a ten-second version of what we've practiced here: acknowledge whatever thoughts and feelings captured your attention, then come back into your body and take control of it, then notice the world around you—where you are, what you're doing. And then refocus your attention on wherever it needs to go in order for you to do what you need to do.

(The therapist briefly discusses this with the client, then goes on to make a further recommendation, as follows.)

Therapist: It's also good to practice this in all those difficult but not *too challenging* situations that keep cropping up throughout the day—you know, when you're stuck in a queue or traffic jam, or you're running late for an appointment, or your kids are taking forever to get ready, or you just made a stupid mistake that you swore you'd never do again, or someone just said something careless that's rubbed you the wrong way. If you practice this a lot when you're mildly anxious or angry or upset, you'll be much better prepared for when those big emotional storms blow up. And conversely, if you don't practice it regularly, you won't be able to do it when you most need it.

Being Creative

The first step in dropping anchor is to acknowledge the thoughts and feelings that are present, whether these are extremely painful, moderately uncomfortable, somewhat neutral, quite pleasant, or even just a feeling of numbness.

After that, the sky's the limit for the next two steps. To help the client regain control of his body, you can invite him to mindfully drink a glass of water, stand up and walk around the room, eat a snack, stretch, change his posture, twiddle his thumbs, nod his head, grab an object (e.g., a book, a pen, an ornament) and explore the surface with his fingers, touch the chair beneath him, gently lay a hand over his heart (which can segue into a lovely self-compassion exercise, as we'll see in chapter 18), run his tongue over his teeth, and so on.

And to help him engage with the world, you can ask him to notice anything he can hear, see, touch, taste, and smell; how he's breathing; how he's sitting; the feeling of tears in his eyes or running down his cheek; the air against his face; the straightness of his spine; the position of his body; the sound of the air conditioner; and so on.

So be creative. Improvise away to your heart's delight, as long as you return—again and again and again—to acknowledging the thoughts and feelings that are present. Why is this so important? Because we want the client to learn that he can respond flexibly to even the most difficult thoughts and feelings; he can mindfully acknowledge their presence, take control of his actions, and focus his attention where it matters most.

So What Do I Do After I've Dropped Anchor?

Sometimes clients will ask you a version of the above question. We would reply something like this:

Therapist: That's a good question. The idea is, once you've anchored yourself, go and do something effective, something that's going to make your life better. Ask yourself, *Am I doing a towards move right now?* If the answer is no, then stop whatever you're doing, and go do a towards move instead. If the answer is yes—you are doing a towards move—then give it your full attention; engage in what you're doing.

Client: What if I can't think of any towards moves?

Therapist: Well, over the next few sessions, we're going to spend quite a bit of time on that: figuring out the sort of person you want to be, and how you want to live your life, so it shouldn't be a problem to think of towards moves; and if it is, we'll address it.

Extra Bits

See chapter 10 in *ACT Made Simple: The Extra Bits* (downloadable from the "Free Stuff" page at http://www.actmindfully.com.au). There you'll find download links for four free recordings of dropping anchor exercises, varying in length from one minute to eleven minutes. You'll also find Q&As on (a) when to "sit" with feelings, (b) how to drop anchor in bed, (c) what to do if the client says it's not working or "I don't get it; what's the point of this?" (d) how to use this with dissociation and flashbacks, and (e) how the ACT Companion smartphone app can assist.

Skilling Up

I encourage you to listen to the dropping anchor exercises mentioned in the Extra Bits section and actively practice them as often as possible. If you make the effort to develop this skill, not only will you be able to teach it better to your clients, but it will also serve you well in those sticky moments of a therapy session when you yourself are fused or overwhelmed. In addition, why not try some or all of the following?

- Read through all the scripts from this chapter (ideally out loud), modifying the language as desired, as if you're doing them with your clients.

- Create your own dropping anchor exercises; write them out and rehearse them.

- Practice dropping anchor throughout the day—both at times when your emotional weather is mild and at other times when it's stormy.

- As soon as possible, start actively doing these exercises in session.

Takeaway

Dropping anchor exercises all follow a repeating three-step structure:

A—Acknowledge your inner experience

C—Come back into your body

E—Engage with the world

Around this structure, you can improvise literally hundreds of different exercises. This practice switches you off autopilot, helps you unhook from or make room for difficult thoughts and feelings, raises your awareness, and gives you conscious control over your actions, making it a very useful skill for (a) "circuit-breaking" impulsive, compulsive, aggressive, addictive, or self-harming behaviors; (b) interrupting cognitive processes such as worrying and ruminating; and (c) responding effectively to overwhelming feelings, extreme fusion, and dissociation.

CHAPTER 11

Notice That Thought

The Big Problem

From an ACT perspective, what's the single biggest problem clients struggle with? (Yeah, I know you already know; just seemed like a good question to start the chapter.) Cognitive fusion is the overarching clinical problem. (Many newbies get the false idea that experiential avoidance is the number one issue in ACT, so I want to remind you: experiential avoidance is often but not always a problem, and it's rarely—if ever—the only problem.)

Defusion in a Nutshell

In Plain Language: *Fusion* means your cognitions dominate your behavior. They dominate your actions (overt behavior) or your attention (covert behavior) or both. *Defusion* means responding flexibly to your cognitions so they *can influence* but do *not dominate* your behavior.

Aims: To see the true nature of cognitions: that they are nothing more or less than constructions of words and pictures. To respond to cognitions more flexibly, in terms of workability rather than literality (that is, in terms of how helpful they are rather than how true or false or positive or negative they are).

Synonyms: Deliteralization (this term is now rarely used); distancing.

Method: We pay attention to our cognitions with:

Curiosity: See their true nature, as constructions of words and pictures.

Openness: Explore whether they are helpful or not.

Flexibility: If our cognitions are helpful, we let them guide us; if not, we let them be.

When to Use: When cognitions dominate behavior (overt or covert) to such an extent that it gets in the way of effective, values-based living.

Defusion involves learning to:

- Step out of the content of cognitions (it's not about true/false/positive/negative)

- Stop fighting with or trying to avoid cognitions (they are not threats or obstacles)

- Stop obeying cognitions (they are not commands or laws we must obey)

- Stop holding on tightly to cognitions (they are not something we have to cling to or dwell on)

- Stop giving all your attention to cognitions (they are only one aspect of your here and now experience)

Remember these two important points about cognition:

1. When we use the word "thought" in ACT, we mean any type of cognition: beliefs, attitudes, assumptions, schemas, fantasies, memories, images, meanings, and desires, as well as the cognitive aspects of urges, cravings, feelings, emotions, and so on.

2. Cognition is an integral element of all emotion; there's no such thing as emotion *without* cognition. (This is why I often talk about "fusion with thoughts and feelings.")

How Do We Get Started with Defusion?

If we want to explicitly focus on defusion in a session, we can lead into it in many ways. For example, suppose we choose to kick off therapy by focusing on towards moves: we identify values and set some goals, but the client doesn't take action. We could now ask questions such as "What's getting in the way?" "How's your mind talking you out of this?" "What's stopping you from acting on these values/ achieving these goals/being the person you want to be/building the relationships you want?" "What's your mind telling you that holds you back/keeps you stuck/makes this difficult for you?"

Alternatively, suppose we choose to start therapy with a focus on learning "unhooking skills." We might then introduce simple defusion techniques, like the ones in this chapter, as the first skills we actively teach. (However, in my experience, "dropping anchor" exercises are easier for most people to learn, so I prefer to start with those.) And yet another option is to lead into defusion after creative hopelessness and dropping the struggle: developing the willingness to have difficult thoughts, rather than fighting or fleeing them.

Now the first thing we need to know when we actively start with defusion is…

What's Hooking You?

We plant the seeds for defusion from the very first session, simply through the questions we ask when we take a history. For example, one of my standard questions is: "If I could listen in to your mind when it's beating you up, telling you all the things that aren't good enough about you or your life, what are the meanest, nastiest, or most judgmental things I would I hear it saying?"

I hope you can see the defusion implicit in this kind of questioning: ideas such as "listening in" to the mind and noticing what "it is saying" (and even just talking about "the mind" or "your mind") can facilitate a little defusion. Usually, this way of speaking helps clients attend to their cognitions in a new way, with more curiosity and openness. And we can vary these questions enormously. For example, if anxiety is an issue, we might ask, "What does your mind say when it wants to get you really anxious?" Or if aggression is an issue, "What does your mind say to get you really angry about this?" Or for depression, "If I could listen in to your mind when it's doing its utmost to make you feel hopeless, what are the most discouraging things I'd hear it saying to you?"

These kinds of questions help us identify the main categories of cognition the client is fusing with. (Remember the six broad patterns of fusion: past, future, self-concept, reasons, rules, judgments? If not, revisit chapter 2.) Furthermore, if we listen carefully, we'll hear the client reveal a lot of her fusion as she criticizes herself (self-concept), or tells you she doesn't want to feel anxious (emotional avoidance), or reveals what she's worried about (future), or explains why she can't do what she wants to do (reason giving), or tells you what she thinks about others (judgment), or comes out with perfectionistic ideas (rules), or details all the times she has failed (past), and so on.

And of course, if your client has completed a homework task like the one at the end of chapter 7—where he's actively noticed the thoughts and feelings that hook him and the "away moves" that result—then you'll have a wealth of valuable information to work with.

In addition to all the above, at any point in any session we can ask questions such as these:

- "So what's your mind telling you now?"

- "And what does your mind have to say about that?"

- "Can you notice what you're thinking right now?"

- "If I could listen in to your mind right now, what would I hear?"

All of the questions we've covered so far are useful for identifying the *content* of cognitions. But far more important is the next step: identifying the *function* of the cognitions (that is, the effects they have on overt or covert behavior). I playfully call this next step…

Make the Link

We want to help clients "make the link" between fusion with cognitions and the way this changes their behavior. In other words, we want to identify what actually happens when the cognitions in question dominate behavior: what problematic changes in (overt or covert) behavior result? If you skip this step, you will almost certainly get stuck. Why? Because if your client doesn't see how fusion negatively impacts his behavior, he's not likely to be interested in learning defusion skills.

Questions to make the link between fusion and overt behavior (actions) may include:

- When you get hooked by those thoughts, what happens next? (What do you do or stop doing? How does your behavior change? What do you say and do differently?)

- If a film crew were following you, filming 24/7, and I got to watch the video footage later, what would I see or hear you doing that would show me these thoughts have hooked you?

- When these thoughts push you around/jerk you around/run your life/call the shots, what do you do differently? What do you start or stop or do more of or less of?

- When you get caught up/entangled/lost in these thoughts, what happens next? What do you do? What do you stop doing or put off until later?

- When you act on these thoughts, let them guide what you say and do, what do you tend to do? What would that look like or sound like on a video?

- How are you different with your partner/child/friend/parent/employer/employees/coworkers when you're hooked by these thoughts? What do you say and do differently?

It's usually trickier to identify changes in covert behavior (e.g., disengaging, focusing on your thoughts and feelings instead of on what you are doing, being inattentive or absentminded with loved ones, doing things on automatic pilot), so we'll often need to ask "leading questions," such as:
When you get hooked by these thoughts and feelings…

- Who (or what) do you cut off from/disconnect from/disengage from?

- What (or who) is it hard to focus on?

- Who is it hard to be present with/engage with?

- What important stuff do you tend do poorly or get easily distracted from?

Note that all the questions above readily map onto a choice point diagram. The difficult cognitions go at the bottom, and when one fuses with them (hooked arrow) there are problematic changes in both overt and covert behavior (away moves).

> **Practical Tip**   All the above questions mention "thoughts," but you can substitute words such as worries, self-judgments, fears, predictions, "not good enough" stories, revenge fantasies, "doom and gloom" scenarios, angry thoughts, anxious thoughts, and so on. You can also ask the very same questions about feelings, urges, impulses, cravings, emotions, images, and memories.

After we've discovered "what's hooking you" and we "make the link," we can then go on to…

Offer a New Skill

Again and again and again (and again and again), ACT newbies ask me some version of this question: "How do I sell mindfulness/defusion/acceptance/self-compassion to the client?" And my answer is always: "Don't." Don't try to "sell" this stuff to your clients; instead, "offer it." First, find out what your client's issues are, and then reframe them into an ACT formulation. Then offer the client skills that he can clearly see are directly relevant to and useful for his specific issues. No "selling" is required when we do this.

For example, if a client is "depressed" and a therapist says "mindfulness can help," the fit between the problem (depression) and the solution (mindfulness) is so vague, it's unlikely to interest the client. But suppose the therapist says something like this:

Therapist: So can I summarize it this way? There are several different aspects to your depression, and we want to address them all, but I'm thinking maybe the best one to start with is the way your mind keeps beating you up—telling you what a loser you are, how hopeless life is, how everyone hates you, how there's no point in trying, and there's basically no future. Seems like when you get hooked by those thoughts, you tend to do things that don't take your life in the direction you want; you tend to drink and smoke dope and stay in your bedroom and avoid people and give up on doing the stuff you used to enjoy. Have I got that right?

Client: Yeah, pretty much.

Therapist: (*compassionately*) That sounds really rough. You've been suffering a lot, for a long time.

Client: That's why I'm here.

Therapist: Well as long as you keep getting hooked by these thoughts, that suffering is going to continue. So I'm wondering if you'd be interested in learning some new skills here; learning how to unhook from these difficult thoughts? How to take their power away, so they don't keep jerking you around and bringing you down and holding you back?

* * *

Please read the transcript again and notice how the therapist:

A. briefly summarizes the main content of fusion ("What's hooking you?"),

B. identifies the relationship between fusion and problematic behavior ("makes the link"), and

C. offers the possibility of learning a specific new skill as an antidote to fusion (without ever using the term "mindfulness").

Without this kind of clarity, we can expect confusion, uncertainty, lack of enthusiasm, or even outright resistance from many clients.

In the next transcript, the therapist runs through the same three steps, but in this case the behavior change is predominantly covert:

Therapist: Can I just have a go at summarizing this? Obviously, worrying is a big issue for you.

Client: You got that right.

Therapist: And when you get hooked by all those anxious thoughts, it makes it very hard for you to engage in what you're doing, or focus on the task at hand, or appreciate what is happening, or really be present with your loved ones. And this is having a big impact on you; you're suffering.

Client: I am.

Therapist: Of course. And as long as you keep getting hooked by those anxious thoughts, this is going to keep happening. So I'm wondering if you'd be open to learning a new skill here.

Client: What do you mean?

Therapist: I mean, learning how to unhook from all those anxious thoughts, so instead of getting all caught up in them, you can learn to let them go, engage in life, focus better, and be more present with the people you love. How does that sound?

* * *

Notice how the therapist reframes worrying as "getting hooked by anxious thoughts"? This is a very useful reframe for worrying, catastrophizing, predicting the worst, and so on. After all, anxiety and worrying are not the same thing. Anxiety is an emotion; "worrying" is fusing with cognitions about bad things that might happen. We can't stop anxiety from arising, but we can learn to defuse from anxious thoughts, make room for anxious feelings, and refocus our attention on what we are doing; this is the antidote to worrying.

At this point, hopefully the client is open to and interested in learning defusion skills. But what if she's not? What if she says it won't work, or she's tried before and failed, or she just wants to get rid of the thoughts, or she's too depressed to learn new skills, or that's not what she came here for, or she wants to think positively, or all she wants is to stop feeling bad? We'll answer all these questions (and more) in chapter 14: Barriers to Defusion. For now, though, let's assume the client is ready and willing. Typically, then, the next stages will involve:

A. A metaphor for defusion

B. Practicing defusion skills

C. Setting defusion homework

We'll get into B and C in the next two chapters, and we'll look at A very shortly in this chapter—but first let's briefly look at a very important practice. This is something that starts in the first session, continues in all subsequent sessions, and plays a huge "background role" in encouraging defusion.

Normalize and Validate Thoughts

When we normalize and validate difficult thoughts, this facilitates both acceptance and defusion. Clients become more willing to have their thoughts and less intent on getting rid of them. And they often feel a huge sense of relief, just knowing they're "normal." There are many ways we can do this, in any session, and one of my favorites is to say things (authentically) such as…

YOUR MIND IS A LOT LIKE MINE

Therapist: You know, your mind sounds a lot like mine.

Client: (*surprised*) Really?

Therapist: Yeah, all these things your mind says to you—how you're not good enough, how you've screwed up, how other people don't like you—my mind says stuff like that to me, too.

Client: That surprises me.

Therapist: Why?

Client: Well, I just thought, you know, you're a therapist, you're trained in this…

Therapist: Sure, and my mind has evolved in exactly the same way as yours.

If the therapist has already explored how the human mind has evolved, she may wish to briefly recap the highlights. If she hasn't yet introduced this topic, now is a good time. You'll find many different versions of this evolutionary spiel in ACT. I collectively refer to them all as…

"CAVEMAN MIND" METAPHORS

(Sorry, I know that's not politically correct. I should call them "caveman and cavewoman" metaphors, or "caveperson" metaphors—but somehow those terms just don't have the same snappy ring. I hope you'll forgive me.) We can use versions of this narrative to normalize virtually any difficult pattern of cognition. Here's an example:

Therapist: So you've told me some of the difficult thoughts that tend to hold you back or make life harder when they hook you. And if your mind is anything like my mind, then it's got no shortage of this stuff; spouts it all the time.

Client: (*nodding*) Oh yeah!

Therapist: There's actually a good reason for this. Is it okay if we take a moment to discuss it?

Client: Sure.

Therapist: Well, it's got to do with the way the human mind has evolved. See, our primitive ancestors lived in a world of constant danger—big critters with big teeth lurked around every corner. So back then, your mind had to constantly be on the lookout for danger, antici-pating anything that could hurt you or harm you in any way: *Watch out. There could be a bear in that cave. There could be a wolf in those bushes. Is that person in the distance a friend or an enemy?* If you were a caveman and your mind didn't do this job well, you'd soon be dead. And that's what we've inherited from our ancestors; our modern mind is basically a "don't get harmed" machine. It's constantly trying to warn you of anything that could possibly hurt or harm you in any way: *You'll get fat, You'll screw up the exam, He might reject you.* This is normal. Everyone's mind does this. It's just our mind trying to do its number one job: to protect us and keep us alive.

* * *

We're sending a powerful message with this metaphor: "Your mind's not dysfunctional; it's just doing what all minds do. Our minds have evolved to judge and evaluate, dwell on the past, worry about the future, find problems, compare us to others. Your mind's not defective; it's just doing its job."

> **Practical Tip**   Not everyone believes in evolution. If your client doesn't, then modify the metaphor; leave out the evolutionary/caveman/prehistoric aspects and just say things like "Your mind's top job is to keep you safe, protect you, stop you from getting hurt."

Another version of the "caveman mind" spiel looks at the inevitability of comparison. It is written below as we might deliver it to clients, except in real life we would pause from time to time and check in with the client: "Does this sound a bit like your mind?"

HOW YOUR MIND EVOLVED TO COMPARE YOU TO OTHERS

Therapist: We've already talked a bit about how our mind has evolved, but there's more to it. You see, in prehistoric times, one absolute essential for survival was belonging to the group. If the group kicked you out, it wouldn't be long before the wolves ate you. So how does the mind prevent that from happening? It compares you to every member of the tribe: *Am I fitting in? Am I doing the right thing? Am I doing it well enough? Am I doing anything that could get me thrown out?* As a result, our modern-day mind always compares us to others. But now, there's not just a small group or tribe. Now we can compare ourselves to everyone on the planet—the rich, famous, and beautiful; movie stars; top athletes; even fictitious superheroes. And we don't have to look far before we find someone who is "better" than us in some way—richer, taller, older, younger, more hair, better skin, more status, smarter clothes, bigger car, and so on. As a result of all this comparing, we're all walking around with some version of the "I'm not good enough" story. For most of us, it starts in childhood; for a few people, it doesn't start until the teenage years. And it's the best-kept secret on the planet. Everyone's got multiple versions of this story—"I'm too old/fat/stupid/boring/fake/unlikeable/lazy/incompetent, blah, blah, blah" or "I'm not smart enough/rich enough/slim enough, and so on." We've all got this story, but almost no one talks about it.

Introduce a Metaphor for Defusion

Before we start to actively practice defusion skills, it's useful to introduce a metaphor that conveys the costs of fusion and the benefits of defusion. This helps the client to understand the purpose of defusion and how learning defusion skills can help him. My favorite metaphor for this purpose is the Hands as Thoughts and Feelings exercise. I took you through an ultrabrief version of this in chapter 2; what follows is a longer, more detailed version. Typically, this would take around four minutes to do with a client. I encourage you to read it aloud and act it out as if doing it with a client.

THE HANDS AS THOUGHTS AND FEELINGS METAPHOR—EXTENDED VERSION

This exercise is predominantly a metaphor for fusion and defusion. It's evolved from my earlier Hands as Thoughts exercise (Harris, 2009a), and the instructions overlap a lot with the Pushing Away Paper exercise detailed in chapter 9. The script that follows is a generic version, suitable for just about anyone. It's much more powerful if we make it specific to each unique client, so instead of saying things like "all the people you care about," we'd say, for example, "your husband, Michael, and your teenage daughter, Sarah."

When I do this, I usually carry my chair over to the client, and we sit side by side, with our backs to the wall, facing the room, and we both do all the actions simultaneously. You don't have to do it this way, of course; like any exercise in ACT, you can modify and adapt it freely to suit yourself; I've just found it more powerful to do so.

I also like to do two lovely variants on this exercise. One option is to write down some relevant thoughts and feelings on a sheet of paper, and use this instead of one's hands. Another option is to write them down with an indelible all-surface marker on something thin, flexible, and transparent such as bubble wrap, acetate, cellophane, or a clear plastic page protector.

Therapist: (*sitting side by side with the client, both facing the room*) Imagine that out there in front of you (*gesturing to the contents of the room and the far wall*) is everything that really matters to you, deep in your heart; everything that makes your life meaningful (*or used to, in the past*); all the people, places, and activities you love; all your favorite foods and drinks and music and books and movies; all the things you like to do; and all the people you care about and want to spend time with.

But that's not all. Also over there are all the problems and challenges you need to deal with in your life today, such as…(*therapist gives some examples based on the client's history, such as "your conflict with your son," "your financial issues," "your health problems," "your court case," "your search for a job," "your chemotherapy for your cancer"*).

And also over there are all the tasks you need to do on a regular basis to make your life work: shopping, cooking, cleaning, driving, doing your tax return, and so on.

Now, please copy me as we do this exercise. Let's imagine that our hands are our thoughts and feelings, and let's put them together like this. (*Therapist places his hands together, side by side, palms upward, as if they are the pages of a book. The client copies him.*) Now, let's see what happens when we get hooked by our thoughts. (*Therapist slowly raises his hands toward his face, until they are covering his eyes. The client copies him. Both keep their hands over their eyes as the next section of the exercise unfolds.*)

Now, notice three things. First, how much are you missing out on right now? How disconnected and disengaged are you from the people and things that matter? If the person you love were right there in front of you, how disconnected would you be? If your favorite movie were playing on a screen over there, how much would you miss out on?

Second, notice how difficult it is to focus your attention on what you need to do. If there's an important task in front of you right now, how hard is it to focus on it? If there's a problem you need to address or a challenge you need to tackle, how hard is it to give it your full attention?

Third, notice how difficult it is, like this, to take action, to do the things that make your life work, such as…(*therapist gives some examples based on the client's history, such as "to cook dinner," "to drive your car," "to cuddle your baby," "to type on your computer," "to hug the person you love"*). So notice how difficult life is when we're hooked. We're missing out, we're cut off and disconnected, it's hard to focus, and it's hard to do the things that make life work.

Now, let's see what happens as we unhook from our thoughts and feelings. (*Therapist now slowly removes his hands from his face and lowers them until they drop into his lap. The client copies him.*) So notice what happens as we unhook. What's your view of the room like now? How much easier is it to engage and connect? If your favorite person were in front of you right now, how much more connected would you be? If there were a task you needed to do or a problem you needed to address, how much easier would it be to focus on it, like this? Now move your arms and hands about (*therapist gently shakes his arms and hands around; client copies*). How much easier is it now to take action: to drive a car, cuddle a baby, cook dinner, type on a computer, hug the person you love? (*Therapist mimes these activities as he says them; the client usually will not copy this part, but that doesn't matter.*)

Now notice these things (*therapist indicates his hands, now once more resting in his lap*) haven't disappeared. We haven't chopped them off and gotten rid of them. They're still here. So if there's something useful we can do with them, we can use them. You see, even really painful thoughts and feelings often have useful information that can help us, even if it's just pointing us toward problems we need to address or things we need to do differently, or simply reminding us to be kinder to ourselves. And if there's nothing useful we can do with them, we just let them sit there.

Extra Bits

See chapter 11 in *ACT Made Simple: The Extra Bits* (downloadable from the "Free Stuff" page at http://www.actmindfully.com.au). There you'll find sections on (a) tricky reactions to the Hands as Thoughts and Feelings metaphor and how to handle them, (b) how to "make the link" when you see fusion showing up in your client during the session, and (c) how to shatter the illusion that our thoughts control us.

Skilling Up

Now that you know the ins and outs and ups and down and this ways and that ways of defusion, you're ready to actually knuckle on down to doing it. So here's your mission:

- Practice all the scripts and spiels in this chapter, adapting and modifying the language.

- Run through the Hands as Thoughts and Feelings metaphor at least twice; there are so many bits and pieces to it, it takes some practice.

- Pick two or three questions that you really like from the "Make the Link" section and memorize them or come up with alternatives of your own. Rehearse them aloud or mentally a few times, and then try them out in session as soon as possible.

- Think of two or three clients. Imagine how you might (a) briefly summarize what they are fusing with, (b) describe the problematic behavior changes (overt and covert) that result from the fusion, and (c) introduce the idea of a specific new skill that could help. Once you've rehearsed this a few times (out loud or mentally), try it out for real with your clients.

Takeaway

To "set the scene" for defusion, there are five basic steps: (1) find out "What's hooking you?" (identify the cognitive content the client is fusing with); (2) make the link (make the connection between fusion and problematic behaviors); (3) offer a new skill (offer defusion as a solution to the problems identified above); (4) normalize and validate difficult thoughts; and (5) introduce a metaphor to summarize the problems of fusion and the benefits of defusion.

CHAPTER 12

Deeper into Defusion

A Treasure Trove Awaits

Once you have permission from the client to do an experiential exercise, there's a treasure trove of options for defusion. (So many, in fact, that it can be overwhelming—see chapter 16: "Technique Overload" and Other Perils.) In the next chapter, we'll look at transcripts of therapy sessions, but in this one I want you to practice defusion on yourself (always the best person to practice ACT on).

As you read on and do these exercises, keep this in mind: there's a potential danger in referring to the client's thoughts as "stories" or doing playful defusion techniques such as singing thoughts. If we do this work carelessly, it can easily come across as invalidating, uncaring, trivializing, or demeaning.

So it's important that we compassionately join with the client: we connect with his suffering and validate how much pain he's experienced. From a stance of empathy, kindness, equality, and respect, we form an alliance; we work together as a team to find a new way of responding to these thoughts and to develop a new attitude that enables mindful, values-based living.

A Taste of Defusion

I'm now going to take you through several defusion techniques, which is typically what I do next with my clients, after the work outlined in the previous chapter. So pull out a scrap of paper and write down two or three negative, self-judgmental thoughts your mind throws up from time to time to give you a good thrashing. You'll need these to work with during the exercises.

Have you done that? Okay, now pick the thought that bothers you the most and use it to work through the following exercises. (At the start of each exercise, I'll ask you to fuse with your thought for ten seconds. You generally won't need to ask your clients to do that as they'll already be fused!)

Do This as an Experiment

When we do these kinds of exercises with our clients, it's useful to say, "Can we do this as an experiment? I'm expecting it to be helpful, but I never know for sure what will happen." This helps both client and therapist to tap into an attitude of openness and curiosity. And the same applies to you as you try the exercises that follow; regard them as experiments, and be open to unexpected results. Some of these exercises will have no effect at all; your level of fusion won't alter. Some may give rise to just a little bit of defusion; others to a massive amount. Some may even create a bit of fusion, ramp it up a notch. So be curious; see what happens.

Now for Some Techniques

Let's start with the first defusion technique I usually formally teach after laying the groundwork in the previous chapter.

I'M HAVING THE THOUGHT THAT...

This is a quick and simple exercise (adapted from Hayes et al., 1999) that gives an experience of defusion to almost everyone. It goes like this:

Put your negative self-judgment into a short sentence—in the form "I am X." For example, *I'm a loser* or *I'm not smart enough.*

Now fuse with this thought for ten seconds. In other words, get all caught up in it and believe it as much as you possibly can.

Now silently replay the thought with this phrase in front of it: "I'm having the thought that..." For example, *I'm having the thought that I'm a loser.*

Now replay it one more time, but this time add this phrase "I notice I'm having the thought that..." For example, *I notice I'm having the thought that I'm a loser.*

* * *

What happened? Did you notice a sense of separation or distance from the thought? If not, run through the exercise again with a different thought.

In a therapy session, you could follow up as below:

Therapist: So what happened to the thought?

Client: It sort of lost some of its sting.

Therapist: Did you get some sense of separation or distance from it?

Client: Yeah. It sort of backed off a bit.

Therapist: Could you just show me with your hands and your arms where the thought seemed to move to?

Client: Out here. (*The client stretches his arms out in front of his chest.*)

Therapist: So that's part of what we mean by unhooking: you start to separate from your thoughts and give them some space to move around in.

You could follow up in other ways, too. For example, you could ask the client, "I wonder if you'd be willing to try talking this way in our sessions. Suppose you have some sort of distressing, painful, or unhelpful thought like *This is all too hard*. When you have a thought like that, could you say to me, 'I'm having the thought that this is all too hard?'"

Once this convention is established, you can come back to it again and again and play with it as a brief intervention. Here are two examples:

Client: I can't handle this.

Therapist: So you're having the thought that you can't handle this?

* * *

Therapist: Could you say that again, but this time, preface it with "I'm having the thought that…"?

Client: I'm having the thought that I'm a stupid idiot.

Therapist: Did you notice any difference?

Client: Yes, it didn't bother me so much the second time.

Practical Tip   You can use the "I'm having a…" technique with emotions, urges, memories, sensations, and so on: "I'm having a feeling of anxiety" or "I'm having the urge to run away." A good alternative phrase is "I'm noticing…," for example, "I'm noticing a bad memory" or "I'm noticing tightness in my chest."

SINGING AND SILLY VOICES

For these two exercises (from Hayes et al., 1999), use the same negative self-judgment as you used above, or try a new one if the old one has lost its impact:

Put your negative self-judgment into a short sentence—in the form "I am X"—and fuse with it for ten seconds.

Now, inside your head, silently sing the thought to the tune "Happy Birthday."

Now, inside your head, hear it in the voice of a cartoon character, movie character, or sports commentator.

* * *

What happened that time? Did you notice a sense of separation or distance from the thought? If not, run through the exercise again with a different thought.

Variations on the theme include singing the thoughts out loud, saying them out loud in a silly voice, or saying them in exaggerated slow motion (for example, "I'mmmmmm stuuuuuuupiiid-dddddddd"). Keep in mind that in the right context, zany techniques like these can be very powerful, but in the wrong context, they can be invalidating or demeaning. For example, you wouldn't ask a client with terminal cancer to sing her thoughts about dying to the tune "Happy Birthday."

COMPUTER SCREEN

This exercise (Harris, 2007) is particularly useful for people who are good at visualizing. The script calls for using an imaginary computer screen, but you can also do this on a real computer (type it out in a PowerPoint or Keynote presentation on a laptop, tablet, or iPad), on paper with colored pens, or using one of the many smartphone apps for sketching, drawing, or painting. These are the steps:

Fuse with your negative self-judgment for ten seconds.

Now imagine a computer screen and imagine your thought written up there as plain black text.

Now in your mind's eye, play around with the formatting. Space the words out, make large gaps between them; then run them together, all one word with no gaps; and then run them vertically down the screen.

Now in your imagination, play around with the color. See it written in green, then blue, then yellow.

Now play around with the font. See it written in italics, then in stylish graphics, then in one of those big playful fonts you see on the covers of children's books.

Now put it back as plain black text, and this time, animate the words like those cartoons on Sesame Street. Have the words jump up and down, or wriggle like a caterpillar, or spin in a circle.

Now put it back as plain black text, and this time imagine a karaoke ball bouncing from word to word. (And if you like, at the same time, hear it sung to "Happy Birthday.")

* * *

So what happened? Did you get a sense of distance or detachment from the thoughts? Did they lose some of their impact?

A Closer Look at Defusion

Now that you've had a taste of defusion, let's explore some common reactions, misconceptions, and distinctions.

Invalidation?

Did any of those exercises feel dismissive, trivializing, mocking? If so, my sincere apologies. That was not the intent at all. There are plenty of people in the world who will readily dismiss or trivialize your issues, but I am not one of them. So if that was your reaction, I'm genuinely sorry, and it means that that particular exercise is not right for you.

The paragraph above is pretty much how I respond to any client who reacts negatively to an exercise. Let's be quick to apologize, clarify the real intent, and drop the particular technique that backfired (at least for now).

But It's True!

When you did those exercises, did your mind protest, "But it's true! I really am XYZ"? From time to time, your clients will resist or criticize a defusion technique on these very grounds. I would usually respond to this in terms of workability: "The thing is, in this approach, it's not about whether your thoughts are true or false; it's about what happens if you let these thoughts run your life. If you hold this thought tightly, or let it dictate what you do, will that help you to live the life you want? To achieve your goals, improve your relationships, act like the person you want to be?"

Below is an example from a therapy session:

Client: But it's true. I am a bad mother.

Therapist: Well, one thing I never intend to do here is debate with you about what's true and what's false. What we're interested in is, would it be helpful to let this thought guide you? You know, when you get all caught up in it, does it help you to be the sort of mother you'd like to be?

Client: Sometimes it kicks my butt into action.

Therapist: Sometimes, yes it does. However, most of the time it seems to just drag you down, doesn't it?

Client: Yes.

Therapist: And once it's dragged you down into the depths, that's when you're most likely to neglect the kids, right? So most of the time, when this thought hooks you, it doesn't help you to be the mother you want to be.

Client: No.

Therapist: So can we put aside the issue of how true it is, and instead work on learning to unhook from it, so you can put your energy into being the sort of mother you really want to be?

Fusion vs. Believability

Fusion isn't the same as believability. You can fuse with thoughts you don't believe (e.g., you can get all caught up in a compelling revenge fantasy without believing you are actually going to do it), and you can defuse from thoughts that you do believe. At a workshop I once gave, one of the attendees—let's call her Naomi—came up to me at the morning coffee break and told me that she had a malignant brain tumor. The tumor was incurable. Naomi had gone through conventional medical and surgical treatment, as well as a mind-boggling range of alternative medicine and treatments—and nothing had worked. She had a few months to live at best, possibly only weeks. She came to the workshop for personal reasons: to help cope with her fear and come to terms with her impending death. Naomi told me it was hard to stay focused in the workshop. She kept thinking about dying: losing her loved ones, the tumor spreading through her brain, the inevitable deterioration to paralysis, coma, then death.

Now clearly, if you have a terminal illness there's a time and a place when it's useful to think about dying: if you're writing a will, planning a funeral, making medical care arrangements, or sharing your fears with a loved one. But if you're attending a workshop for personal growth, it's not useful to be so caught up in your thoughts about dying that you're missing out on the workshop. So after listening compassionately and validating her fears, I talked to Naomi about naming the story, and she chose this title: the "scary death" story.

I asked her to practice naming the "scary death" story throughout the workshop. By midway through the second day, she had significantly defused from those thoughts about death and dying. They had not altered in believability one tiny bit—and we wouldn't expect them to because they were 100% true—but she was now able to let them come and go without getting caught up in them.

When we defuse from thoughts, they often do reduce in believability—but from an ACT perspective, that's not really important. After all, believing a thought simply means taking it to be true. In ACT, we're interested not in whether a thought is true or false, but in whether we can use it for guidance in acting effectively and building the life we want.

The Power of Flexible Thinking

Keep in mind, not only do we help clients to defuse from unhelpful cognitive repertoires, we also help them learn to think more flexibly. This is known as *cognitive flexibility*. Most commonly, we help clients develop cognitive flexibility through problem solving, action planning, strategizing, reframing, thought experiments, and perspective taking. We'll touch on different aspects of cognitive flexibility in many chapters, and near the end of the book, there's a whole chapter (27) on this topic.

Common Misconceptions

Clients often have misconceptions about defusion, as do many new ACT therapists. They may think the point of defusion is to get rid of painful thoughts, images, or memories or to reduce the painful feelings associated with them. But please remember:

- The aim of defusion is NOT to feel better or to get rid of unwanted thoughts.

- The aim of defusion IS to reduce the problematic dominance of cognitions over behavior, and to facilitate being psychologically present and engaged in experience.

- In other words, the aim of defusion is to enable mindful, values-based living.

Clients often find that when they defuse from a painful thought, it disappears, or they feel better, or both. When this happens, the therapist needs to clarify that (1) this is merely a bonus, not the primary purpose, and (2) it won't always happen, so don't expect it. If the therapist doesn't do this, clients will start using defusion to try to control their thoughts and feelings. And then, of course, it no longer functions as a mindfulness technique but as an emotional control technique. And then it's only a matter of time before the client becomes frustrated or disappointed (and comes back to say, "It's not working"). Here are two examples of how the therapist may handle this:

Client: That was great. The thought just went away.

Therapist: Interesting. You know, sometimes that happens, and sometimes it doesn't. Sometimes a thought just keeps on hanging around. Our aim is not to try and make it go away; our aim is to stop getting caught up in it, make some room for it, allow it to be there without struggling—so that if and when it does hang around, it doesn't stop you from doing what matters and engaging fully in your life.

* * *

Client: That's good. I feel less anxious now.

Therapist: Interesting. That quite often happens, but certainly not all the time. Please don't think of this as a way to control your feelings. The aim of it is to disentangle yourself from your thoughts so that you can be in the present moment and do the things you consider important. So if you feel better, by all means enjoy it. But please, consider it a bonus, not the main intention. If you start using these techniques to control how you feel, I guarantee you'll soon be disappointed.

* * *

If your client seems disappointed or surprised when you say this, it means she has misunderstood the purpose of defusion, in which case you'll need to recap it—and you may need to visit (or revisit) creative hopelessness. One way to do a quick recap is to "replay" the Hands as Thoughts and Feelings metaphor (chapter 11) and highlight the last section about how the thoughts and feelings are still there.

Defusing Is Not Dismissing

We want to respond to our cognitions with openness and curiosity—not dismiss them. Even the most difficult cognitions and cognitive processes usually have something useful to offer us. For example, our anxious thoughts often point us toward important issues we need to address, and self-judgmental thoughts often point us toward values we are neglecting. In later chapters, we'll look at how we can "extract the good stuff" from unhelpful thoughts.

Sometimes therapists get the idea that we aren't interested in the content of thoughts in ACT. Again, this is a major misunderstanding. We won't directly challenge or dispute the content, or judge whether it's positive or negative, but we are interested in it. After all, in order to assess a thought in terms of workability, we do first need to know the content.

When Defusion Backfires

Occasionally, we'll take a client through a defusion technique, and it'll have the opposite effect to what we intended: our client will become even more fused than before. Luckily, this won't happen often, but when it does, it's not a major problem. First, we apply ACT to ourselves: drop anchor, unhook from the "I'm a lousy therapist" story, make room for our anxiety, and refocus on the client. And then we apologize and turn it into an opportunity to help our client discriminate between fusion and defusion. For example:

Therapist: I'm sorry. That didn't turn out the way I expected. Usually that exercise helps people step back and get some distance from their thoughts, but in this case it seems to have had the opposite effect. However, given that this has happened, let's learn from it. Notice how you're even more caught up in that thought than before. Notice the impact it's having on you. This is what we mean by "hooked."

Extra Bits

See chapter 12 in *ACT Made Simple: The Extra Bits* (downloadable from the "Free Stuff" page at http://www.actmindfully.com.au). There you'll find (a) how to tell when your clients are defusing and (b) a popular defusion technique called Titchener's Repetition.

Skilling Up

Is this the end of defusion? No way. In the next chapter, we'll look at the defusion smorgasbord, and in the chapter after that, we'll look at common barriers to defusion. But before reading on, some suggestions to develop your skills are:

- Go back and try out any of the above defusion techniques you skipped.

- Read all the exercises out loud as if taking a client through them (or at least, vividly imagine doing so).

- Pick your favorite technique and use it during the week ahead. When you realize you've been hooked, drop anchor, and notice the thought that hooked you. If you're still entangled in it after dropping anchor, then use your chosen technique to play around with it, and notice what happens.

Takeaway

There are zillions of defusion techniques, and the ones in this chapter are but a few. When you introduce them to clients, always do so with great empathy and respect, and make sure you've first established a clear rationale (see "Make the Link" in chapter 11) to avoid the risk of confusion or invalidation.

Do everything as an experiment—because you never know for sure what will happen. And be alert for common misconceptions, such as thinking the aim is to feel good or to get rid of unwanted thoughts.

CHAPTER 13

The Defusion Smorgasbord

So Many Choices!

Conventional wisdom has it there are many ways to skin a cat. I can't personally vouch for the truth of this assertion, as I've never actually skinned a cat (nor do I intend to). But regardless of the veracity of this aphorism (how's that for a couple of big words?), it's a useful segue to the idea that there are literally hundreds of different ways for us to model, instigate, and reinforce defusion in a session. It's hardly surprising that many ACT newbies get overwhelmed by the vast range of techniques available. So let's see if I can make things a little bit simpler.

The Three Ns of Defusion

There is no fixed sequence (or number) of steps for defusion. However, all defusion techniques begin with "noticing" a cognition, and most of them combine this with "naming" the cognition. In addition, many defusion techniques also include "neutralizing" the cognition. Let's look at the "three Ns of defusion" more closely:

Notice

The basic first step in any type of defusion intervention is to notice what cognitions are present. To help clients notice their cognitions, a therapist might say, "Notice what you're thinking," "Notice what your mind is doing," "Notice what thoughts are popping up," "What's your mind saying to you?", "What's hooking you?", "What's your mind doing?", and so on.

Name

To name the cognition or cognitive process is usually the second step in defusion. Naming can be simple (e.g., "thinking," "worrying," "self-judgment," "black-and-white thinking," "predicting the worst"). It can be playful (e.g., "the not-good-enough story," "radio doom and gloom," "mind chatter," "the inner critic mouthing off again"). It can be self-referential (e.g., "I'm having the thought that…" or "there goes my mind"). And it can include words or phrases that acknowledge its recurrence, such as "Aha!" "Here it is again," "I know this one."

Neutralize

Most defusion techniques include a step that I call "neutralizing." (This is not an official ACT term, but it's one I find helpful for training therapists.) This term means that you put your cognitions into a new context that neutralizes their influence, disarms them. The simplest way to neutralize a cognition is to look at it in terms of workability: "If you act on this thought/let it guide or advise you/dwell on it/buy into it/get caught up in it/obey it/hold it tightly/let it dictate your choices…will it take you toward or away from the life you want to live/help you to be the sort of person you want to be/help you to act effectively?"

In addition to workability, neutralizing can also involve any combination of the following strategies (many of which overlap with each other):

Observe the thought as if it were an object. Notice the words or images the thought is composed of; notice its size and location; notice how it comes and goes—its movement, speed, direction.

Describe the thought. Describe the nature or properties of the thought in terms of the words or images it contains; its size, location, movement, speed, or direction; and other symbolic properties (e.g., "hot thoughts," "heavy thoughts," "sticky thoughts," "hooky thoughts").

Play with the properties of the thought. Play around with its:

- visual properties—shape, size, color, texture, solidity, brightness

- auditory properties—volume, speed, voice, tone, pitch; sing it, say it slowly or quickly or in different voices, add music

- kinesthetic properties—position, movement, direction, speed, location

Depict the thought. Write it out, draw it, paint it, type it, sculpt it, dance it, act it out, sing it, mime it, text it, represent it through photography or collage.

Transpose the thought. Imagine placing your thoughts onto other objects in your imagination (e.g., leaves on a stream, suitcases on a conveyor belt, clouds drifting across the sky, labels on items in a shop window), putting them onto objects in the room (e.g., place them on a chair or a bookcase, or project them onto the wall), or transposing them into another medium (e.g., see them as subtitles on a TV or text messages on a smartphone, or hear them as broadcasts from a radio).

Give the cognitive process a character. For example, characterize a pattern of harsh self-judgment as the "inner critic" or a pattern of worrying, catastrophizing, and predicting the worst as "radio doom and gloom."

Defusion: A Therapy Session Transcript

The transcript that follows illustrates a small number of the many different ways to help clients defuse. The client is a twenty-four-year-old single, female chiropractor. She and her therapist are about twenty minutes into session two, following (a) a brief dropping anchor exercise to start the session, (b) a quick review of the previous session (exploring how much the client has practiced dropping anchor and the benefits thereof), and (c) a quick discussion of how the human mind evolved.

Introducing Defusion: Part 1

Therapist: So one thing we identified last week, a big part of the problem, is that you often get hooked by thoughts about being worthless or useless.

Client: Yeah, I do. I feel like I'm a waste of space. I don't even know why you're wasting your time with me.

Therapist: And I notice that as you're saying that, you're slumping down—almost as if you're sinking into the chair. I'm getting a sense that these thoughts really drag you down. (*Client nods.*) That must hurt. (*The client nods again, and her eyes tear up.*) What're you feeling right now?

Client: (*shaking her head*) It's silly.

Therapist: What's silly?

Client: I am. This is. (*wiping her eyes*) I don't think you can help me.

Therapist: Well, that's a perfectly natural thought to have. Lots of people have thoughts like that, especially at the start of therapy. And the truth is I can't actually guarantee that it will help. But I can guarantee that I'll do my very best to help you create a better life. So, how about we give it a go, even though you're having the thought that it's hopeless, and let's see what happens?

Client: Okay.

Therapist: Okay, well, we agreed last session that one of your goals here is to learn new ways to handle difficult thoughts and feelings, so they don't jerk you around so much. Is that still important to you?

Client: Yeah.

Therapist: Okay. (*He pulls out a white index card.*) Well, what I'd like to do, if it's okay with you, is jot down some of your thoughts on this card so we've got something to work with. Would that be okay with you?

Client: Sure.

Therapist: Thanks. So, when your mind is really beating you up, really getting stuck into you about what's wrong with you, and what's wrong with your life—if I could listen in at those times, sort of plug into your mind and listen in to what it's saying, what it's telling you, what would I hear?

Client: Oh. Um. Just really negative stuff, like, um, you're stupid, you're lazy, nobody likes you.

Therapist: Okay. So let me get this down. (*He starts writing the thoughts down on the index card.*) Your mind says, "I'm stupid... I'm lazy... Nobody likes me." What else?

Client: I don't know.

Therapist: Well, you mentioned "silly" and "waste of space" today, and "worthless" and "useless" last week. Are those names your mind often calls you?

Client: Yeah.

Therapist: (*writing them down*) Okay. So your mind tells you "I'm silly... I'm worthless... I'm useless... I'm a waste of space." What else?

Client: (*chuckles*) Isn't that enough?

Therapist: Yes, it is—but I was just wondering if your mind tells you any really dark or scary stories about the future? You know, when it really wants to make you feel hopeless, what are the scariest things it says to you?

Client: Um. Just that I'm f***ed. There is no future. Life is f***ed and then you die.

Therapist: Okay, so your mind likes to swear a bit. Let's get that down. (*He writes the words down as he speaks them aloud*). "I'm f***ed... There is no future... Life is f***ed and then you die!" And, I know we touched on this last session, but just remind me: when you get hooked by these thoughts, what kind of away moves do you do?

Now let's unpack that. Before continuing with this chapter, read through the above transcript again and identify the various ways the therapist subtly establishes a context of defusion: normalizing and allowing thoughts, treating the mind as an "entity," listening to the mind, writing thoughts down, reading thoughts aloud, describing thoughts as "stories," and "making the link." Let's take a quick look at each of these.

Normalizing and allowing thoughts. Notice how the therapist responds to "I don't think you can help me" by saying "Well, that's a perfectly natural thought to have." We facilitate defusion when we describe a thought as normal, natural, typical, or common and make no attempt to judge it, dispute it, correct it or get rid of it.

Treating the mind as an "entity." Defusion involves separating from your thoughts, so in ACT we often find it useful to talk about the mind, playfully and metaphorically, as if it's a separate entity. For example, the therapist talks about the mind "getting stuck into you," "beating you up," and "calling you names" and also humorously notes that "your mind likes to swear."

Listening to the mind. Many defusion techniques involve noticing or playing with the auditory properties of thoughts. Here, the therapist talks about "listening in to the mind" and "hearing what it is saying" and "what it sounds like."

Writing thoughts down. One of the simplest ways of separating from thoughts is to write them down. This helps you to take a step back and see the thoughts for what they are: strings of words. The therapist can do the writing and then pass it on to the client, or the client can write the thoughts down.

Reading thoughts aloud. The therapist reads the client's thoughts aloud (always prefaced with the words "I am" and not "you are"). This often adds to a sense of separation, as if the therapist is reading out his own thoughts.

Describing thoughts as stories. In ACT, we often talk about thoughts as "stories." This ties in nicely to metaphors about the mind as a storyteller and getting absorbed or lost in the story. The therapist specifically asks about any "dark or scary stories" about the future.

Making the link. At the very end, the therapist starts to lead into "making the link" with the useful question "When you get hooked by these thoughts, what kind of away moves do you do?"

Introducing Defusion: Part 2

The therapist now spends about three minutes quickly "making the link" (chapter 11). The therapist discovers that when she is hooked, the client withdraws socially, binge watches TV shows, smokes marijuana, becomes snappy and irritable with her family, stays in bed excessively, rings in sick instead of going to work, procrastinates on applying for a better job, and eats lots of junk food.

After gathering this information, the therapist offers a new skill, as follows:

Therapist: So when you get hooked by these thoughts, they pull you into doing all sorts of stuff that only adds to your problems, makes your life worse?

Client: Yeah. I told you, I'm f***ed!

Therapist: I heard you say that, and I've written it down, right here. (*pointing to the card*) So would you be interested in learning how to unhook from this stuff?

Client: Yes, but I don't know if I can.

Therapist: Well, we'll soon find out. (*handing the card to the client*) So this is the sort of stuff your mind says to you when it's beating you up?

Client: (*looking down at the card*) Yeah.

The therapist now takes the client through the Hands as Thoughts and Feelings metaphor with one big change from the version in chapter 11: instead of asking the client to use her hands, the therapist asks her to use the index card. The client lifts the card up in front of her eyes (to represent fusion) and then lowers it down and rests it on her lap (to represent defusion).

Introducing Defusion: Part 3

This transcript continues from the end of the Hands as Thoughts and Feelings metaphor. The card now rests on the client's lap, with the writing face up so the transcribed thoughts are clearly visible to both client and therapist.

Therapist: Okay, so that's the basic idea of unhooking, and I'm going to ask you to do a couple of experiments now, to help you learn how to actually do that. I call them "experiments" because although I'm expecting this to be helpful for you, I never know for sure exactly how it's going to go. So the idea is we approach this with a sense of curiosity, and see how it goes.

Client: Okay.

Therapist: Okay, so (*pointing at the card*) notice those thoughts haven't gone away. They're still right there, in your lap. And if you want to, you can let them hook you. Check it out for yourself. Look down at the card and give it all your attention, and see if you can let those thoughts reel you in. (*Client looks down at the card in her lap.*) And notice how, as you get pulled into those thoughts, you cut off from me—and you lose touch with the world around you. (*Client nods.*) Can you feel them sucking the life out of you? (*Client nods*) Now look back at me. (*Client looks up at the therapist.*) So notice, there's you and me here, working together. And come back into your body, push your feet into the floor, have a stretch, and straighten your back. And notice the room around you—notice what you can see and hear. (*Client looks around the room.*) So there's a stack of difficult thoughts there, and you've got a body around those thoughts, and a room around your body, and you and me here, doing this work. Now which do you prefer—to get sucked into your thoughts down there (*points to the thoughts on her lap*) or to be out here in the world interacting with me?

Client: (*smiling*) I prefer this.

Therapist: Me too.

Client: But I keep wanting to look at it.

Therapist: Of course you do. Our minds train us to believe that everything they say to us is super important and we must give it our full attention. But the thing is, there's nothing written on that card that's new, is there? I mean you've had those thoughts, what, hundreds, thousands of times?

Client: Try millions.

Therapist: So notice, you have a choice here. You can look down and get hooked into that stuff, or you can just let it sit there and you engage with the world around you. The choice is yours. Which do you choose?

Client: Um… (*She seems unsure. She glances down at the card.*)

Therapist: (*warmly, humorously*) Oh, I've lost you. (*Client looks up again at the therapist.*) Ahh, you're back again. See how easily those thoughts hook you?

Client: Yeah. I know. That happens all the time.

Therapist: Yeah—to you, me, and everyone else on the planet. That's what we're up against. That's what minds do. They hook you. So one way to unhook is with this dropping anchor stuff. But there's lots of other ways to unhook too. So what I'd like to do, if you're willing, is take you through some of these other techniques—and again, they are experiments— and see how they work for you. Would that be okay?

Client: Okay.

Now let's unpack that some more. When we write thoughts down on a card and then turn the card into a physical metaphor, that is a defusion technique in itself. There is some psychoeducation going on here too; the exercise helps the client to experience how defusion enables her to be present and engage with the therapist, whereas fusion interferes with this. (The exercise is, of course, a variant on dropping anchor.)

At the end of the transcript, the therapist asks whether the client would be willing to go through some other techniques, and the client answers, "Okay." The therapist can now take the client through any defusion technique(s) he prefers. As a general rule, it's best to start with some quick and easy techniques rather than the longer, more meditative ones.

But suppose the client is not so willing. Suppose she says she doesn't want to let the thoughts just sit there—she wants to get rid of them! Or suppose she says okay, but her tone of voice and body language suggest that she's really not keen on the idea. What might be a good response from the therapist?

You got it. In both cases, the therapist would likely do a quick creative hopelessness intervention: run through everything she's tried to get rid of these thoughts, assess how well it worked in the long term, and look at what it has cost her; and from there, go on to ask something like "So given that you've been trying for years to get rid of these thoughts, and clearly it hasn't worked, are you open to exploring a different approach?"

Introducing Defusion: Part 4

The fourth and final part of this transcript picks up about fifteen minutes after the end of part 3. In the interim, the therapist took the client through several of the brief defusion techniques you tried in the previous chapter, working with specific thoughts written on the card. During all that time, the client left the card sitting on her lap, an ongoing metaphor for both defusion and acceptance. Occasionally she would look down at the card, and the therapist would ask, "Hooked?" The client would immediately look up again, at which point the therapist would make a lighthearted comment like "Ah. You're back again."

Now, in part 4, the therapist ties the whole session together with another defusion technique called Naming the Story (Harris, 2007), which neatly doubles up as homework.

Therapist: So let's come back to all these thoughts on the card there. I'm going to ask you something and it may seem a bit odd.

Client: I'm getting used to it.

Therapist: There's a lot of painful thoughts, feelings, emotions, and memories tied into this issue, going all the way back to your early childhood, when your mom first left home. And suppose we took all those thoughts, feelings, and memories, and we somehow managed to put them all into a documentary of your life, or an autobiography—so we create this video or special book that contains them all—and you might never share it with anyone, or you might just share it with a few people you really trust. And suppose you give it a title that goes on the cover, a title that summarizes the whole thing. Ideally a short one. So, you know, the catch-all title is the "not good enough" story; it's always that someone or something or some aspect of life is not, or was not, or will not be good enough. So we can call it the "not good enough" story, or you can come up with your own title, like maybe the "worthless" story or the "I'm f***ed!" story.

Client: (*thinking*) Ummmm.

Therapist: Take your time. It can be a humorous title if you want, as long as it doesn't trivialize it or make light of it.

Client: Um. How about the "useless Jane" story?

Therapist: Okay. That sounds good to me. You're quite sure that title acknowledges your suffering and doesn't trivialize it?

Client: Yeah.

Therapist: Okay. Can I have the card back for a moment? (*The client passes it over.*) I'm going to write a few words on the back here. (*The therapist flips the card over and starts writing. As he writes, he reads out the words, slowly.*) So here's what I'm writing: "Aha! Here it is again! The 'useless Jane' story! I know this one."

Client: Okay.

Therapist: So here's the next experiment. If you're willing to do this, I'm going to ask you to read through all of these difficult thoughts on this side, and really let them hook you. And when you feel well and truly hooked, flip the card over and read what's written on the back. Then push your feet into the floor, drop anchor, and check in with me, and tell me what happened and whether it was useful or not. Okay?

Client: Do you mean read it out loud?

Therapist: No. Just do it in your head. And I honestly don't know what will happen. I hope it will be useful, but remember, we're doing this as an experiment, okay?

Client: Sure. (*The therapist passes the card to the client. She silently reads through all the negative thoughts, a frown on her face. Then she flips the card over and silently reads the words on the back: "Aha! Here it is again! The 'useless Jane' story! I know this one." Then she grins and looks up at the therapist.*)

Therapist: You're smiling. How come?

Client: It's like you said. I can see it as a story. That's what it is. It's the "useless Jane" story.

Therapist: And are you hooked by this story?

Client: No. It's—this card sort of contains it.

Therapist: So show me what happened during that experiment. If this (*therapist puts his hands over his eyes*) is totally hooked, and this (*therapist rests his hands on his lap*) is totally unhooked, what was it like at the start, and what is it like now?

Client: I guess, when I was really hooked at the start, it was like this (*holds the card in front of her eyes*), and now it's like this (*lowers the card so it's about halfway between her face and her lap—about level with the lower end of her rib cage*).

Therapist: Cool. So a successful experiment then. You can't get rid of the story—not without major brain surgery anyway—but you can learn to unhook.

Client:	Well, I can do it in here. But I don't know about outside.
Therapist:	I'm glad you said that. Because this is a skill, and it needs practice. Like I said last time, if you want to become a good guitarist, you need to practice in between your guitar lessons. So if you want to get better at doing this, would you be willing to practice a couple of things between this session and the next?
Client:	Like what?
Therapist:	Well, the first thing is to practice naming the story. Anytime a thought, feeling, or memory that is linked to this story shows up, the moment you notice it, say to yourself, *Aha! There's the "useless Jane" story* or something like that. That's all you do. Just name it. Sometimes it'll hook you before you know it. That's normal. We expect it. As soon as you realize it's happened, say to yourself, *Oh. Just got hooked by the "useless Jane" story.* Then drop anchor; engage with the world around you. Does that sound doable?
Client:	Yeah. I'll give it a go.
Therapist:	There's another thing too. And this may seem a bit odd, so please feel free to say no if you don't want to do it.
Client:	Okay.
Therapist:	Okay. Can I have the card back? (*takes back the card and folds it up into quarters*) So would you be willing to put this card into your purse and carry it around with you, wherever you go, whatever you do, for, let's say, the next month? And pull it out at least three or four times a day, and unfold it, and read through all these difficult thoughts, and then flip the card over and read what's written on the back?
Client:	I hope no one gets into my purse.
Therapist:	(*chuckles*) I just want to be crystal clear with you about the purpose here. One thing is, it reminds you that you can take these thoughts and feelings around with you, but that doesn't have to stop you from living your life and doing the things that matter. Two, by pulling it out and reading all these thoughts, it reminds you that you can—and will—get hooked by them repeatedly; but when you fold it up, it reminds you that you can unhook. And when you put it back in your purse, it reminds you that unhooking isn't a way to get rid of them; it's a way to take the power out of them. So would you be willing to do that? It's fine if you don't want to. There are plenty of other things I can suggest.
Client:	No. That's fine.
Therapist:	Great.

Now before we wrap up, let's unpack that yet again. Here are a few things to consider:

1. It doesn't always go that smoothly. This client readily embraced defusion. A few may find it difficult or miss the point. Others may return to the agenda of trying to get rid of the thoughts; if so, your best bet is to jump back to creative hopelessness.

2. The therapist can use any number of defusion techniques in a session like this. There's nothing essential about writing thoughts on a card or naming the story. However, as you've probably guessed, the therapist is me—and this double-combo is my personal favorite. I particularly like using an index card (or a sheet of paper) because (a) it provides a great physical metaphor to work with in session; (b) when your client takes it away, it reminds him of the session and jogs his memory about homework; and (c) carrying the card (or paper) around in a purse or wallet is an ongoing metaphor for defusion and acceptance.

3. Suppose the client is reluctant to take the card away. Suppose she says, "No, I don't want it. That might make it worse." That would indicate both fusion and experiential avoidance, so you would say, "Right, well, I think in that case, this wouldn't be a good thing for you to do after all. So let's try something else." You would then set a different homework task and put the card away in her file and bring it out again in the next session.

Techniques Galore

There are well over a hundred different defusion techniques documented in ACT textbooks and self-help books, and there's plenty of opportunity for you or your clients to create new ones. You can do anything that puts the thought into a new context, where you can see it for what it is: a chain of words and pictures; nothing you need to fight with, flee from, cling to, or obey.

.For example, you might visualize the thought as a caption on a greeting card, written in frosting on a birthday cake, or popping up inside the speech bubble of a comic book character. Or you might imagine the thought coming from a radio or cell phone, or hear it in the voice of a well-known politician or sports commentator. Or you might imagine yourself dancing with the thought, walking hand in hand with it down the street, or bouncing it up and down like a ball. You might draw or paint the thought, write it out in different colors, or sculpt it in clay. You might visualize it on the T-shirt of a jogger, imagine it as a text message on your cell phone, or see it as a pop-up on your computer. You might sing it in different musical styles (for example, opera, jazz, rock 'n' roll), say it in an outrageous foreign accent, or have a hand puppet say it out loud. The options are endless. So before reading on, see if you can think up a few techniques of your own. And have some fun with it. (How often do you hear that in a textbook?!)

Following is a summary of many (but nowhere even close to all) common defusion techniques. We'll cover most of these techniques in this book; you can find the few that we don't in Extra Bits.

PRAGMATISM

If you go along with that thought, buy into it, and let it control you, where does that leave you? What do you get for buying into it? Where do you go from here? Can you give it a go anyway, even though your mind says it won't work?

INTERESTED

That's an interesting thought.

MEDITATIVE

Let your thoughts come and go like: passing clouds, cars driving past your house, etc.

YOUR MIND IS LIKE....

- a "don't get killed" machine
- a word machine
- radio "doom and gloom"
- a masterful salesperson
- the world's greatest storyteller
- a fascist dictator
- a judgment factory

BULLYING REFRAME

What's it like to be pushed around by that thought/belief/idea? Do you want to have it run your life, tell you what to do all the time?

PROBLEM SOLVING

This is just your mind problem solving. You're in pain, so your mind tries to figure out a way to stop the pain. Your mind evolved to solve problems. This is its job. It's not defective; it's doing what it evolved to do. But some of those solutions are not very effective.
Your job is to assess whether your mind's solutions are effective: do they give you a rich and full life in the long run?

WORKABILITY

If you let that thought dictate what you do and hook you, where does it take you: toward or away from the life you want? If you let this thought guide or advise you, will that help you to behave like the person you want to be?

THOUGHTS

THE CLASSICS

I'm having the thought that...
Say it in a silly voice.
Sing it.
Say it very slowly.
Repeat it quickly over and over.
Write thoughts on cards.
Passengers on the Bus Metaphor.
Thank your mind for that thought.
Who's talking here: you or your mind?
Leaves on a Stream Exercise.
How old is that story?

SECONDARY GAINS

When this thought shows up, if you take it at face value/go along with it/let it tell you what to do, what feelings, thoughts, or situations might it help you avoid or escape from (in the short run)?

FORM AND LOCATION

What does that thought look like? How big is it? What does it sound like? Your voice or someone else's? Close your eyes and tell me, where is it located in space? Is it moving or still? If moving, in what direction and at what speed?

COMPUTER SCREEN

Imagine this thought on a computer screen. Change the font, color, and format. Animate the words. Add in a bouncing ball.

INSIGHT

When you buy into this thought, or give it all your attention, how does your behavior change? What do you start or stop doing when it shows up?

NAMING THE STORY

If all these thoughts and feelings were put into a book or movie, titled "the *something something* story," what would you call it? Each time this story shows up, name it: "Aha, there's the XYZ story again!"

NOTICING

Notice what your mind is telling you right now.
Notice what you're thinking.

THE NOTICING SELF

Take a step back and look at this thought from your noticing self.

Summary of Common Defusion Techniques

Metaphors Galore

We can also use all sorts of metaphors to help with defusion. We can compare the mind to

- a word machine: it manufactures a never-ending stream of words;

- radio "doom and gloom": it likes to broadcast a lot of gloom about the past, a lot of doom about the future, and a lot of dissatisfaction with the present;

- a spoiled brat: it makes all sorts of demands and throws a tantrum if it doesn't get its way;

- a reason-giving machine: it churns out an endless list of reasons why you can't or shouldn't change;

- a fascist dictator: it constantly orders you about and tells you what you can and can't do; or

- a judgment factory: it spends all day making judgments.

And so on and so forth. Once you've used these metaphors with a client, you can come back to them again and again in subsequent sessions as brief defusion interventions. For example, in response to a client who comes out with a whole stream of negative self-judgments, you might say, "There goes the judgment factory again; it's really pumping them out today." Or in response to a client who keeps saying, "I should do X, I have to do Y!" you might say, "Wow! Seems like that little fascist dictator inside your head is really laying down the law today."

You probably already know quite a few metaphors for the mind: for example, the "chatterbox" and the "inner critic" are both in common usage. Before reading on, why not take a few moments to see if you can come up with a metaphor or two of your own?

Keeping Defusion Simple

As we've seen, there are all sorts of defusion techniques, and you can certainly have a lot of fun inventing your own and getting your clients to do so. However, there are plenty of times when, for one reason or another, I just like to keep it all very simple. So here are a few of the simplest defusion interventions I know:

"Notice what your mind is telling you right now." This simple phrase—or the shorter version, "Notice that thought"—is usually instantly defusing. It immediately gets your client to notice his thoughts rather than being caught up in them. Sure, it may not give him a huge degree of defusion, but it rapidly creates a little distance from his thoughts. This can then be increased by adding in any number of brief defusion techniques. For example, you can ask questions like "If you let this thought guide you, where will it take you? Will it help you?" "How old is this story?" "What would happen if you allowed yourself to get all caught up in this thought? Would it be a good use of your time and energy?"

Notice the form. You can ask your client to notice the form of the thought: "Is it made up of words, sounds, or pictures? Do you see it or hear it or just sense it?" You may choose to focus on the sound: "What does that thought sound like in your head? Is it your own voice or somebody else's? Is it loud or soft? What emotion can you hear in that voice?" Or you may focus on location and movement: "Just close your eyes for a moment and notice where that thought seems to be: Is it in front of you, above you, behind you, inside your head, inside your body? Is it moving or still? If moving, in what direction and at what speed is it moving?"

"That's an interesting thought." This is what I say when I'm a bit thrown or taken aback. When a client says something that throws me, triggers a strong reaction, or sets my mind in a frenzy trying to figure out how to respond, I find this little phrase stops me from rushing in and getting caught up in the content. It's a simple phrase that reminds both me and the client that no matter what she has just said, what we're dealing with is a thought. And it invites us both to stop and look at the thought rather than leaping straight into the content of the thought. I usually follow this statement with a long pause (at least ten seconds long), which allows me to center myself so I can respond effectively and mindfully.

Thank your mind. Encourage your client to thank his mind for its input (Hayes et al., 1999). This needs to be done playfully, with a sense of humor. You might say, "Whatever your mind says to you, no matter how nasty or scary, see if you can simply reply, with a sense of humor, *Oh, thanks, mind! Thanks for sharing.*" (If you use this method with a client, make sure you emphasize the need for playfulness and humor; specify that "the idea is to help you not take the thought so seriously.")

Short phrases. When your client expresses a particularly negative, critical, or unhelpful thought, you could say "Nice one!" with a sort of nonchalant, humorous openness. Or you can use other words such as "lovely," "neat," "beautiful," or "very creative." Once the client "gets" the concept, purpose, and experience of defusion—and provided there is a good therapeutic rapport so there's no chance of the client feeling invalidated or belittled—then you can say these words in response to a wide variety of harsh criticisms, judgments, catastrophic thoughts, or other "nasty stories." Accompanied by a compassionate grimace, saying "Ouch!" can also work well.

Don't Forget About the Client

When I was new to ACT, there were times when I got so caught up in playing around with all these wonderful new defusion techniques that I forgot about the human being in front of me. So we need to remember: we do techniques *with* clients, not *on* clients. And ACT is not about delivering techniques: it's about building a vital, meaningful life.

So a mindful, attuned connection with the client is essential in all this work. We need to be watchful of our clients, respectful of where they are at, and open to their responses. And if we get so caught up in delivering techniques that we neglect the relationship, then as soon as we notice it, we should apologize: "Whoa! I'm so sorry. I just realized what I've been doing here. I got so caught up in my own enthusiasm, I lost touch with you. Can we just pause and rewind a little, back to before I started bombarding you with all this stuff?"

These sorts of interactions not only build a trusting and open relationship; they also allow us to model self-awareness and self-acceptance. And they demonstrate that we're in the same boat as our clients: that we too can get caught up in our heads and lose touch with the present moment—and we can bring ourselves back to the present and act effectively!

Homework and the Next Session

Homework is essential. Defusion, like any skill, requires practice. This could involve a quick technique to practice intermittently throughout the day—like naming the story. Alternatively, if you take the client through Leaves on a Stream (chapter 15) or a similar meditative exercise, you could ask him to practice that each day, or several times a week. Yet another type of homework assignment involves asking clients to fill in a worksheet such as the Getting Hooked worksheet (see Extra Bits).

For a more informal homework task, we might say something like:

Therapist: I wonder if you'd be willing to practice a few things. First, learn more about how your mind hooks you. In what situations does it happen? What sort of things does it say to you? And as soon as you realize you've been hooked, just acknowledge it: "Aha! Hooked again." Second, would you be willing to play around with one of those defusion techniques we covered? (*Select one or ask the client to pick one.*) As soon as you realize you're hooked, identify the thought that's hooked you—and try the technique. And third, notice any times that your mind tries to hook you but you don't take the bait.

In the next session, we review the homework and find out what happened. We may need to do more work around defusion, or if the client has fallen into the emotional control agenda, we may need to move to creative hopelessness. With most of my clients, if they've already done dropping anchor and are making good progress with defusion, I tend to move to values next—however, you can move to any other part of the hexaflex.

Extra Bits

See chapter 13 in *ACT Made Simple: The Extra Bits* (downloadable from the "Free Stuff" page at http://www.actmindfully.com.au). There you'll find (a) a printable version of the "Summary of Common Defusion Techniques," with descriptions of the few methods we don't cover in the main textbook, (b) a description of fusion in everyday language, (c) the Getting Hooked worksheet, and (d) how to use the ACT Companion app for defusion.

Skilling Up

To get yourself up to speed on defusion techniques:

- Think of two or three current clients, and consider what technique(s) from this chapter you might use with them.

- Read all the exercises and metaphors out loud, or if not, then at least mentally rehearse them.

- Run through the thoughts on cards intervention (illustrated in the transcripts in this chapter) with an imaginary client; act it out or vividly imagine it. Then try it for real in session.

Takeaway

After you've paved the way to start working explicitly on defusion skills with clients (using the principles covered in chapter 11), the next steps are to (a) actively practice skills in session, (b) debrief each exercise and ask how it could be helpful with the client's issues, and (c) assign further practice for homework.

When it comes to learning defusion skills, here are a few rules of thumb:

- Start with quick and easy techniques before moving on to more challenging meditative exercises, such as those in chapter 15.

- Be alert for the possibility of invalidation; err on the side of caution with the techniques you use.

- Remember, defusion is a process, not a technique. There are quinzillions of techniques for instigating and reinforcing this process, and the aim is to find ones that suit both yourself and your clients.

CHAPTER 14

Barriers to Defusion

Anything That Can Go Wrong…

ACT newbies often ask me questions such as "When you do that (defusion technique), is it possible the client may take offense/feel shamed/get angry/feel stupid/get upset/feel invalidated?" My answer is always a resounding "yes." This is the only valid answer to any question that asks "Might the client think, feel, say, or do X?" As the old saying goes, "Anything that can go wrong, will go wrong!" You can guarantee that sooner or later even your greatest all-time-favorite-tried-true-and-trusted defusion interventions will fail or backfire in ways you never imagined.

So in this chapter, we're going to look at common barriers to defusion. (Of course, you probably guessed that from the title, but hey—it never hurts to repeat a key point.) As you work through this chapter, keep in mind that many of the barriers to defusion also obstruct other core processes, and most of the strategies we cover here can readily be used in those situations too. We'll kick off with a very important topic: invalidation.

Invalidation

As we discussed in chapter 5 (and will explore further in chapter 30), a strong therapeutic relationship is fundamental to doing ACT well. So if a therapist says and does things that make the client feel invalidated, that's going to prevent effective therapeutic work (of any sort, not just defusion). That's why it's a good idea to…

First Dance in the Dark, Then Lead to the Light

In *ACT Questions and Answers* (Harris, 2018), I coined the phrase "First dance in the dark, then lead to the light" to convey the importance of a calm, patient, empathic approach for helping highly fused clients to gently defuse. When our clients are stumbling around in a thick, black, impenetrable smog of fusion, we naturally feel an urge to flick on the high beams of defusion and light up a path out of the darkness. The problem is, if we rush into defusion techniques without first taking the time to truly empathize, see things from the client's perspective, and validate her pain and suffering, then it's not likely to go down well. Rather, it's likely to invalidate the client and ramp up her fusion. And this is especially likely if we use playful techniques that are inappropriate for such situations (like singing thoughts or thanking the mind).

For example, suppose your client says, "I can't stand it any longer. My boss is always picking on me. She's always looking over my shoulder, checking up on me. Never gives me any credit for what I do. And she's even taken my ideas and told people they're hers. And any time I slip up or anything's less than f***ing perfect, she rips into me. I'm so f***ing sick of it. I keep hoping something really bad happens to her—like a car accident or cancer or something. I know that sounds bad. But I just hate her."

Imagine what would happen if the therapist now smiles and chirpily says, "Aha, there's your 'bad boss' story," or "Thank your mind for those thoughts," or "Let's try singing 'My job sucks' to the tune Happy Birthday." Would not get a good reaction, right?

So if a client is very fused, let's first "dance in the dark" for a while and then gently and respectfully "lead her to the light." In other words, let's acknowledge and allow the fusion for a while; sit with it compassionately instead of rushing in to disperse it. Let's take the time to get a sense of what the client is experiencing, to see things from her perspective, to empathize with her predicament and acknowledge how painful it is. Dancing in the dark would involve:

A. Listening with openness and curiosity

B. Seeing things from the client's perspective

C. Empathizing, normalizing, and validating

For example, we might say something like "That's really rough. I'd feel angry too. It's especially hurtful given how hard you work and how much you put into it. And stealing your ideas—if someone did that to me, I'd be furious too! And you know, when people are making my life difficult, I also have thoughts about hoping they get hurt in some way, get a taste of their own medicine. Almost everyone does. That's how our minds work; the default setting is, if someone hurts us, we want them to hurt too."

It goes without saying that as we do this, we don't want to trot out some formulaic empathic statement. We want to respond genuinely, from the heart—speaking to the client with our own authentic voice. And take the time necessary to help the client feel heard, understood, and validated. How much time does this take? Not very long. If we listen mindfully and validate compassionately, usually this will take no more than a few minutes. (So if you're spending most of your session doing this kind of work, you're in danger of moving away from ACT into supportive counseling, and there's a real risk of reinforcing client fusion.)

Once we've danced in the dark long enough for the client to feel understood and validated and to trust us as a dance partner, we want to gently lead her to the light. In other words, we want to gently introduce any of the six core processes to help her move to a more psychologically flexible place.

For example, we can often dig up important values that got buried beneath the avalanche of fusion. In this client, for example, underneath her anger, fury, and sense of unfairness we're likely to find important values such as fairness, justice, and respect.

On the other hand, we may dance over to committed action. We may explore what action the client wants to take: be more assertive, lodge a formal complaint, or look around for a different job.

Then again, we could explore acceptance and self-compassion: help her to notice and name her emotions, acknowledge her suffering, and respond to herself with kindness.

Or we might move to dropping anchor: practice staying grounded when intense emotions arise.

And, last but not least, we may go directly into defusion. For example, we could begin with some compassionate acknowledgment of what the mind is doing: "You know, your mind is a lot like mine. When life is tough and we're struggling with really difficult feelings, our minds often tell us stuff that doesn't actually help us to deal with it very well—stuff that, you know, often just makes things harder than they already are. So would it be okay if we take a look at what your mind is telling you about all this, and see what it's got to say that's helpful, and also maybe what's not so helpful?"

So any time you're working with a highly fused client and you find his fusion is thickening rather than dispersing, take a moment to reflect: have you flicked on the defusion beams too quickly? If so, flick them off again. And gently step back into the darkness with your client. And dance there for a while. Then, kindly, calmly, patiently lead him, step-by-step, toward the light.

Many Ways to Invalidate

There are numerous ways a therapist can unintentionally invalidate a client's experience. The best antidote to unintentional invalidation is to embody ACT in session; live your values of compassion, respect, openness, and authenticity, and mindfully appreciate your client—see her as a rainbow, not a roadblock. And be alert in yourself for the following common traps.

"STORY"

The word "story," if used wisely and appropriately, with compassion, empathy, and respect, is very useful for defusion with most clients. However, if we use it flippantly, or without genuine empathy or compassion, it can come across as dismissive or trivializing. If you suspect that your client might not respond well to the word, don't use it; stick to terms like "thoughts," "cognitions," "worries," and so on.

If you ever do use the word "story" and your client does feel upset or offended ("It's not a story!"), then immediately apologize. Say something like "I'm so sorry. I didn't mean to offend you. By 'story' I didn't mean it's made up or untrue. I just meant it's a string of words that come together to convey information or tell a narrative. I use the phrase simply because most people find it helps them to unhook. If you prefer, I can use the word 'cognition' or 'thought' instead. Would that be better?"

PLAYFUL DEFUSION TECHNIQUES

In the right context, playful defusion techniques, such as singing your thoughts, thanking your mind, and saying thoughts in silly voices, are very powerful (and a lot of fun). In the wrong context, they are completely invalidating. For example, imagine a client arrives in overwhelming grief because the person she loves most has just died, and the therapist asks her to sing her thoughts to Happy Birthday; or imagine a client reveals some horrible memories of childhood sexual abuse, and the therapist says, "Thank your mind for those thoughts." We can see how insensitive and inappropriate these interventions are, yet all of us will at some point, inadvertently, despite our best intentions, say something that invalidates a client. When this happens, ACT advocates immediately taking responsibility: owning up to it, apologizing, and repairing. (We explore this in more depth in chapter 16.)

LACK OF EMPATHY

Fusion creates a huge amount of suffering. If the therapist fails to empathize with the huge amount of pain, difficulty, and suffering that fusion has caused, then defusion interventions may come across as dismissive or trivializing. This often triggers a client response such as "You don't understand" or "You don't know what it's like for me!" This commonly occurs when a therapist says, "It's just a thought." This will almost always come across as trivializing the thought. It may be "just a thought" to the therapist, but that's not how it feels to the client in this moment, so this kind of comment from the therapist conveys a lack of empathy. (On the other hand, when a client spontaneously says, about her own cognition, "It's just a thought," this usually indicates defusion.)

NEGLECTING FEELINGS

Suppose you start working with defusion and painful emotions arise. Usually, you'll want to put defusion on hold and work with the emotions: dropping anchor, acceptance, self-compassion. If you keep banging away at defusion and ignoring the huge emotional pain that's arising, not only is this likely to be ineffective, but it can easily come across as uncaring or invalidating.

LACK OF CLARITY

It's crucial to prepare the ground for actively learning defusion skills by (a) making the link between fusion and unworkable behavior, (b) clarifying the purpose of defusion, and (c) teasing out how this skill will be useful and relevant to the client's therapy goals. Therapists often fail to do some or all of the above before moving into active work on defusion, and clients then quite naturally get confused or upset. And sometimes the reason for such failure is actually the therapist's own fusion, as we'll explore next.

Therapist Barriers to Defusion

Let's begin with a look at our own fusion. (Remember: the best person to practice ACT on is yourself.)

Fusion with Self-Doubt and Fear of Failure

When we're new to ACT, almost all of us get hooked by our own unhelpful stories: *I can't do this, I'll screw it up, It'll go wrong, It won't work, It'll upset the client, It'll backfire, It'll destroy rapport,* and so on. And of course, these thoughts are completely normal and natural; it's our "caveman mind" being overly helpful, trying to protect us from harm. And we don't want to totally dismiss these thoughts: they can be useful reminders of the need to actively practice our new therapy skills so we can do them competently; the need to be attuned to our clients, compassionate, and respectful, rather than leaping in and pushing them into ACT when they aren't ready; and the need to always be clear about the purpose of the skills we're bringing in and how specifically they can be helpful with the client's issues.

But while we do want to "extract the wisdom" from our fears and doubts, we don't want to fuse with them. Because if we do, we will stay in our comfort zone and stick to what makes us feel safe: listening empathically, being supportive, talking compassionately about clients' problems and feelings—and actively avoiding doing the experiential work of building new skills. In other words, we end up…

Talking About ACT Instead of Actually Doing ACT

This is the single most common mistake made by ACT newbies (a mistake I've made many times myself). It's easy to talk about ACT because there are so many cool metaphors and interesting bits of psychoeducation. It's so much harder to actively *do* ACT: to initiate and practice new ACT skills in session. I know when my supervisees have been talking about rather than doing ACT because they say things like "We discussed defusion" or "We did the Hands as Thoughts and Feelings metaphor." It's okay to discuss what defusion is and how it can help, and to illustrate what it involves by means of a metaphor—but this is not the same as actively practicing defusion skills, such as "I'm having the thought that…," Leaves on a Stream, naming the story, singing thoughts, or thanking your mind.

TOO MANY METAPHORS?

When therapists get stuck in "talking about ACT" mode, they often do something that we humorously call "metaphor abuse." This is when a client comes into therapy and the therapist (hooked by self-doubt, anxiety, and uncertainty) goes over to her bookcase and takes down a huge can of metaphors. She takes off the lid, starts pulling out metaphors by the handful, and flings them at the client, one after another, hoping one or two of them will stick. At the end of the session, the client leaves the therapy room dripping with metaphors.

The main reasons we use metaphors in ACT are that (a) they convey a lot of information in a short time, (b) clients tend to accept them because they are truisms, and (c) clients tend to remember them after a session. However, we can easily overuse them, and we're most likely to do this when we don't fully understand their purpose or when we're avoiding doing active skills building in session.

SO…UNHOOK, LESS TALK, MORE ACTION!

The take-home message is this: recognize when you've been hooked by your own fears and doubts (we are in the same boat as our clients, right?) and practice defusion on yourself. Notice and name that scary story that's holding you back; unhook from it. Cut back on "talking about" defusion and ramp up actively practicing it in session.

Client Barriers to Defusion

Learning to recognize and unhook from our own barriers to defusion is only half the battle; the other half involves looking out for—and gently dismantling—our clients' barriers. Here are some of the most common ones.

I Have to Get Rid of These Thoughts!

Very often, clients will try hard to avoid or get rid of their thoughts—especially unpleasant thoughts such as harsh self-judgments, painful memories of hurt and failure, and worries about the future. This tendency toward experiential avoidance is usually because they see these thoughts as bad (e.g., signs of mental illness, character deficiency, a weak mind, or being a bad person), dangerous (e.g., a threat to health or sanity), or simply abnormal (no one else has these thoughts). In addition, they may believe their thoughts control their behavior, so in order to change what they do (e.g., stop an addiction, break a bad habit), they must get rid of these thoughts. (Quick reminder: excessive experiential avoidance is due to (a) fusion with judgments—*these thoughts and feelings are bad*—and (b) fusion with rules—*I have to get rid of them; I can't have a good life until they are gone*.)

As you read in chapter 11, we address these issues by lots of normalizing and validating the client's difficult thoughts (e.g., self-disclosure, caveman mind metaphors) and shattering the illusion that thoughts control actions. But if your client remains fixated on avoiding his thoughts, he's unlikely to be interested in genuine defusion. What he's likely to do is pseudo-defusion.

Pseudo-defusion (not an official ACT term) refers to a common scenario where a client misuses a defusion technique to try to avoid or get rid of his unwanted thoughts (usually with the hope this will make him feel better). If this happens, you will soon know, because your client will say, "It's not working!" You will then inquire, "What do you mean, when you say it's not working?" And he will reply something like "I'm not feeling any better" or "These thoughts aren't going away."

When clients are intent on avoiding or getting rid of unwanted thoughts, you will need to do some creative hopelessness (chapter 8); either introduce it for the first time or revisit it if you've done it before. Go through all the ways he's tried to get rid of these thoughts; explore how it worked and what it has cost him; be extremely compassionate to however he reacts; and then see if he's interested in learning a new way. If so, run through the Hands as Thoughts and Feelings metaphor again and really emphasize the end bit, where the hands are still there, resting on the lap.

But I Have Real Problems!

Sometimes when we introduce defusion, a client may get the wrong idea. He may think you're saying it's all in his mind. He's then likely to protest, "It's not just my thoughts. I have real problems here!" Almost always, this happens because the therapist has not (a) validated the very real problems and difficulties the client is facing and (b) clarified how fusion makes these problems worse rather than better. The Hands as Thoughts and Feelings metaphor (extended version) is the best way I know to prevent such misunderstandings because it:

- clearly acknowledges and names the client's problems and challenges: "Out there in front of you are all the problems you need to address, all the challenges you need to face up to, such as (*therapist names the client's biggest issues, e.g., health, relationship, social, work, financial problems*)";

- separates the client's problems from her thoughts and feelings *about* the problems;

- makes it clear that in the face of these problems, she can fuse with or defuse from her thoughts and feelings; and

- clarifies that when defused, it's much easier to deal effectively with these problems.

(At this point, I highly recommend you stop reading and go back and rehearse the extended Hands as Thoughts and Feelings metaphor in chapter 11 again, making sure you have included all these key elements. Alternatively, if you don't like this exercise, rehearse your own way of making these key points without it.)

If, despite your best efforts, this kind of client reaction (i.e., "But I have real problems") happens, your best bet is usually to apologize straight away and clarify your intentions: "I'm so sorry. That's not what I meant. You do have very real problems, such as…(*name the client's main issues, and if they are written on a choice point, simultaneously point to them*). What I'm hoping to do here is help you take action to address these problems. It's very hard for most of us to do that when we're hooked by difficult thoughts, so I thought it would be useful to work on unhooking skills. But we don't have to. If you like, we can work on problem solving and taking action to deal with these issues." If this is what the client prefers, then you can shift to "doing what matters"—values, goals, action planning, and skills training—and then return to defusion later, when fusion shows up as a barrier to values or committed action.

I'm Not Fully Unhooked

Clients and therapists often get the idea that you have to be totally unhooked—100 percent defused—in order to do towards moves. Not so! Even a little bit of unhooking is enough to help you get moving. If you can switch off autopilot, become a bit more aware of where you are and what you're doing and what's been hooking you up until this moment, that's often enough to get you started. With this increased awareness, you can choose towards moves and throw yourself into them, and, as you get more focused on your new values-guided activity, you will progressively unhook from your difficult thoughts and feelings.

Sometimes clients (and therapists) get the idea that you are only defused from a thought when you no longer believe it or are no longer upset by it. Neither of these ideas is correct. Often, defusion does reduce the believability or emotional discomfort of a thought—but not always. Such outcomes are bonuses or by-products; by all means appreciate them when they happen, but do not seek or expect them. The aim of defusion is to reduce the domination of cognitions over overt or covert behavior, and this can happen even while you still believe the thought or are still upset by it.

Seven Strategies for Hopelessness and Reason-Giving

Many clients—especially those suffering from depression—come into therapy feeling hopeless. Typically, they fuse with all sorts of reasons why therapy won't work. And this reason-giving frequently overlaps with many other categories of fusion: the past (I've tried before and failed), the future (It will never work), self-concept (I'm a hopeless case; I don't deserve to get better; I've always been this way; this is who I am; I'm too depressed; I'm too anxious; I'm an addict; I've got no willpower/discipline/motivation; I've been diagnosed with W; I've been permanently damaged by X), judgments (It's too hard; this is bullshit, my life is Y; other people are Z; I'm too A; I'm not B enough; therapy is useless), and rules (I can't do anything difficult when I feel so bad; I have to feel good before I can take action; I should be able to do this by myself).

When this kind of fusion shows up at the very start of therapy, it often throws therapists. After all, you're just taking a history and building rapport with the client, so how are you supposed to help her defuse from this? Well, the beautiful thing is, you can introduce defusion even at this early stage, without needing to be explicit about it. Here are some ideas for how we might do this. You can use some or all of the following seven strategies, in any combination or order, and modify them in many different ways, as suits your needs:

Strategy 1: Notice and Name

Luckily, in ACT, we don't get into challenging the content or validity of cognitions (i.e., assessing whether they are true or false, valid or invalid, positive or negative, right or wrong, appropriate or inappropriate, warranted or unwarranted). If we had to try to convince clients that their doubts about therapy are false, invalid, or unwarranted, we'd be in trouble!

Doubts about therapy are perfectly natural, and only to be expected. However, if clients (or their therapists) fuse with these doubts, it will get in the way of effective work. Thus, such cognitions are good candidates for defusion, right from the word go. We aim to create, as fast as possible, a context of defusion: a space where we can allow unhelpful cognitions to be present, and see them for what they are. We also want to facilitate a context of acceptance, where there is no fighting with or challenging of thoughts, no trying to invalidate or get rid of them.

A good first step is the simple but effective strategy of *noticing and naming*: noticing the presence of cognitions and nonjudgmentally naming them. For example, you might say, "I can see there's a bunch of thoughts showing up for you right now about why this won't work for you." (Remember to modify all language to suit the needs of yourself and your clients. Instead of thoughts, you may talk of concerns, worries, doubts, fears, objections, and so on.)

Strategy 2: Validate and Normalize

As therapists, it's vital that we validate such cognitions. They are commonplace—among both clients who are new to therapy and those who have experienced a lot of it. And they are completely normal and natural thoughts to have. So I tend to say something like "Those are all very common thoughts (or concerns, worries, doubts, fears, objections, and so on). Many of my clients have similar thoughts when we first start working. It's perfectly natural. And to be honest, I expect they'll crop up again and again."

A big part of both defusion and acceptance in ACT is helping clients understand that their mind is not irrational, weird, or defective; it's basically just trying to help. This is both normalizing and validating for clients. You might say something like "These thoughts are just your mind trying to look out for you, do you a favor. It's basically trying to save you from something that might fail or go wrong or be unpleasant. What your mind is saying is *Hey, are you sure you want to do this? You might just be wasting your time, money, and energy. This might even make things even worse for you.* And you know, the truth is, there's probably nothing I can say that will stop your mind from doing that. It's just doing its job—just trying to protect you."

Note how this spiel plants seeds for caveman mind metaphors that may come later.

Strategy 3: Declare "No Guarantees"

You could then go on to say something like this:

"You know, there's a part of me that really wants to reassure you; to say, 'Hey! This will work for you!' But the truth is, I can't guarantee that it will work. And if you ever go to any type of health professional who guarantees you 'This will work!'—my advice would be don't go back, because they are either lying or deluded. Because no one can ever guarantee that.

"I mean, sure, I could show you all the research. There's over a thousand papers published on the ACT model; it's helped hundreds of thousands of people around the world. But that wouldn't guarantee it will work for you. And I could tell you about all my other clients it's helped—but again that won't guarantee it will work for you. But there are two things I will guarantee. I guarantee I'll do my best to help you. And I guarantee, if we give up because your mind has doubts, we won't get anywhere. So even though your mind will keep coming up with reasons why this can't or won't work for you—can we go ahead with it anyway?"

By this point, many clients will be unhooking from their doubts, concerns, objections, and other barriers to therapy. But what if this isn't happening? What if the client continues to insist that therapy can't or won't help? We'll explore that shortly, but first, two important cautions to keep in mind:

- First, as for any type of intervention in any model of therapy, the therapist must be compassionate, respectful, and incredibly validating of the client's experience. If the techniques that follow are delivered in a dismissive, impatient, uncaring, or otherwise invalidating manner, this will obviously offend or upset the client.

- Second, there is not one intervention in any model of therapy that works predictably and favorably with all clients. So if you apply anything from this book (or from any other ACT textbook or training) and it's not having the effect intended, then be flexible. Consider: do you need to modify what you're doing in some way? Or are you better to cease doing it and do something else instead?

Strategy 4: Write Thoughts Down

If the previously mentioned strategies fail to help the client unhook from her objections, doubts, concerns, or other cognitions that act as barriers to therapy, a good next step is to write those thoughts down. Doing this usually makes it a whole lot easier for any of us to "take a step back" and "look at" our thoughts, instead of "getting caught up" in them.

I recommend you ask for permission to write the thoughts down: "So you have some real and valid concerns about whether this will work for you. And I think we need to address these concerns right now, or we're not going to get anywhere. So is it okay if, as a first step, I quickly jot them all down, so I can make sure we address them all?"

The therapist now writes the thoughts down—every objection or concern the client has about why this won't work: I've tried before, I can't do it, and so on.

As the therapist is doing this, ideally she'll repeat some of her previous comments: "I just want to reiterate, these are all very common... Many of my clients have similar thoughts when we first start working... It's perfectly natural—your mind is trying to help, to save you from something that might be unpleasant... So really, we can expect these kinds of thoughts to keep cropping up, again and again."

Strategy 5: Refuse to Convince

It's often useful to say something like "You know, I don't think I'll be able to persuade you or convince you that this approach is the right one for you. In fact, my guess is, the harder I try to convince you, the more those thoughts are going to show up. What do you think?"

At this point, most clients will reply along the lines of "Yeah, I guess you're right." Often there's a hint of amusement in this response, which is usually indicative of some defusion. The door is now wide open to usher in the concept of workability: the client has choices about how to respond to these thoughts, and some of these choices are more workable than others.

Strategy 6: The "Three Choices" Strategy

The therapist could now say something like:

"So here's the thing. These thoughts (pointing to the thoughts written on the paper) are going to show up again and again and again as we do this work together. I have no idea how to stop that from happening. And each time they do, we have a choice to make about how we respond to them. One choice is: we give up. We let your mind call the shots. Your mind says *This won't work*, so we go along with that—we call it a day and we pack it in.

"A second choice is: we get into a debate. I try hard to convince your mind to stop thinking this way; I try to prove your thoughts are false and to convince you that this approach will work. The problem is, that kind of debating will eat up our valuable session time, and I can pretty much guarantee your mind will win the debate anyway—so we won't be any better off.

"A third choice is: we can let your mind say this stuff, and we can just carry on…we just keep on working together as a team…working away here, to help you build a better life…and even though your mind will keep saying all this (pointing to the thoughts on the paper), we just keep on working."

Finally, the therapist asks, "So which of those options would you prefer?"

If the client now agrees to option three, well, that's defusion, right there: the thoughts are present, but they are no longer dominating the client's behavior in self-defeating ways. And the client is also consciously allowing the thoughts to be present: a gentle first step toward acceptance. If our client later comes up with more objections, we can add them to the list, and then repeat the same three choices.

If our client tries to debate, we can notice and name it: "So it seems like you want me to debate this with you. But there's just no point. I won't win. I won't convince your mind. I won't be able to get rid of your doubts or concerns. We really have just two choices here: we give up and pack it in because your mind says it won't work, or we let your mind say all this stuff and we carry on working." If the client now agrees to option three—again, that's defusion, right there!

I've only ever twice had a client choose option one. Both times, I replied, "Okay. I get that's the choice you'd like to make. But given that you're already here, it seems a shame to give up now. Can we at least finish this one session, given you're here? And for this one session, can we not get into a debate about these thoughts? Can we just let your mind say this stuff, and carry on?" Both times, the client agreed. (Obviously, this strategy may not work with a mandated client, but that's a different issue, beyond the scope of this textbook. I discuss how to work with mandated clients in my advanced-level textbook: *Getting Unstuck in ACT* [Harris, 2013].)

Strategy 7: Acknowledge Recurring Thoughts

The therapist can now use the above methods for ongoing defusion and acceptance, throughout the session. For example, when new objections occur, the therapist can write them down and again ask the client to choose how to respond. But when a previously noted objection recurs, the therapist can respectfully and compassionately acknowledge it and point to the paper: "We've got that one down already. So again, there's a choice to make here…"

Alternatively (and more powerfully, in my opinion), you give the sheet to the client with a pen, and ask her to mark each thought as it recurs. The therapist can respectfully and compassionately acknowledge it each time: "Keeps showing up. So do we give up, or waste time debating, or do we acknowledge the thought just popped up again and carry on?"

If you're using this strategy, it's often helpful for you to keep the paper, and on the next session, present it to the client: "I expect these will all show up again today. Any of them showing up right now? Most of them? Cool. Can we let them be there, and carry on? Great. And let's see if your mind comes up with any new ones today."

Note just how much we've covered here in terms of defusion. We now have a wealth of strategies to draw on repeatedly and develop further in subsequent sessions. And all of these strategies involve some combination of the "three Ns": noticing, naming, and neutralizing. (Remember, the easiest step in neutralizing is to look at thoughts in terms of workability: if you let this thought dictate what you do, where does that get you?) Note too that all of this could be done on the very first session if necessary—yes, even as we're getting to know the client and taking our initial history.

Therapists often see fusion with hopelessness and reason-giving as a barrier to therapy. I hope that you will now reframe it: it's not a barrier to therapy but a golden opportunity to actively DO therapy. It gives us the chance to actively build defusion skills in session (instead of just talking about them).

Adapting These Strategies to Other Cognitive Processes

With a little imagination, you can easily adapt strategies 1, 2, 4, and 7 outlined above to deal with just about any problematic cognitive process that interferes with progress in a session: blaming, ruminating, obsessing, revenge fantasies, worrying, catastrophizing, and so on.

For example, suppose a client keeps blaming everyone else for her problems. Strategy 1 is notice and name, so we might say, "Do you notice what your mind is doing here? There are a lot of people in your life who aren't behaving the way you want—which is really upsetting for you—and your mind keeps reminding you of that." (Note how this way of speaking avoids using the term "blaming," as this might be invalidating.)

Strategy 2 is validate and normalize, so we might say, "And this is perfectly natural. When there are things going on in our lives that upset us, our mind keeps reminding us about them because it wants us to do something about it. Your mind's job is to look after you, make your life better, so it's alerting you to problems you need to deal with."

After this, we'd establish (or reestablish) behavioral goals (chapter 6). We might say, "So given your mind wants you to do something about this, can we take a moment to get clear on what you want from our sessions? Do you want to look at how to deal with your feelings when others behave that way? Or do you want to look at how you can influence their behavior in constructive ways that help build healthy relationships? Or do you want to learn how to unhook yourself and refocus when your mind keeps pulling you into thinking about this stuff?"

If the client wants to learn how to handle her thoughts and feelings better, we can then look at what happens when her mind starts blaming and help her learn to unhook. As part of this work, it could be very useful to bring in strategy 4: write thoughts down. We could write down all the client's "blaming" thoughts (without ever using the word "blaming") and explore: "What happens when you get hooked by these thoughts? What do you say? What do you do? Where does your attention go to? Does that help you to be the person you want to be or influence others effectively?"

If the client wants to learn how to influence others more effectively, we can now look at how to do so, through assertiveness and communication skills, positive reinforcement, and shaping behavior (see chapter 29: Flexible Relationships). We can also bring in strategy 7: acknowledge recurring thoughts; each time blaming recurs in session, we can say, "So here's your mind reminding you yet again about all these difficult relationships in your life." The thought-marking strategy will usually work very well here. After marking a recurrent thought, the therapist can ask, "So do we carry on with XYZ (where XYZ = the behavioral goals just established), or do we let this thought pull us off track?"

Practical Tip   For strategy 7 to work, you must clearly establish behavioral goals for therapy. If you don't, there's no motivation for the client to unhook. The client will only be interested in unhooking if she can see that getting hooked interferes with her behavioral goals.

Skilling Up

Time for another reminder to practice, practice, practice. Are you able to clearly "make the link" between fusion and problematic behavior? Are you able to clarify the purpose of defusion? Please read through the scripts and rehearse the seven strategies for working with hopelessness and reason-giving:

- Notice and name

- Validate and normalize

- Declare "no guarantees"

- Write thoughts down

- Refuse to convince

- The "three choices" strategy

- Acknowledge recurring thoughts

Practice in your head or out aloud with imaginary clients, willing friends, colleagues, coworkers, or other members of an ACT interest group in order to build up your skill levels.

Takeaway

I hope and trust you now have a lot of ideas for overcoming barriers to defusion. There are four main take-home messages: First, practice defusion on yourself: unhook from your own fears and doubts, and start actively doing ACT, not just talking about it. Second, model ACT for your clients. Live your values and be mindful in each session. Infuse your work with empathy, respect, and compassion. And see your clients as rainbows, not roadblocks. Third, dance in the dark before you lead to the light. And finally, validate, validate, validate! If you think a given intervention may be invalidating, then don't do it; there are always many alternatives. And if you ever do accidentally invalidate a client, then immediately apologize and clarify what your real intentions were.

CHAPTER 15

Leaves, Streams, Clouds, and Sky

Meditative Defusion

"Don't give me that hippy bullshit!" Have you ever had a client say something like that to you? I certainly have, on several occasions—and always in response to the word "meditation." The problem is, "meditation" is such a loaded term; it conjures up images of hippies chanting "Om," incense sticks and lighted candles, gurus and Buddhist monks; or it's heavily linked to other words such as "boring" and "difficult." That's why I now talk about unhooking skills rather than mindfulness meditation.

As we discussed in chapter 3, from an ACT perspective, formal meditation is only one way among hundreds of learning the core mindfulness skills: defusion, acceptance, flexible attention, and self-as-context. If clients want to take up meditation or other formal mindfulness practices such as yoga or tai chi, that's great—when it comes to learning new skills, the more practice the better—but it's definitely not something we expect or ask for.

Having said that, some defusion techniques are clearly meditative in nature. These are longer exercises, where we notice our thoughts with openness and curiosity; we notice them come and stay and go in their own good time, without judging them, clinging to them, or pushing them away. Meditation-style defusion is much harder for most people than the brief interventions we've covered so far, so if we want clients to practice it, then we really need to clarify…

How Will This Help?

How do these longer, more challenging, meditative exercises help our clients with the issues that brought them into therapy? Here's the way I tend to explain it:

Therapist: You're spending a lot of time lost in your head worrying (or *ruminating, obsessing, dwelling on the past, or whatever cognitive processes the client is struggling with*). And it seems like as soon as these thoughts show up, they instantly hook you. You get lost in them. You get so caught up in them you're no longer able to give your attention to GHI or engage in JKL or focus on MNO. (*GHI, JKL, and MNO are specific activities that the client has difficulty engaging in or focusing on when worrying, ruminating, obsessing, and so forth, such as being present with the kids or focusing on a task at work.*) What if you could get to a point where these thoughts show up and you can let them float on by, instead of getting pulled into them, or holding onto them—so that instead, you can give your full attention to GHI and JKL?

Client: That would be good.

Therapist: Well, the aim of this exercise is to help you do just that: learn how to step back and notice your thoughts, and watch them come and go, without getting pulled into them or holding on to them.

Client: Okay, that makes sense.

Therapist: It also builds the other unhooking skills we've been working on, makes them more effective, and easier for you to do. It's a bit like working out at the gym. The exercises we've done so far are like the light weights you lift to warm up your muscles; this one is the heavy lifting.

Planting Seeds for Self-as-Context

Self-as-context, better known as the *noticing self* or *observing self*, is intimately connected with defusion. The first step in defusion is always to notice your thoughts; so what is this aspect of you that does the noticing? This "part that notices" is implicit in all mindfulness exercises, not just defusion, because they all, at their core, involve noticing. So we can start planting the seeds for explicit self-as-context (SAC) work early on in therapy, without making a big deal out of it. We can then water these seeds in later sessions if we want them to sprout.

One way to plant these seeds early is to mention SAC in the form of a passing comment, as part of some other intervention. For example, as I'm doing the first dropping anchor exercise with a client, after I've asked her to "notice X, notice Y, notice Z," I'll casually mention, "So there's a part of you that can notice everything."

I'll often then add, "And we're going to be using that part of you throughout our work together… to help you in various ways."

The client will usually nod or say "uh-huh." On occasion, she may look blank or confused, but I don't mind; at this point, I'm not wanting to explore SAC, I'm just planting seeds for later work. So unless the client protests, "I don't know what you mean!" or something like that, I won't try to clarify; I'll just carry on with whatever exercise we are in the midst of doing.

We can easily plant SAC seeds while doing any type of mindfulness exercise, whether it's defusion, acceptance, or contacting the present moment, by using phrases like these:

- "As you notice X, be aware you're noticing."

- "There's X and there's a part of you noticing X."

I'll have more to say on this topic later in the book. For now, I'll just ask you to take note of these "seeds for SAC" as you encounter them "implanted" into many of the scripts that follow in this and later chapters.

Setting Up for Leaves on a Stream

The Leaves on a Stream exercise often seems simple at first sight. You visualize a gently flowing stream with leaves on the surface of the water, and you place your thoughts onto the leaves and allow them to float on by. However, it's easy to run into problems with this exercise, so I want to give you a few pointers to make it more effective.

OFFER NONVISUAL OPTIONS

First, given that the exercise involves visualization, it's a good idea to ask your clients whether this is something they can readily do. About one in ten people finds visualization extremely difficult if not impossible (I'm in that group myself), in which case, we need to offer a nonvisual alternative. One good option is simply to close your eyes, and instead of trying to picture a stream and leaves, just use the black space behind your eyelids. (Another option is to do the Hearing Your Thoughts exercise instead, discussed later this chapter.)

LET IT COME AND STAY AND GO

The phrase "let it go" is often misunderstood (by clients and therapists) to mean "let it go *away*"; there's an assumption that the thought will pass on by, disappear. And yes, that does often happen; most thoughts come and go pretty quickly. But sometimes, thoughts hang around for quite a while. Defusion doesn't mean they disappear; it means they aren't dominating us. For this reason, I recommend instead of using the phrase "let it go," you say things like "Let your thoughts come *and stay* and go, in their own good time, as they please."

Remember, the aim of the exercise is to learn how to step back and watch the flow of your thoughts, not to make them go away. So if the client starts speeding up the stream, trying to wash the thoughts away, this exercise turns from mindfulness into experiential avoidance. That's why I like to add comments like, "It's okay if the leaves hang around and pile up, or the river stops flowing; just keep watching."

INCLUDE POSITIVE AND NEGATIVE

Emphasize that during this exercise, we are aiming to put all our thoughts onto leaves or black space: positive and negative, optimistic and pessimistic, happy and sad. You might say to the client, "The skill we're learning is how to observe the stream of our thoughts without getting pulled into it, how to watch them come and go without holding onto them. So if a positive or happy thought shows up and you go, 'Oh, I'm not going to put that one on a leaf; I don't want it to float away,' then you're not truly learning the skill of watching your thoughts."

INVITE CREATIVITY

Invite clients to creatively modify the exercise: they may prefer to use suitcases on a conveyor belt, clouds in the sky, platters on a sushi train, or carriages on a train. One of my clients was a *Star Wars* fan, and you know how the letters float up the screen in the opening credits of those movies? Well, that's what he did with his thoughts. Another of my clients had so many thoughts rushing through her head, leaves couldn't handle it, so she changed it to tree trunks floating down a stream!

DON'T DO THIS IN A BUSINESS MEETING!

With any meditation-style exercise, it's wise to say something like "Of course, this wouldn't go down well in the middle of a business meeting, or social event, or challenging situation at work or at home. This is something you practice outside of those difficult situations, to build up your unhooking skills. When you're in those situations, the idea is that you rapidly unhook, ground yourself, and refocus on the task at hand. That will be much easier to do if you practice these skills outside of those situations."

CONSIDER DROPPING ANCHOR AND PLANTING SEEDS

We can easily top and tail any formal meditative exercise with dropping anchor, and at the same time, plant seeds for self-as-context. This is optional of course, but I encourage you to try it out and see what happens. Below, you'll find an example of how to do this, and after that we'll get to the main exercise. Where you see an ellipsis (…), this indicates a pause of three to five seconds; longer pauses are indicated with time in brackets. (Note: All timings are merely rough indications. The idea is to be flexible—shorten or lengthen the pauses as required.)

Therapist: I invite you to sit up straight … and let your shoulders drop … and straighten your spine … and sit slightly forward in your chair, supporting your own back … and either close your eyes or fix them on a spot in front of you … and tap into a sense of curiosity … as if you are a curious child doing something you've never done before, embarking on an adventure and wondering what you will discover …

And with that sense of curiosity, take a moment to notice what thoughts and feelings are present … and just acknowledge they are present, without trying to change them in any way … and again, with curiosity, notice how you are sitting … connect with your body … notice where your feet are … and your hands … and your shoulders … and your neck … notice your spine, and whether or not it is straight … and whether your eyes are open or closed, notice what you can see … and notice what you can hear … and notice what you can taste and smell, or the sensations in your nose and mouth … and notice where your hands are and what they are touching … and notice what your mind is doing … is it silent or chattering? … and notice what you are feeling … and notice what you are doing …

(*Planting seeds for self-as-context*) So there's a part of you that notices everything … everything that you see, hear, touch, taste, smell, think, feel, and do in any moment … and you're going to use that part of you in this exercise, to take a step back and watch your mind in action … to watch your thoughts coming and staying and going … and to help you do that, I invite you to imagine a gently flowing stream …

* * *

If you don't want to plant seeds for SAC, then you can leave out the bit about the part that notices.

Now for the Exercise Itself…(and an Alternative One)

Whether or not you use the introduction above, the main exercise is as follows.

The Leaves on a Stream Exercise

1. Find a comfortable position, and either close your eyes or fix your eyes on a spot.

2. Imagine you're sitting by the side of a gently flowing stream, and there are leaves flowing past on the surface of the stream. Imagine it however you like—it's your imagination. (*Pause 10 seconds.*)

3. Now, for the next few minutes, notice each of your thoughts as it pops into your head … then place it onto a leaf, and allow it to come and stay and go in its own good time … Don't try to make it float away, just notice what it does … It may float on by quickly, or it may go very slowly, or it may hang around … Do this regardless of whether the thoughts are positive or negative, pleasurable or painful … even if they're the most wonderful thoughts, place them onto a leaf … and allow them to come and stay and go, in their own good time … they may float by quickly, or slowly, or they may hang around … simply notice what happens, without trying to alter it. (*Pause 10 seconds.*)

4. If your thoughts stop, just watch the stream. Sooner or later, your thoughts will start up again. (*Pause 20 seconds.*)

5. Allow the stream to flow at its own rate. Don't speed it up. You're not trying to wash the leaves away—you're allowing them to come and go in their own good time. (*Pause 20 seconds.*)

6. If your mind says, *This is stupid* or *I can't do it*, place those thoughts on a leaf. (*Pause 20 seconds.*)

7. If a leaf gets stuck, let it hang around. Don't force it to float away. (*Pause 20 seconds.*)

8. (*An optional add-in: introducing acceptance*) If a difficult feeling arises, such as boredom or impatience, simply acknowledge it. Say to yourself, *Here's a feeling of boredom* or *Here's a feeling of impatience.* Then place those words onto a leaf.

9. From time to time, your thoughts will hook you, and pull you out of the exercise, so you lose track of what you are doing. This is normal and natural, and it will keep happening. As soon as you realize it's happened, gently acknowledge it and then start the exercise again.

After instruction 9, continue the exercise for several minutes or so, periodically punctuating the silence with this reminder: "Again and again, your thoughts will hook you. This is normal. As soon as you realize it, start up the exercise again."

You can end the exercise with another round of dropping anchor, or with a simple instruction such as this: "And now, bring the exercise to an end … and sit up in your chair … and open your eyes. Look around the room … and notice what you can see and hear … and take a stretch. Welcome back!"

After doing Leaves on a Stream, debrief the exercise with the client: What sort of thoughts hooked her? What was it like to let thoughts come and stay and go without holding on? Was it hard to unhook from any thoughts in particular? Did she speed up the stream, trying to wash the thoughts away? (If so, we need to clarify: we aren't trying to make these thoughts go away; we're simply watching what they do.) Does she see how this is the opposite of rumination, worrying, obsessing, and how it can therefore be useful in disrupting those habits?

A shorter, simpler alternative to Leaves on a Stream is to simply…

Watch Your Thinking

This exercise begins with a brief round of dropping anchor and the curious child metaphor, as above (and, if desired, a similar "planting seeds" instruction). Once the client is grounded and paying attention with curiosity, the next instructions are:

1. Now bring that curious attention to your thoughts, and see if you can notice: Where are your thoughts? … Where do they seem to be located in space? (*Pause 10 seconds.*) If your thoughts

are like a voice, where is that voice located? ... Is it in the center of your head or top or bottom or to one side? (*Pause 10 seconds.*)

2. Notice the form of your thoughts: Are they more like pictures, words, or sounds? (*Pause 10 seconds.*)

3. Are your thoughts moving or still? ... If moving, at what speed and in what direction? ... If still, where are they hovering?

4. What is above and below your thoughts? ... Are there any gaps in between them?

5. For the next few minutes, observe your thoughts coming and going as if you're a curious child who has never encountered anything like this before.

* * *

The rest of the instructions, and the debriefing afterward, are pretty much the same as for Leaves on a Stream.

Creativity with Exercises

In any meditative exercise or practice, we can accentuate whichever core mindfulness process we wish to emphasize: defusion, acceptance, contacting the present moment, or the noticing self. We can accentuate defusion in any mindfulness exercise by (a) adding comments such as "Notice how your mind hooks you" or "As soon as you realize you've been hooked, acknowledge it, unhook yourself, and refocus" and (b) adding metaphors about "letting your thoughts come and stay and go," as in the examples below.

Allow your thoughts to freely come and stay and go, like:

*   passing cars, driving past outside your house;

*   clouds drifting across the sky;

*   people walking by on the other side of the street;

*   waves washing gently onto the beach;

*   birds flying across the sky; or

*   trains pulling in and out of the station.

How Long Do Meditative Exercises Go For?

Make your exercises in ACT as short or as long as they need to be to (a) meet the demands of the situation and (b) accommodate the capabilities of the client. If you don't have a clue as to how the client will cope, start with a four- to five-minute version as a test, and subsequently modify it depending on the client's response. But if you suspect that your client will struggle with an exercise this long, make it shorter, and if you think she can handle a longer exercise, then you can extend it. All the meditative exercises in ACT can be shortened to two or three minutes or expanded to twenty or thirty minutes.

Extra Bits

If you or your clients have difficulty "visualizing" or "seeing" your thoughts, an alternative is to practice "hearing" them: you notice them as if listening to someone's voice, and you pay curious attention to auditory qualities like volume, pitch, tone, and emotionality. See chapter 15 in ACT *Made Simple: The Extra Bits* (at http://www.actmindfully.com.au), where you'll find a link to download a free audio recording of the Hearing Your Thoughts exercise.

Skilling Up

Homework time for you again. Before you do these exercises with clients, it's important that you know them inside out. So your mission, should you choose to accept it, is to:

- rehearse these scripts (at the very least, mentally, but ideally, out loud) so you can get a feel for the language, and modify them to suit your style; and

- try these practices out on yourself, so you know what's involved—because whatever difficulties you have with these exercises will probably be similar to those of your clients.

Takeaway

It's often useful to give clients meditative exercises that involve "thought watching" (or "thought listening") as an antidote to rumination, worrying, and the like. But we must always be clear about the purpose—how will it specifically help the client with his issues? And we should always adapt the exercise to suit the client: make it shorter or longer, change the metaphor, or shift the emphasis from seeing thoughts to hearing thoughts. We always want to debrief the exercise carefully afterward and make sure the client can link it to his issues. And finally, assuming the client sees the potential benefits of the exercise, we then want to encourage him to practice it between sessions. (We'll look at how to do this in the next chapter.)

CHAPTER 16

"Technique Overload" and Other Perils

Too Much of a Good Thing

Have you ever experienced "technique overload"? It's quite overwhelming. You're in session and it feels like you have a googazillion techniques floating around in your head, and you don't know which one to use. Your session gets clunkier and clunkier, and your mind starts saying, *I'm a lousy therapist, I don't know what I'm doing, I'm screwing this up*. At this point, many therapists give up on ACT and fall back into supportive counseling or other models of therapy that they find easier.

We'll kick off this chapter by looking at a terrific way to avoid technique overload. Then we'll run through a whole stack of practical tips that apply to all experiential exercises and mindfulness practices. If I added these tips to every chapter, this book would get very repetitive and rather thick (a bit like me, some might say). So I'm going to clump them all together in this chapter.

First off, let's tackle technique overload. Here's a great tip I picked up from Kirk Strosahl, one of the original pioneers of ACT. For each of the six core processes, pick three main techniques—tools, worksheets, exercises, metaphors, practices, questions, and so on—and use them over and over until you are really familiar with them. This will give you a core set of eighteen interventions that can be mixed and matched, adapted and co-opted for a myriad of different issues. (With a bit of imagination, most techniques can be used for several different processes.) These eighteen interventions will become your very own personalized ACT tool kit.

Below, I've given you my personal tool kit, not to proclaim that it is "right" or "better" than anyone else's, but purely to provide an example. (At this point in the book, we've only covered a few of these techniques, but don't worry—by the end, you'll know them all.)

CORE PROCESS	TECHNIQUES		
DEFUSION	Naming the Story	Hands as Thoughts and Feelings	"I'm having the thought that…"
ACCEPTANCE	Pushing Away Paper	Observe, Breathe, Expand, & Allow	Compassionate Hand
CONTACTING THE PRESENT MOMENT	Notice X	Mindfulness of the Hand	Dropping Anchor
SELF-AS-CONTEXT	Stage Show of Life	Sky and Weather	Notice That You Are Noticing
VALUES	Flavoring & Savoring	The Bull's Eye	Values Cards
COMMITTED ACTION	SMART Goals	The Choice Point	Towards Moves

I encourage you to create your own version of the table above and fill it in as you work through the book: identify your favorite metaphors, worksheets, and exercises for the six core processes. I recommend you do it on a computer rather than on paper because you'll probably change your mind quite a few times. (There's a printable version in Extra Bits.) For at least a few weeks, see if you can largely limit your practice to playing around with these eighteen interventions, until they are so familiar to you that they come naturally and fluidly.

Once you've done this, feel free to add new techniques to your repertoire, one at a time, and see how they work and how you like them. The lovely thing with ACT is there is no need for you to ever get bored with any given tool or technique, as there are countless alternatives available.

Practical Tips for Experiential Exercises

What follows next are practical tips relevant to just about every experiential exercise you ever do. I hope you come back to this chapter repeatedly, as soon as you run into trouble with experiential work.

Check In with Your Clients

If you're doing exercises one-on-one with your clients, check in with them periodically (especially with longer practices): "How are you doing with this? What's showing up for you? Is your mind on board or interfering? Are we okay to keep going?" If your client is struggling, then pause the exercise and explore her reaction, as discussed below in "When Things Go Awry."

Go Slowly

When you're taking your clients through an exercise, it's easy to go too fast but almost impossible to go too slow. So go slower than you think you need to. And if in doubt, ask your client: "Am I going too fast or too slow for you, or is it about right?"

Play, Adapt, Create

As you learn all these new ACT skills, I really hope you have some fun with it. The idea is that you "play" with these techniques; you adapt, modify, reinvent them. Change the words, change the imagery, change the objects used. If you don't like mindfully focusing on the breath, there are about 10,000 other things you could focus on instead. I fell in love with the ACT model instantly—but I didn't fall in love with many of the "classic" techniques (i.e., the ones used in the earliest ACT protocols). For example, as an ACT newbie, I rapidly stopped using classics such as Man in the Hole and Passengers on the Bus for the simple reason that I found these metaphors to be too long and complex for my liking. But that's just me; the ACT world is full of people who love these classics, and you'll find them in the vast majority of textbooks and protocols, so we each need to find what works for us. Instead, I started creating my own techniques, modifying existing ones, and taking ones from other models but adapting them so they became ACT-congruent; I adapted everything to suit my own way of speaking and my own style of working. And I really, really, really, encourage you to do the same thing (yes, really!).

(By the way, I did actually use Passengers on the Bus in the first edition of my first book, *The Happiness Trap*. That's because when I chopped it up into little bits and pieces and delivered it over the length of a book, it didn't feel long or complex. But even then, I changed it to "Demons on the Boat," just for the fun of being creative. Similarly, the idea of seeing clients as "rainbows not roadblocks" is my version of psychologist Kelly Wilson's classic metaphor about seeing our clients as "sunsets not math problems." So please adapt and modify to your heart's delight.)

Improvise

All ACT textbooks contain scripts for exercises. Please DON'T read word for word from the script; it will sound stilted, odd, or artificial. Improvise around the script; use it as a reference but put everything into your own words. If you have phrases, terms, imagery, or metaphors that seem better or more natural to you than the ones in the script, use those instead.

Mix and Match

You can take parts of one exercise or technique and add them to another. For example, in dropping anchor exercises, after an instruction such as "Notice A and B and C and D and E," you could add "So there's a part of you that notices everything," which plants seeds for future work on self-as-context. Similarly, it's often useful to end longer mindfulness exercises with a bit of dropping anchor or a brief connection to values.

Record Your Exercises

You can easily find a stack of prerecorded mindfulness and values exercises to share with your clients. (For example, I have quite a few free ones you can listen to on the smartphone app "ACT Companion" and plenty more you can purchase as MP3s from http://www.actmindfully.com.au. However, it's far better for you to record your own exercises and give them to your clients because they will usually have a much deeper connection to your voice than to that of someone they've never met. You can prerecord exercises outside of sessions, or you can record them as you do them in the session. You can easily do this on almost any smartphone or laptop. Just google "record audio on" followed by the name of the device you use, and you'll find out how. You can then give it to your client via email, text message, or a flash stick. (Please feel free to use any of the scripts in this book or *ACT Made Simple: The Extra Bits* as the basis for your recordings.)

Ensure Clarity

You may have noticed that I keep harping on the importance of clarity. I do this because it's such a huge issue among ACT newbies and old timers alike. All too often, therapists ask clients to do unusual exercises (that are often difficult and challenging) without a clear rationale. It's worth taking the time to clearly link these interventions to the client's specific issues to ensure the client understands how this is relevant to and helpful for solving his problems and achieving his therapy goals.

For any technique you intend to use, check: Are you clear on its purpose? What specific client goals is this likely to help with, and how? Would you be able to answer these questions if the client were to ask you? If not, you have some homework to do; you shouldn't be using these techniques until you yourself are clear about them.

The same caution applies to metaphors: what specific insight are you hoping for the client to achieve, and how does that link to her therapy goals? Watch out for a common therapist trap that's playfully called "metaphor abuse." This is when the therapist, who is not really clear about what he is aiming to achieve, throws metaphor after metaphor at the clients, hoping one will stick. This rarely leads anywhere useful. Use your metaphors sparingly and precisely, aligned with clients' therapy goals.

Debrief the Exercise

It's very important to debrief experiential exercises after they've finished. Useful questions to ask include:

- What was that like for you?

- What happened there?

- What feelings showed up? Did you struggle with them? Did they hook you?

- What did your mind do? What did it say? Was it helpful or a hindrance?

- Did you get hooked at any point? By what? And what happened then? Did you manage to unhook again? How did you do that?

- What was useful or helpful for you in this?

- Do you see any link between this and ABC? (ABC = a client issue, problem, or therapy goal previously specified.)

- How might this help you with ABC?

The last question above—"How might this help you with… (specific issue, problem, or therapy goal)?"—is very important. If the client says, "I don't know!", then you need to take the time to make it clear.

Turn an Exercise into "Homework"

Reminder: don't use the word "homework" with clients; almost nobody likes it. Use words like "practice," "try it out," "experiment," "play around with it," or "give it a go." Now, as you know, after we've done experiential exercises in session, we debrief them, and we ask, "How can this help you with ABC?" If the client comes out with a good answer that shows he understands the aim of the exercise and its potential to help with his therapy goals, then often we can set this exercise, or something similar, as a homework task. For example, if the exercise was mindful breathing or a body scan or Leaves on a Stream, we may ask:

"So given this could help you with ABC, would you be willing to practice it outside of these sessions?" If the answer is yes, we can go on to explore: "When will you do it? Where will you do it? For how long? How often?" and so on. And if the client is willing, it's a good idea to get her to record her practice on a worksheet or in her journal.

Create a Context for Experiments and Curiosity

When introducing experiential exercises, it's a good idea to use the language of "experiments." The reality is, we never know for sure what the outcome will be of any exercise, technique, or practice, so let's be open about that with our clients. We could say, prior to an exercise, "I'm asking you to try this because I think it will be helpful with ABC. However, there's no way to know for sure exactly what will happen; it's always an experiment. Can we try it out, see what happens?" This facilitates an open, curious mindset (in both client and therapist). If we liberally use the language of "experiments," it's much easier to handle those unfortunate situations.

When Things Go Awry

Sooner or later, you'll be doing some sort of work with defusion, acceptance, or flexible attention, and your client will complain that an exercise isn't working; or even worse, your intervention will completely backfire. But don't fret, you can use these moments as opportunities to learn, and then quickly get back on track. Let's look at each of these scenarios more closely.

When It's Not Working

When a client complains, "It's not working," we always want to respond with openness and curiosity (which usually means we'll need to drop anchor, make room for our own anxiety, and unhook from our own unhelpful thoughts). We might say something like "Oh, I'm sorry to hear that. Can you tell me what's happening?"

The client will usually then give an answer that clearly reveals the emotional control agenda: "I'm not feeling any better," "The thoughts aren't going away," "My anxiety is getting worse," "I'm still feeling angry," "The memory is still there," "I'm not relaxing," "I'm still upset."

The therapist may then gently inquire, "So if I get you right, you were expecting this exercise to get rid of this memory/thought/feeling/sensation?" The client will usually answer yes (often with a bit of irritation or frustration). The therapist may then reply, "I'm so sorry. I obviously wasn't clear about the purpose of this. It's not a way to get rid of unwanted thoughts and feelings/control how you feel/relax you/make you feel good." The therapist then recaps the purpose of the exercise. For defusion and flexible attention techniques, the best way I know to do this is the Hands as Thoughts and Feelings metaphor (chapter 11), and for acceptance and self-compassion, it's the Pushing Away Paper exercise (chapter 9) or the Struggle Switch metaphor (which we'll get to in chapter 22). We particularly emphasize, as we recap these metaphors, that the thought/feeling/memory doesn't disappear; instead we learn a new way of responding to it that frees us up to engage in life and invest energy in doing meaningful things.

We might also say, "There will be times you do these exercises and those thoughts/feelings rapidly change, reduce, or disappear. By all means, enjoy that when it happens—but please don't expect it. It's a pleasant bonus, but it's not the main aim. If you turn this technique into a way to control how you feel or get rid of unwanted thoughts and feelings, then you'll be right back here telling me 'It's not working.'"

Obviously, if the client has a negative reaction to this, we will need to revisit creative hopelessness (or bring it in now if we previously skipped it).

When Things Go Horribly Wrong

But what do we do if an exercise fails or backfires? For sure, we can reduce the risk of this through clarity about the purpose of the exercise (linking it to therapy goals) and setting it up as an experiment. But sooner or later, no matter how experienced and skillful we may be, our interventions are going to go wrong.

At this point, a few words of advice: when anything in a therapy session fails, goes wrong, or backfires, stay calm! We won't *feel* calm, of course. But we can *act* calmly. We may feel anxious, sad, frustrated, guilty, fearful, or angry; we may have all sorts of unhelpful thoughts about ourselves, the client, the exercise, or even the ACT model itself. But even with all those thoughts and feelings present, we can still act calmly.

In other words, let's use ACT on ourselves in these situations: defuse from our thoughts about screwing it up, make room for our feelings of anxiety (chapter 22), drop anchor, and get fully present. And even though we don't feel calm, we can model the quality of calmness through our voice, our words, our body posture, and our actions.

And not only do we drop anchor for ourselves, we help our clients to do likewise. If the client is upset or fused or struggling in any way—sad, angry, frightened, shaken, disappointed, frustrated, dissociated, overwhelmed—we can help him drop anchor. (If we haven't yet introduced this, now is a good time to do so.) After grounding, we can model openness and curiosity as we explore what just happened. If we have set it up as an experiment, we can now say, "Well that experiment didn't go the way I'd hoped. I'm sorry; looks like you've had a bad reaction—not what I'd expected."

After this, we want to explore what actually did happen, with the aim of finding something useful in the experience: either something directly relevant to the client's therapy goals or something more generally useful for developing psychological flexibility. Useful questions could include:

- What happened just then?

- What thoughts, feelings, memories showed up?

- What did your mind hook you with?

- What feelings are showing up for you now?

- What's your mind saying now?

We also want to consider whether an apology is warranted. If so, let's be quick and genuine. For example, we might say, "I'm sorry. I didn't expect that to happen. I can see that you're upset. I hope this hasn't put you off working this way."

It's generally useful at this point to remind the client of the rationale for the exercise. We might say, for example, "I'm sorry. As I said to you before we started the exercise, I was hoping it would help you unhook from difficult thoughts, but unfortunately, it looks like you ended up more hooked than before." Or "I'm sorry. I was hoping that exercise would help you stop struggling with difficult feelings, but it looks like you actually ended up struggling even more than before."

After all that, we can now say something like "I didn't want or expect this to happen, but given it has happened, can we look at this as a learning opportunity?"

Among other things, we can learn:

- more of the ways your mind can hook you,

- more of the ways you can get pulled into a struggle with thoughts and feelings, and

- how our minds easily make life difficult for us—and can interfere with anything we try to do.

Let's look at an example of putting this into practice.

Mark, aged thirty-four, an army veteran, has PTSD related to wartime events. He often gets hooked by harsh self-criticism, and while working on defusion in session two, he labeled this pattern of thinking as "the dictator." In sessions one to three, he repeatedly participated in dropping anchor exercises to good effect, and he has also practiced it between sessions. This transcript takes place near the start of session four. The therapist has just finished a three-minute dropping anchor exercise and is now about to debrief it.

Therapist: So, what was that like for you?

Client: (*long pause, then laughs cynically*) Pretty f***ing stupid.

Therapist: (*surprised*) Stupid?

Client: Yup.

Therapist: Okay. Anything else, apart from stupid?

Client: Irritating.

Therapist: Irritating?

Client: To be honest, it was really irritating me.

Therapist: (*accepting his own reactions of anxiety and disappointment, and remaining open and curious*) Okay. So it was irritating, and stupid.

Client: Yup.

Therapist: Okay. So can I ask…this part of you that's judging the exercise as irritating and stupid… is that the same part of you that we've been calling "the dictator"?

Client:	Maybe. Yeah, maybe. He sits in a little black box about there (taps on his right temple). I guess it's the same guy.
Therapist:	Okay, so the dictator just kind of piped up and started calling this irritating and stupid?
Client:	Yeah you could say that.
Therapist:	Well, that's to be expected, right? I mean, we already know this part of your mind is going to interject and interfere throughout every session. Look how many times that happened last week.
Client:	True.
Therapist:	And I'm wondering if during active duty there were times when guns were going off or explosions, and even though there was all this loud noise around you, you were able to focus on the tasks you needed to do?
Client:	(*nodding thoughtfully*) Yeah, sure. That's what we were trained to do.
Therapist:	So you've got training in this stuff—being able to focus on the task and not get distracted. And it's a bit like that in here. As you and I work together, your mind's going to chip in with all these judgments and comments, and the challenge is to treat them the same way as all those distractions when you're out in the field. Don't let those thoughts hook you. And if they do, unhook, and come back to what we're doing.
Client:	(*engaging in the session now, nodding*) Got it.
Therapist:	And remember last time we talked about the caring part of you? The part of you that cares enough to bring you in here to see me, even when your dictator does everything possible to talk you out of coming?
Client:	Yeah.
Therapist:	So let's see if we can notice how those two parts play out in today's session. I'm expecting them to keep jostling for the head position. Right now, which one's on top?
Client:	I think the caring part is stepping up.
Therapist:	Interesting. What's the dictator doing?
Client:	He's still there saying this is f***ing bullshit. But um, yeah, he's a bit quieter.
Therapist:	Cool. Was there anything in particular that I said or did in that exercise that triggered your reaction?

* * *

A few things to highlight in the above transcript:

1. The therapist feels anxious and disappointed at the client's negative reaction. He defuses from his own worries and self-judgment, accepts his anxiety and disappointment, grounds himself, and taps into a sense of openness and curiosity (thus the need to practice ACT on ourselves if we want to do it well with our clients).

2. The client is obviously fused, so the therapist shifts the process from flexible attention (dropping anchor) to defusion (noticing and naming the cognitions).

3. The therapist validates the client's negative response as natural and normal and anticipates that it will keep happening. Later in session, if a similar reaction occurs, the therapist might humorously say something like "Aha. There goes the dictator again. Knew he wouldn't be quiet for long."

4. The client is settling into the session now, defusing and engaging, so at this point the therapist wants to explore, with genuine openness and curiosity, if there was anything he said or did that specifically triggered this reaction.

Things will inevitably go wrong at times. However, if we can defuse, accept, ground ourselves, and remain open and curious, we can usually turn these events into useful learning experiences.

Technique vs. Process

A *technique* is something you say and do with your clients in a session. This might include asking your client to notice where in her body she is feeling this or inviting her to drink a glass of water mindfully or asking her what sort of mother she wants to be, deep in her heart, and so on. A *process* is the underlying change mechanism you are hoping to elicit with these techniques. For example:

Technique: I'm having the thought that… (chapter 12)

Process: Defusion

Technique: Mindfully notice your hand (chapter 17)

Process: Flexible attention (contacting the present moment)

Technique: The Ten Years from Now, Looking Back exercise (chapter 19)

Process: Values

As you know, ACT has six core processes, which together make up psychological flexibility. And we have a truly vast number of techniques at our disposal—including metaphors, worksheets, questions, experiential exercises, mindfulness practices, and so on—that we can use to instigate and reinforce any core process(es). Because of this, quite a few ACT trainers talk about the dangers of "relying on technique" and emphasize the greater importance of "working with process." However, I find this way of speaking potentially confusing because the only way of "working with process" is through the use of techniques.

Now clearly, some techniques are far more flexible than others. For example, consider the "notice X" technique (chapters 3, 10, 17). Common to all mindfulness-based therapies, this simple technique is just what it sounds like: the therapist encourages the client to notice X (with openness and curiosity). X might be thoughts, if the desired process is defusion. X might be painful emotions, if the desired process is acceptance. X might be what you can see and hear and touch and taste and smell, if the desired process is engaging with the world around you. So far, in every single transcript, demonstration, and video I've ever seen that is described as "working with process," the therapist relies heavily on the "notice X" technique: "Notice what you're feeling," "Notice what you're thinking," "Do you notice what you're doing?" "Do you notice what you just did?" "Can we slow down here for a moment, and can I ask you to just check in and notice what's showing up for you?" "Notice what your mind is saying," "Do you notice how you just skipped over my question and changed the topic?"

"Notice X" is a very flexible technique (and by the end of the book, you'll see you can effectively use it for all six core processes). On the other hand, techniques such as singing your thoughts to Happy Birthday or thanking your mind are much less flexible. They are useful for the process of defusion, but not for any other core process. And even with defusion, you have to carefully limit when and where you use these interventions, so as to be sure you don't invalidate the client. Likewise, some metaphors are useful for several different processes (e.g., the Stage Show metaphor, chapter 25, readily lends itself to defusion, acceptance, flexible attention, and self-as-context), whereas other metaphors are largely limited to just one process.

If you go on to do advanced training in ACT (as I hope you do), you're likely to hear a lot about "technique versus process." If so, please keep in mind there is simply no way to instigate any core process without using some type of technique. The real issue is not "technique versus process"; the issue is "flexibility with technique." The salient questions are:

- Can we be flexible enough with the techniques we use to successfully foster the desired core process(es)?

- Are we able to choose a technique that is appropriate, at this point in the session, with this unique client, to foster the process(es) we want?

- Are we able to modify or adapt a technique "on the fly," improvising or adjusting it to better fit the client, so it's effective in fostering the process(es) we want?

- Are we able to shift to other techniques if the one we've chosen isn't working, in order to foster the desired process(es)?

Flexibility with technique is harder than it sounds. We will all find our favorite techniques, and it's easy to overrely on them. But no technique (in any model of therapy) always works as desired, so we really do need to be flexible. To help yourself in this endeavor, when you fill in your tool kit above, include at least a few very flexible techniques (i.e., ones you can readily use to foster at least two or three different processes, such as "notice X").

Extra Bits

See chapter 16 in *ACT Made Simple: The Extra Bits* (downloadable from the "Free Stuff" page at http://www.actmindfully.com.au), where you'll find a document for creating your own ACT tool kit.

Skilling Up

We've covered a stack of tips in this chapter. It's a lot to take in, so please do review and practice them regularly to hone your skills. In particular, aim to do the following:

- Create your own ACT tool kit as outlined above.

- Start playing around with the language of experiments in session with your clients. Introduce each new exercise explicitly as "an experiment" and tap into that sense of curiosity.

Takeaway

Be creative with your techniques. Mix and match, adapt and modify, and if you're up for fun, invent your own. The more unusual or challenging the technique, the more important it is to be clear about its purpose; explicitly link it to the client's issues or therapy goals. Remember to debrief each exercise afterward and ask the client how it is relevant to her issues or useful for her therapy goals. If the client has found it helpful and sees its relevance, see if you can turn it into a homework activity.

Finally, be flexible with your techniques. Before you launch into them, consider these questions: What core process are you hoping to foster? Does this particular technique seem likely to help this unique client, at this point in the session, to experience the desired process? Either stop using or adapt and modify a technique if it isn't helping to foster the process you want.

CHAPTER 17

Being Present

The Only Time Is Now

Leo Tolstoy, the great Russian author, wrote: "There is only one time that is important—NOW! It is the most important time because it is the only time that we have any power." Tolstoy's famous quote reminds us that life happens now—in this moment. The past and future only exist as thoughts occurring in the present. We can plan for or predict the future, but that planning and predicting happens here and now. We can reflect on and learn from the past, but that reflection happens in the present. This moment is all we ever have.

Contacting the Present Moment in a Nutshell

In Plain Language: *Contacting the present moment* is the ability to flexibly notice your here-and-now experience and to narrow, broaden, sustain, or redirect your focus, as desired.

Aims: To enhance awareness so we can perceive more accurately what's happening and gather important information about whether to change or persist in behavior. To engage fully in whatever we're doing for more satisfaction and fulfillment. To train attention so we can perform better or act more effectively.

Synonyms: Flexible attention, being present, connection, awareness, focusing, engaging, noticing, observing.

Method: Notice—with curiosity and openness—what is happening here and now; learn to discriminate between *directly noticing* your experience and *thinking about* your experience; pay attention flexibly to both the inner psychological world and the outer material world.

When to Use: When clients are disengaged, disconnected from their own thoughts and feelings, easily distracted, lacking self-awareness, in need of grounding, cut off from or missing out on important aspects of experience, or fused with any type of cognitive content. It's an essential first step and a "core component" of the other three mindfulness processes: defusion, acceptance, and self-as-context.

Paying attention, with openness, curiosity, and flexibility, lies at the heart of all mindfulness. It is the starting point for all defusion, acceptance, and self-as-context techniques. And it plays a major role in values-based living. If you're acting on your values but not fully engaged in what you're doing, then you're missing out. Being present adds richness and fullness to your experience. It also enables effective action: it's hard to do anything effectively when you don't pay attention to what you're doing.

When doing values work, many clients will mention something like "living in the moment," "appreciating what I've got," or "stopping and smelling the roses," and almost everyone will talk about wanting to cultivate loving or caring relationships. These activities all require us to be present. And, of course, if we want to know whether or not we're living by our values, and whether or not our behavior is workable, we need to be aware of what we're doing and notice the consequences of our actions.

Flexible attention is also essential for self-awareness and self-knowledge. The more in touch we are with our own thoughts and feelings, the better we're able to regulate our behavior and make wise choices that take our life in the direction we want to go.

The Costs of Inflexible Attention

What's the point of learning how to flexibly pay attention? How will it help your client to solve his problems, deal with his issues, achieve his therapy goals? If you want your client to practice these new skills in and between sessions, you will need to ensure he has the answers to these questions. To help make this clear, it's often useful to discuss what happens when we lack (or don't utilize) these skills. There are three main adverse consequences: we cut off, we miss out, and we do things poorly.

Cutting off. We "cut off" from the people we're interacting with; we're talking and listening but we're not fully present; we're not giving them our full attention with genuine openness and curiosity. Because of this, there's no real sense of connection; it feels like we're going through the motions.

Missing out. We "miss out" on important aspects of our experience; we fail to savor or appreciate important or enjoyable elements of what we're doing, so it becomes dissatisfying or unfulfilling. It's a bit like trying to watch your favorite movie while wearing dark sunglasses, or have a massage while wearing a wetsuit, or eat some delicious food while your tongue is still numb from your visit to the dentist.

Doing things poorly. If you want to do any activity well—from playing guitar to driving a car to making love to cooking dinner to reading a book—you need to stay focused, to keep your attention on what you are doing. The more distracted or unfocused you are, the more poorly you will do whatever it is you're doing.

You can easily emphasize these overlapping, interconnected issues with the Hands as Thoughts and Feelings metaphor (chapter 11). Any category of cognitive fusion—past, future, self-concept, reasons, rules, judgments—can result in cutting off, missing out, or doing things poorly. Experiential avoidance can also result in any or all of these things, and you can highlight this with the Pushing Away Paper exercise. To put it simply, when your thoughts and feelings hook you (that is, when you respond to them with fusion or avoidance), they pull your attention away from the rest of your life.

Your client may not relate to all three of the issues mentioned above, but she will surely connect with at least one or two of them. The transcript that follows shows how you can introduce these concepts. The client says he is still actively socializing, not avoiding it, and to everyone else he appears normal, but he doesn't enjoy it anymore; he just "goes through the motions," feeling anxious and depressed.

Therapist: So while you're talking to your friend, what's your mind saying?

Client: You know, why aren't I enjoying this? What's wrong with me? I'm boring. Or you know, just thinking about all my other problems.

Therapist: And when you're hooked by those thoughts, I'm guessing it's hard to focus on your friend?

Client: I can still focus.

Therapist: By "focus" I don't just mean look and listen and respond. I mean, are you paying attention with genuine curiosity? Are you truly interested in what he has to say? Are you really engaged in the conversation?

Client: No. (*looks sad*) No, I used to be like that.

Therapist: It's so hard to do that when you're hooked by all these thoughts.

Client: But it's not just my thoughts. I feel really shitty. I feel depressed.

Therapist: Yeah, and that makes it all the harder, right? Because your attention goes inward to all those unpleasant feelings in your body. Hard to focus on your friend when you're focused on how shitty you feel.

Client: What are you saying? Just ignore how I feel?

Therapist: Not at all. Have you ever tried ignoring a loud voice in a restaurant, or a radio playing in the background? (*Client nods.*) And what happened?

Client: Bugged me even more.

Therapist: You've already tried ignoring these feelings. And distracting yourself. And if I recall correctly about a zillion and one other things to try and get rid of them (*therapist is referring to an earlier creative hopelessness intervention*).

Client: So what am I supposed to do? Just suck it up and get on with it?

Therapist: You've tried doing that too, many times. And it's exhausting, isn't it? So you don't want to do more of that.

Client: So what can I do?

Therapist: Good question. The way it is right now, these thoughts and feelings keep showing up... and usually when they do, they hook you...and they pull you out of whatever you're doing, so you can't engage in it. So when you're with your friends and family, it's like you're cut off: you're so hooked by what's going on inside you, you can't engage with what's going on around you.

Client: (*nodding*) It's awful.

Therapist: So what if you could learn how to really engage in things—instead of getting hooked?

Client: How do I do that?

Therapist: Well, it involves learning something we call "engaging skills."

* * *

Note the gentle reframing throughout the above transcript. The client's viewpoint is "My thoughts and feelings are the problem." From this perspective, the solution will always be "Get rid of these thoughts and feelings." The therapist can gently reframe this: "When you are *hooked by* your thoughts and feelings, you can't engage or connect with others." The solution ACT offers to this problem is to unhook from these thoughts and feelings and actively engage with others rather than "cutting off."

Similarly, when "missing out" is a significant client issue, the therapist can reframe the problem as this: *When we're hooked by* our thoughts and feelings, we miss out on enjoyable, pleasurable, or satisfying aspects of the experience—and so it becomes dissatisfying or unfulfilling.

And if "doing things poorly" is the issue, the therapist can reframe the problem as this: *When we're hooked by* our thoughts and feelings, we can't focus properly on what we are doing; we get distracted, our attention wanders, and we don't do things properly or well.

Fostering Flexible Attention

Once you've introduced these concepts and have helped the client see the costs of inflexible attention, the hope is he'll be more open to the skills we'll cover next.

Engaging, Savoring, and Focusing

The three antidotes to cutting off, missing out, and doing things poorly are engaging, savoring, and focusing. I find it useful to think of these as three broad classes of skills:

Engaging skills. The aim of these skills is to engage fully in your current activity and connect deeply with whomever or whatever is involved.

Savoring skills. The aim is to savor, enjoy, and appreciate your current activity (if it is something potentially pleasurable or enjoyable).

Focusing skills. The aim is to focus fully on whatever aspects of your current activity are most important (in order to do it well) while narrowing, broadening, sustaining, or refocusing your attention as required.

Obviously, these categories overlap enormously and are somewhat interchangeable, and most formal exercises foster at least two if not all three of them. Whether you class a particular skill as engaging, savoring, or focusing will depend to a large degree on (a) what you emphasize during the exercise and (b) how you link it to the client's issues.

Keep in mind, though, that savoring skills only apply to activities that are potentially pleasurable: drinking a cup of tea, eating a snack, listening to music, smelling flowers, looking at beautiful scenery or objects. In stark contrast, we can engage and focus even when there's nothing even remotely pleasurable about the current activity, such as when taking action in challenging, stressful situations or doing formal exposure to fear-evoking stimuli.

When it comes to teaching savoring skills, I like mindfully eating a raisin or drinking water, and for focusing skills, I often use the classic mindfulness of the breath exercise or a body scan; for scripts and explanations of these exercises, see Extra Bits. To teach engaging skills, my favorite exercise is Notice Your Hand, explained in detail below.

TEACHING ENGAGING SKILLS: NOTICE YOUR HAND

Clients use many different expressions to convey that life is not fulfilling. They may talk of boredom, drudgery, tedium, going through the motions, and so on. Often, these complaints center around social interaction with friends, family, and coworkers. So we want to help the client to engage fully in her experience and to genuinely connect with the other person. (Of course, it's not always about people; it may be about connecting with nature or a dog, cat, or kangaroo.) An ideal exercise for this purpose is Notice Your Hand. Although a hand is not a person, the debriefing questions clearly link this exercise to social engagement and pave the way for useful social experiments outside of session.

The Notice Your Hand Exercise

This exercise was inspired by my son, when he was about ten months old and I was watching him discovering his hands. He would hold up one tiny hand in front of his face and wiggle his tiny fingers around, utterly fascinated by their movements. And I thought, *Wow. That would make a great mindfulness exercise*. It's impossible to appreciate the beauty and simplicity of this exercise purely through reading the script, so please download and listen to the free recording of it in Extra Bits.

Therapist: In a moment, I'm going to ask you to notice your hand. And I mean really notice it, as if you've never seen one before. And I'm going to ask you to look at it for five minutes. But before we do that, I'd like to know, what's your mind predicting about the next five minutes?

Client: Seems like a long time.

Therapist: Yeah. And—just guessing here—is your mind predicting it's going to be boring, tedious, difficult—something like that?

Client: (*laughs*) Yeah, it sounds pretty boring.

Therapist: Okay. So let's check it out and see if that's the case. Sometimes our mind is spot on at predicting things. Gets it absolutely right. But very often, its predictions are a bit off mark. So let's see what happens—see if it really is slow, tedious, and boooooring.

(In the rest of this transcript, the ellipses indicate pauses of about five seconds.)

Therapist: I invite you to get into a comfortable position. And just turn one of your hands palm upward, and hold it a comfortable distance from your face. And tap into a sense of curiosity. For the next few minutes, the aim is to observe your hand as if you're a curious child who has never seen a hand before.

Let's start with the shape of it. Mentally trace the outline of your hand, starting at the base of the thumb, and tracing around all the fingers … and notice the shapes of the spaces in between the fingers … and notice where your hand tapers in at the wrist.

And now, notice the color of your skin … notice it's not just one color … there are different tones and shades, and dappled areas … and ever so slowly, stretch your fingers out, and push them as far back as they will go, and notice how the color changes in your skin … and then slowly release the tension, and notice how the color returns … and do that once more, ever so slowly, noticing the color disappear … and then return …

And now, notice the large lines on your palm … notice the shapes they make where they come together or diverge or intersect … and zoom in on one of those lines and notice how there are many smaller lines feeding into it and branching out of it …

And now shift your attention to one of your fingertips … and notice the spiral pattern there … the pattern that you always see on fingerprints … and notice how the pattern doesn't stop in your fingertip … it carries on down your finger … and trace it right on down and notice how it continues into your palm …

And now ever so slowly, bring your little finger toward your thumb … and notice how the flesh in your palm scrunches up … and now slowly release … and notice the flesh resume its normal contours …

And now turn your hand to the karate-chop position … and notice the difference between the skin on the palm and the skin on the back … and look at your index finger, and notice there's a sort of dividing line, where those two types of skin meet each other …

And ever so slowly, turn your hand over … and notice the skin on the back … and notice any criticisms or judgments your mind makes … notice any scars, sunspots, blemishes … and notice the different colors in the skin … where it passes over a vein … or over your knuckles …

And ever so slowly, curl your hand into a gentle fist … and notice how the texture of your skin changes … and notice any comments your mind makes about that … and focus in on your knuckles … and gently rotate your fist, and notice the contours and valleys of your knuckles …

And now tighten your fist, and notice what happens to the knuckles … to their color and their prominence … and then ever so slowly open your hand up, straighten your fingers, and notice how your knuckles just disappear …

And now bring your attention to one of your fingernails … and notice the texture of the nail … and the different shades of color … and notice where it disappears under the skin … and the cuticle that seals it in there … and now ever so slowly, ever so gently, wiggle your fingers up and down … and notice the tendons moving under the skin … pumping up and down like pistons and rods …

And that brings us to just over five minutes.

Client: (*amazed*) You're kidding! That was five minutes?

Therapist: Sure was. And was it slow, tedious, boring?

Client: No. It was really interesting.

DEBRIEFING THE NOTICE YOUR HAND EXERCISE

Almost everybody who does that exercise is amazed not only at how quickly time passes—it seems like the blink of an eye—but also at just how fascinating their hand is. We now debrief the exercise. Four lines of questioning are especially useful here:

1. What did you discover about your hand that was new or interesting?

2. Did your attitude toward your hand change in any positive way?

3. Did you get hooked by any negative judgments about your hand? If so, how did that affect your attitude?

4. How is this exercise relevant to your relationships with other people?

In response to question 1, many clients report they have never noticed the dividing line along the index finger, or the way the fingertip spiral goes all the way down the finger, or the way the hand changes color all the time, and so on.

With question 2, many clients report positive shifts toward the hand: they see it as interesting, as opposed to "taking it for granted," and often they experience a sense of appreciation or gratitude. Some people express interest in the complex mechanics of it, whereas others may feel like they want to take care of it—rub in some moisturizing cream. I usually ask, "Do you feel more connected with it?" The client typically says yes, to which I jokingly reply, "Did your other hand feel jealous?"

In reply to question 3, most clients report that at some point, they get hooked by negative judgments—*My hand is fat, old, ugly, something weird and alien*—leading to a sense of disconnection from or dissatisfaction with their hand.

All these lines of query neatly pave the way for question 4, in response to which clients often share insights around:

• how we easily take others for granted, lose interest in them, fail to pay attention to them, or fail to appreciate what they contribute to our lives;

• how easily we get hooked by judgments of others, and how that hurts our relationships; and

• the huge positive difference it makes, and the sense of connection we develop, when we really pay attention to people with genuine curiosity.

It's often useful to extrapolate these realizations to life in general: how we all take things for granted and fail to appreciate them, and how, when we really pay attention, life is so much more interesting and fulfilling.

To turn this exercise into a homework activity, we could ask, "What might happen in your closest relationships if you paid attention to your loved ones in the same way you just did to your hand? Would you be willing to give it a go?" or "Next time you're feeling bored, stressed, anxious, or otherwise caught up in your head, would you be willing to really engage in whatever it is you're doing, like you just did with your hand, and notice what happens?" We can then get into the specifics of when and where and with whom they will do this.

> **Practical Tip**   Curiosity is a key quality of mindfulness, so it's a good idea to make it explicit. Useful metaphors include "Observe it like a curious child," "Observe it like a curious scientist," and "Observe it as if you've never seen something like this before."

Noticing Feelings

Being present also involves noticing our feelings, emotions, sensations, urges, and impulses—which is an essential first step toward acceptance. We're still a few chapters away from exploring how to accept pain and discomfort, and the reason we're taking so long to get there is that it's a very hard thing for most people to do; it will usually be much easier if we first cover dropping anchor, defusion, values, and committed action.

However, we can lay the groundwork for acceptance way in advance, through brief flexible attention interventions, based on the instruction "notice X." Again and again and again throughout our sessions, we can ask questions such as "Do you notice what's happening in your body right now?", "What are you feeling?", "Where are you feeling that?", "What's it like?", "Where is the feeling most intense?", "What's the shape and size of it?", "Is it at the surface or inside you?", and so on. In this way, we repeatedly encourage the client to notice her feelings with openness and curiosity: a small but significant step toward acceptance.

Of course, some clients are unwilling to notice their feelings. This usually indicates high levels of experiential avoidance: if you want to avoid your feelings, then you certainly *don't* want to notice them! Other clients are unable to notice their feelings because of dissociation. But if your clients *can* notice their emotions, the next step is to name them. We might ask, "What is this emotion?", "What would you call this feeling?", or "Are there any other feelings in there, mixed up with it?" And if clients are unable to name their emotions—a skills deficit technically called "alexithymia"—we will need to teach them how to do so.

Narrow Focus or Broad Focus?

Another aspect of developing flexible attention is the broadening and narrowing of focus. For example, if clients are prone to worry and rumination, you may want to encourage a narrower focus: have them engage in some valued activity and focus their attention primarily on that activity. They can let thoughts come and go in peripheral awareness while repeatedly bringing their attention back to the activity itself. In contrast, if the problem is chronic pain, you may want to encourage a broader focus. While pain is acknowledged and accepted, awareness is broadened to encompass the five senses, the surrounding environment, and the current activity. In this way, pain becomes only one aspect of a much broader experience.

In session, we often ask clients to focus primarily on one aspect of their private experience—for example, on their thoughts or on physical sensations in their body. It's important that they realize this is simply to teach them a skill. In the world of everyday living, the idea is that when distressing thoughts and feelings arise, they can be accepted as just one aspect of awareness (one performer among many on a well-lit stage) rather than completely dominating awareness (one performer standing in a spotlight on a darkened stage).

Keeping Clients Present

When we work with people who are high in experiential avoidance or dissociate easily (e.g., many clients with trauma-related issues), it's best to start with exercises that focus on the external world. We ask clients to notice—with curiosity and openness—what they can see and hear and touch in the world around them. If the client is very drowsy or dissociates easily, encourage him to keep his eyes open, and keep the exercise short.

If our client "drifts off" in a session, we bring him back: "I seem to have lost you. Where are you?" or "I may be wrong about this, but I get a sense that you're not fully present right now. You seem a bit distant or preoccupied." Or "Can I just check in with you for a moment? I notice you're staring down at the floor and I think you may have gotten caught up in a story. Am I right?" Once our client is present again, we could ask, "Where did your mind take you just then?" or "So how did it hook you?" We can take these opportunities to point out—compassionately and respectfully—how easily our mind pulls us out of our experience.

When our client keeps drifting into the past or the future—rehashing a story or repeating worries that we've already heard many times—we can respectfully point out what's happening and interrupt it. If we just sit back, say nothing, and allow him to keep going, we're not helping him, or ourselves; he's uselessly fused with his worries or memories, and he's missing out on the present—and meanwhile, we're getting bored or frustrated and missing the opportunity to help him develop a useful skill. Here's an example of how we might do this using the Press Pause metaphor (chapter 5):

Client: That bitch! I'm tellin' ya. I still can't believe it. I can't believe—ten f***ing years, there I am working like a dog, morning, noon, and night—while she's at home f***ing the next-door neighbor. And then—then she has the balls to ask for half the house.

Therapist: Can I press pause here, please? I'm sorry to interrupt you. I can see how painful this is for you, and I can only begin to imagine what that must feel like. At the same time, I'm wondering if you've noticed what's happening here. You've already told me about this several times now in quite some detail. Is there anything helpful or useful in going over it again?

Client: (*long pause*) Not really. No.

Therapist: Can you notice how your mind keeps hooking you here? Pulling you back into the past, back into all that pain. Is that really where you want to be right now?

Client: No. But—I can't stop thinking about it.

Therapist: I'm not surprised. This is very painful for you. It's not like you can just put on a happy face and pretend it never happened.

Client: That's right. My friends say I should get over it, but I'd like to see them try it.

Therapist: So how about this: rather than trying to stop the thoughts, how about we practice unhooking from them?

Creativity

I encourage you to be creative with the exercises you practice in session. Don't just stick to the same old classic mindfulness exercises (such as body scans, breathing, and eating a raisin). These traditional exercises have a place, for sure; however, there are so many other ways we can teach these skills. So be playful and imaginative; think outside the box. For example, in session I've had clients mindfully massaging hand cream into their skin, mindfully popping bubble wrap, mindfully exploring a book (the sound of flipping pages, the smell of the paper, the different textures of the book cover and the pages), mindfully listening to a lawn mower outside the room or the air conditioner inside, mindfully smelling flowers and examining petals, mindfully listening to their favorite music and tracking various instruments, mindfully going for a walk with me outside the building, mindfully stretching—and that's just for starters.

So invent a few mindfulness practices of your own. Spend a few minutes thinking about this: what do you have in your therapy room (including anything the client brings in with him) that could become an "X" to notice?

Homework for Clients

For homework, ask your clients to practice being present. Ask them to mindfully do any activity: wash the dishes, play with the kids, drive the car, do the gardening, work out at the gym, take a shower, give a presentation at work, brush their teeth, and so on. You can emphasize engaging, savoring, or focusing, or any combination thereof, to match your client's main issues.

In addition, you can suggest a formal mindfulness meditation practice, such as mindful breathing or a mindful body scan. And don't forget you can also draw on all the other techniques we covered in earlier chapters, from the choice point to dropping anchor. Last but not least, you can also give your clients a copy of the Engaging, Savoring, and Focusing worksheet, which gives them lots of ideas for converting everyday activities into mindfulness-training opportunities (see Extra Bits).

Extra Bits

See chapter 17 in *ACT Made Simple: The Extra Bits* (downloadable from the "Free Stuff" page at http://www.actmindfully.com.au). There you'll find (a) scripts for mindful breathing, a mindful body scan, and mindfully drinking water; (b) a link to download a recording of Notice Your Hand; (c) the Engaging, Savoring, and Focusing worksheet; (d) a discussion about "The Mindful Therapist"; (e) some tips on applying all this to clients with low mood who ruminate and worry; and (f) how to use the ACT Companion app to foster this process.

Skilling Up

Okay, you know the drill: enough of the chit chat, time for some practice:

- Read all the exercises, metaphors, and other interventions out loud as if taking a client through them (or at least rehearse them mentally).

- Review the cases of two of your clients and identify when and how they're losing touch with the present moment: worrying, ruminating, dissociating, "zoning out" with drugs and alcohol, and so on.

- Reflect on yourself; when and where do you cut off, miss out, or do things poorly? How do you "drift off" during your therapy sessions (like we all do at times)? How does your mind pull your attention away from your client? How often do you get caught up in thinking about what to do next or judging yourself—and thereby disconnect from your client?

- Practice the activities described in the Engaging, Savoring, and Focusing worksheet and notice what happens.

- Dream up some creative mindfulness practices to do in session with your clients.

Takeaway

Contacting the present moment (flexible attention) plays an important role in every session of ACT. To facilitate flexible attention, the basic instruction is "notice X," where X is anything that is here in this moment. This is the first step in both defusion and acceptance: you notice what you are fusing with or avoiding. The main costs of inflexible attention are cutting off, missing out, and doing things poorly, and the skills to reverse this are engaging, savoring, and focusing. It is so rewarding to help our clients make this shift—so notice when this happens, and truly savor it.

CHAPTER 18

Hold Yourself Kindly

The Art of Self-Compassion

Life is hard. The inconvenient truth is, if we live long enough, we're going to experience a huge amount of pain. It visits us repeatedly, dressed in different clothes; but no matter what it's wearing, one thing's for sure: it always hurts. And most of us don't handle our pain well. Most of the time, our default settings are to (a) fight with or avoid the pain, (b) allow it to dominate or defeat us, (c) try to deny or dismiss it, or (d) blame, judge, and criticize ourselves. One response that doesn't come naturally to most of us is to gently acknowledge our pain and treat ourselves with genuine kindness and caring. The name for this way of responding is *self-compassion*.

Now, ACT doesn't tell you what your values should be or which values are "right" or "the best ones"; rather, it helps you identify your own core values from deep within. At the same time, there is one value that infuses every aspect of the ACT model: compassion. Compassion is a huge, complex, multilayered concept, and (just as for "mindfulness") there is not one universally agreed-upon definition of the term. However, if we want to keep things simple, we can define it in just six words: "acknowledge pain and respond with kindness."

In other words, *compassion* means we acknowledge the pain and suffering of others and we respond to it with genuine kindness and caring. These responses may include overt behavior—physically saying and doing things to actively be kind, caring, and supportive to those in pain—or covert behavior, such as praying, doing a loving-kindness meditation, or empathizing and thinking kindly about them. And *self-compassion* means responding in this way to ourselves. (But note: self-compassion is a whole lot more than just "being kind to yourself." It's often very challenging: a huge act of courage.)

In my experience, a fair number of clients react negatively to the term "self-compassion," at least initially. The term may bring up connotations of religion, Buddhism, mysticism, or simply of being "unscientific." It may trigger judgmental thoughts to do with "flower power," "new age," "touchy feely," or "hippy bullshit." It may be judged as a sign of weakness or of being "effeminate." Thus, in order to play it safe, I often don't use the term until clients have learned how to do it. Instead, I often introduce the concept with the Two Friends metaphor.

The Two Friends Metaphor

Therapist: Suppose you're going through a rough patch. A really hard time in your life. There are all sorts of problems and difficulties, and just about everything that can go wrong has gone wrong. In other words, life is pretty shit. Now as you're going through this, what kind of friend would you like by your side?

Would you like the sort of friend who says, "Ah, shut up. Stop your whinging and whining. I don't want to hear about it. What the hell have you got to complain it? There are people out there a lot worse off than you. You're just a big wimpy kid. Suck it up and get on with it"?

Or would you like the sort of friend who says, "This is really rough. With what you're going through right now, anyone would be struggling. So I want you to know I'm here for you. I've got your back. We're in this together. I'm with you every step of the way"?

In my experience, clients always choose the second friend over the first. We can then say, "Of course you would. So the question is, what kind of friend are you being to yourself, as you go through this? Are you more like the first one or the second?"

This simple metaphor readily segues into self-compassion, without ever using the term itself. You can probably think of many ways to go from here; the avenue I often take is this: "Can we take a few moments to discuss the kinds of things you tend to say and do to yourself when you're in pain, and see which category of friendship they fall into—kind and supportive, or harsh and uncaring?"

For many clients, there is little or nothing that falls into the category of "kind and supportive friend"; almost everything they do falls into the category of the harsh, uncaring friend. From time to time, you may encounter some confusion around this, like the client who thinks that getting drunk or stoned or high is a form of self-kindness because it gives him relief from his pain. If your client says something like this, then you want to validate that those behaviors do indeed provide pain relief—but they are not kind ways to treat your body; a truly kind and caring friend will offer you support in ways that don't compromise your health and well-being.

We can then go on to explore, "What are the qualities of a good friend; a true friend who supports you through difficult times while acknowledging how hard things are for you?"

With this line of gentle inquiry, we usually quickly get to values of support, caring, and kindness, as well as other qualities of a "good friend." The next step then is to help the client to put these values into action: to become a good friend to himself in his time of need.

The Six Building Blocks of Self-Compassion

Kristin Neff, the world's foremost researcher on the topic, deconstructs self-compassion into three main elements: mindfulness, kindness, and "common humanity," which is the recognition that our suffering is something we share with all humans (Neff, 2003). When I first attempted to map out self-compassion in terms of ACT, I stuck to Neff's triad, but over the years, I have expanded it from three to six elements, which we can think of as the "building blocks" of self-compassion. In any given session, we may play with just one block—or we may stack several (or even all) of them together. There is no fixed sequence we need to follow, and the potential for different combinations is enormous.

1. Acknowledge the wound.

    Let's take the time to acknowledge that we are hurting: to notice and name our difficult thoughts and feelings and the situations that trigger them. This is an important aspect of flexible attention. All too often, we instantly move into avoidance mode—distracting ourselves, numbing ourselves, or otherwise trying to escape from our pain in maladaptive ways.

2. Be human.

    Let's validate our pain as a natural and normal part of being human. Our painful thoughts and feelings are not a sign of weakness, defectiveness, or mental illness. They are reminders that we are human, and we care. This is what a living, caring human being feels when he or she encounters difficulty in life.

3. Disarm the critic.

    When we fail, get rejected, or make mistakes; when we catch ourselves acting in ways we do not approve of; when we believe that we have contributed to our reality gap, our mind's natural tendency is to beat ourselves up. The mind likes to pull out a big stick and give us a hiding, to kick us when we're already down. It may tell us that we're not being strong enough, or that we should be handling things better, or that others are far worse off than we are, so we really have nothing to complain about. It may tell us to get a grip or sort ourselves out. It may even tell us that we're pathetic or that we only have ourselves to blame for what has happened. So let's bring in our defusion skills to take the power out of all that harsh self-criticism.

4. Hold yourself kindly.

    At the core of self-compassion is the value of kindness. When life is difficult, when we're in great pain, we need support and kindness more than ever. So let's talk to ourselves kindly; give ourselves gentle messages of support and understanding. And let's look after ourselves with genuine kindness—with wise gestures and deeds that help us to get through these difficult times, while also taking care of our health and well-being.

5. Make room for your pain.

   When we practice opening up and making room for our pain (as in chapter 22), this is an act of kindness in itself. It frees up our time and energy so we can invest it in life-enhancing pursuits, rather than in futile struggles with our pain. (And it's so much kinder than many of the self-destructive things we do when trying to escape from our pain.)

6. See yourself in others.

   If we look around with open eyes, we will find that everywhere we turn, people are struggling and suffering in ways very similar to our own. If we can acknowledge and empathize with their pain, recognize that this is part of being human, and appreciate that life hurts everyone (no matter how privileged they may be), then we can develop a sense of "common humanity," a sense that we are not alone in our suffering, a sense that we are a part of something much bigger.

Many Paths to Self-Compassion

Because self-compassion infuses every aspect of ACT, you'll find one or more of the six building blocks amid many of the tools and techniques in most of the chapters. And later, when we look at the many different ways of working with acceptance, you'll see that a lot of them involve self-compassion. There many different techniques for developing self-compassion, and they all involve sending ourselves the same basic message: *I see you're in pain, I care about you, and I want to help.* Next, I'll introduce you to my all-time favorite self-compassion practice, the Kind Hand exercise, and then I'll give you some tips for creating exercises of your own.

THE KIND HAND EXERCISE

The script below is for you to use on yourself, so please don't just read it; actively do it.

A quick reminder: adapt every exercise to suit your clients. Some people might prefer to place two hands on the body: one over the heart, the other on the abdomen. Some might prefer to wrap their arms around themselves, in a self-hug. Some clients may not wish to touch their body—especially if they are fused with harsh self-judgments about it or if self-touch triggers painful feelings (e.g., disgust) or memories (e.g., of sexual abuse). In these cases, they could rest their hands in their lap, or have them hover above the body, and imagine warm, kind energy radiating out from the palms and into their heart, and from there, spreading throughout the body to areas of pain or numbness.

* * *

Therapist: I invite you now to find a comfortable position in which you are grounded and alert. For example, if you're seated in a chair, you could lean slightly forward, straighten your back, drop your shoulders, and press your feet gently onto the floor.

Now bring to mind a problem you are struggling with.

Take a few moments to reflect on the nature of this issue: remember what has happened, consider how it is affecting you, and think about how it might affect your future.

And as you do this, notice what difficult thoughts and feelings arise. Tap into a sense of curiosity, and notice where you feel this pain in your body. (Is it in your head, neck, shoulders, throat, chest, abdomen, arms, legs?) Notice it as if you are a curious child discovering something totally new and fascinating: where exactly is it, and what's it like?

Now pick one of your hands, and turn it palm upward, and take a moment to connect with times you have used this hand in kind ways. Perhaps you have held the hand of a loved one in pain; or rubbed his back, or given him a supportive hug. Or maybe you have cuddled and rocked a crying baby. Or maybe you have used this hand to help out a friend with some difficult task.

See if you can fill this hand right now with that same sense of caring, support, and kindness. Imagine it filling up with warm, kind energy.

Now place this hand, slowly and gently, on whichever part of your body hurts the most. (Perhaps you feel the pain most in your chest or in your head, neck, or stomach?) Wherever it is most intense, lay your hand there.

(If you're numb, lay your hand on the part that feels the numbest. And if you're feeling neither pain nor numbness, then gently rest your hand over your heart.)

Allow your hand to rest there, lightly and gently; feel it against your skin or against your clothes. And feel the warmth flowing from your palm into your body, and spreading in all directions, up and down.

And wherever you find an area of pain or tightness or tension, let that warm, kind energy infuse it, and imagine your body softening around this discomfort: loosening up, softening, and making plenty of space. If you're numb, then soften and loosen around that numbness.

(And if you're neither hurting nor numb, then imagine it any way you like. You might imagine that in some magical sense, your heart is opening, for example.)

Hold your pain or numbness very gently. Hold it as if it is a crying baby, or a whimpering puppy, or a priceless and fragile work of art.

Infuse this gentle action with caring and warmth—as if you are reaching out to someone you care about.

Let the kindness flow from your fingers into your body.

Now use both of your hands in one kind gesture. Place one hand on your chest and the other on your stomach. Let them both gently rest there, and hold yourself kindly.

And as you rest in this space of warmth and kindness, take a moment to consider that this pain (or numbness) is a part of being human. It's not a sign of something wrong with you. It's a sign that you are a living, caring human being. This is what living, caring humans feel when life is difficult; we hurt (or we shut ourselves down and go numb). This is something you have in common with every living human on the planet. It's a part of who you are, a part of being human and having a heart.

Take as long as you wish to sit in this manner, connecting with yourself, caring for yourself, contributing comfort and support. Continue this for as little or as long as you wish: five seconds or five minutes, it doesn't matter. It's the spirit of kindness that counts when you make this gesture, not the duration of it.

* * *

Personally, I love this exercise. I use it frequently on myself, and over the years, I've done it with almost all of my clients, sooner or later. (And if you ever come to one of my workshops, I'll do it with you too!) Once you've practiced the above exercise on yourself (please don't skip it), I recommend you read it through again, and notice how it incorporates all six building blocks.

Of course, this exercise doesn't work for everyone; no tool or technique ever does. If your client, for one reason or another, doesn't manage to tap into a sense of kindness, she will likely stare at you with an unimpressed expression on her face and ask, "Am I supposed to feel something?" If this happens, it usually indicates that self-compassion is an alien concept to this person, and you'll need to work on it bit by bit through brief, gentle interventions as described in the next section.

Creating Your Own Self-Compassion Exercises

Self-compassion exercises can be very brief. They don't have to involve long, formal meditative-style interventions. They can focus on any or all of the six building blocks. Use the suggestions below to get your creative juices flowing, and see if you can come up with your own self-compassion intervention(s).

Kindly acknowledge pain. Acknowledge, with kindness in your words and a warm, caring tone to your inner voice, "This is really painful" or "This is really difficult" or "This hurts" or "I'm noticing sadness" or "I'm having a feeling of shame" or "This is a moment of suffering."

This is probably the quickest and simplest of all self-compassion techniques. Be creative with it. You can use any expression you like that nonjudgmentally acknowledges the presence of pain. After this acknowledgment, the next step is to say something that facilitates kindness to yourself: either a phrase, such as "Go easy on yourself," "Be kind to yourself," or "May I treat myself kindly," or a single word, such as "Gentle" or "Kindness."

Add on a kind gesture. It's easy to add a kind gesture to the previous intervention, for example, laying a hand gently and kindly on top of the pain or numbness; or resting the hand in a soothing manner upon the chest, abdomen, or forehead; or massaging an area of tension in the neck, shoulders, or temples.

Add on acceptance. Alternatively, it's easy to add on a simple acceptance move, such as breathing into and around the pain, or to drop anchor and expand awareness, noticing what else is present *in addition to* the pain (not distracting yourself from it).

Add on defusion. Likewise, it's easy to add on a simple defusion move, such as noticing and naming: "Here's my mind beating me up again. And even so, I'm going to be kind to myself." Or "Aha. There's the not-good-enough story." Or "I'm having the thought that I'm a loser."

Add on kind imagery. There are many self-compassion exercises that involve kind imagery. This may involve:

- imagining warm healing light going into the parts of your body where it hurts, to soothe and heal;

- imagining someone who is a source of love and kindness (e.g., a friend, relative, historical figure such as Gandhi or Mandela, fictional character, or spiritual/religious figure) reaching out to you with compassionate words or gestures; or

- various forms of "inner-child" imagery (see Extra Bits).

Add on a sense of "common humanity." Last but not least, it's easy to add on a simple move that aids connectedness to others: "This is something I have in common with everyone else. Everybody hurts sometimes," or "This shows I'm human. We all screw up and make mistakes/get rejected/fail at things/experience disappointment," or "It's hard to be human at times. So many people on the planet have felt this way at times!" or "This shows I'm human. All humans feel pain when life is tough."

Barriers to Self-Compassion

Like any aspect of the ACT model, we will encounter barriers to self-compassion. As mentioned above, one of these barriers is often negative reactions to the word itself. We can deal with this quite easily by avoiding the term "self-compassion" and making good use of the Two Friends metaphor.

Another barrier is lack of clarity: the client wonders, *How's this going to help me?* Again, we deal with this issue by being clear up front about the purpose and potential benefits, and linking it to the client's therapy goals. The choice point can really help with this, as follows:

Therapist: So when you treat yourself like the harsh, uncaring friend…is that a towards or an away move?

Client: It's away. But I can't help it.

Therapist: Yes, right now, you can't help it. It's an automatic response you've been doing for years. It happens instantly, before you know it. So I'm wondering if maybe you would you like to change that? Learn a different way? I'm wondering, if we could do some work around learning to treat yourself more like the kind, caring friend, would that be useful to you?

Client: I don't know. How will that help me?

Therapist: Good question. Let's look at your experience. Some of the main things you want to get out of our work together are XYZ (*therapist recaps client's behavioral goals for therapy*). Now when you treat yourself like the harsh, uncaring friend, does that usually help you to do these things?

Client: Not usually.

Therapist: So maybe if you try a different approach—treat yourself like a kind, caring friend—you'll find it easier to do those things?

Client: Hmmm. I'm not sure about that.

Therapist: Neither am I, to be honest. As I keep saying, what we do here is an experiment. I never know for sure what will happen. I mean, I can tell you there's a lot of scientific research that shows many people get enormous benefits from learning to treat themselves this way; they become more resilient, cope better with stress, and have a greater sense of well-being. And at the same time…I can't ever guarantee that will happen for you. I hope it will; I believe it will; and…it's always an experiment. Are you willing to give it a go, even though your mind will keep saying that you can't do it and it won't work?

* * *

Sometimes a client insists that being hard on himself is a good form of motivation and worries that if he is kind to himself, he will fall into self-defeating patterns. A useful response to this is the classic metaphor of…

Donkeys, Carrots, and Sticks

Therapist: (*humorously, playfully*) So I'm guessing you've got a pet donkey, right? And each week it carries your load to the market? Yeah, me too. So we've got two ways of motivating our donkeys. One option is to beat your donkey with a stick. This works well. Guaranteed to get any donkey moving. But another option is to motivate your donkey with carrots. He carries the load for a while, he gets a carrot. Carries it a bit more, gets another one. And this works just as well as the stick. But over time, if you use that stick a lot, you end up with a pretty miserable donkey. On the other hand, if you motivate your donkey with carrots, you end up with a happy, healthy donkey (with really good night vision).

Now obviously humans aren't donkeys. But we do often try to motivate ourselves with big sticks. And that's really what you're doing, isn't it? Being hard on yourself, beating yourself up. It motivates you for sure; but don't you sometimes feel a bit like that battered, bruised donkey? The good news is, when it comes to motivation, humans have something that's far more effective than carrots; we have something called "values."

* * *

As you can see, this metaphor readily segues into work on values and committed action. Most other barriers to self-compassion come under the headings of fusion and avoidance:

Fusion. Attempts to foster self-compassion can at times trigger fusion, especially in clients with deeply entrenched self-hatred. This often shows up as an increase in harsh self-judgment or comments such as "I'm unworthy" or "I don't deserve kindness."

Experiential avoidance. Self-compassion often triggers painful emotions, especially anxiety, sadness, guilt, or shame. (And for clients with intense self-hatred, it often elicits extremely high levels of fear and anxiety.) Clients often want to avoid these painful emotions, so in order to do so, they avoid self-compassion itself.

The main antidotes to these barriers, at least early on in therapy, are usually dropping anchor and defusion. Of course, later in therapy, any ACT process can be used to address these barriers, as appropriate.

Extra Bits

Turn to chapter 18 in *ACT Made Simple: The Extra Bits* (at http://www.actmindfully.com.au) for (a) scripts for additional self-compassion exercises, (b) how to handle tricky client reactions, (c) how the ACT Companion app can help, (d) inner-child imagery, and (e) a look at forgiveness.

Skilling Up

Compassion is a huge topic, so if you want to know more about it, I highly recommend the textbook *The ACT Practitioner's Guide to the Science of Compassion* by Dennis Tirch, Benjamin Schoendorff, and Laura R. Silberstein (2014). You may also want to look at *The Reality Slap* (Harris, 2012), my self-help book on the ACT approach to grief and loss, which has a major focus on self-compassion.

I also encourage you to:

- Come up with your own brief self-compassion exercise, incorporating some or all of the six building blocks, and practice it on a daily basis.

- Take a quick "self-compassion break": when you've had one of those really stressful or upsetting therapy sessions (that we all have at times), before getting back into work (making those calls, writing those notes, seeing the next client), take two or three minutes to run through a brief version of your exercise, and notice the difference this makes each time you do it.

Takeaway

Compassion infuses every aspect of ACT, and self-compassion is a vitally important part of therapy. We can think of self-compassion as made up of six building blocks, and we can work with any number of them, in any combination, to help clients develop this powerful skill. As therapists, our work is often challenging and painful, especially when our clients don't respond to our best efforts: when they remain stuck, or get even worse, from session to session. So let's be sure to practice self-compassion on ourselves, as well as help our clients to develop it.

CHAPTER 19

Know What Matters

The Bedrock of ACT

The whole ACT model has one main aim: developing the ability for mindful, values-guided action, technically known as "psychological flexibility." The more we develop this ability, the greater our potential to live a rich and meaningful life. And it's this desired outcome that motivates everything we do in ACT. We wouldn't want someone to accept pain, practice defusion, or expose herself to challenging situations unless it served to make her life richer and fuller. So what, in fact, are values?

Values in a Nutshell

In Plain Language: *Values* are words that describe how we want to behave in this moment and on an ongoing basis. In other words, values are your heart's deepest desires for how you want to behave—how you want to treat yourself, others, and the world around you.

Aim: To clarify our values so we can use them as an ongoing guide, for both overt and covert behavior. We can use them for inspiration, motivation, and guidance to help us do the things that give our lives a sense of meaning or purpose.

Synonyms: Chosen life directions; what you want to stand for; desired personal qualities.

Method: Distinguish values from goals; help clients connect with and clarify their values so they can use them to inspire, motivate, and guide ongoing behavior.

When to Use: When looking for guidance from within; when motivation for action is lacking; as a guide for goal setting and action plans; to facilitate acceptance; to add richness, fulfillment, and meaning to life.

Some ACT protocols do not explicitly work on values until they've first covered defusion, acceptance, present moment, and self-as-context. However, others start with clarifying values up front. There are pros and cons to both approaches. On one hand, work around values often triggers fusion and avoidance; therefore, some clients will be unable or unwilling to explore values in any depth until they first develop defusion and acceptance skills. On the other hand, some clients will not be motivated to do the hard work of therapy unless they first get in touch with their values.

For a sense of the first approach, you may like to read my self-help book *The Happiness Trap* (Harris, 2007), which takes the reader step by step along the more traditional route of creative hopelessness first, followed by mindfulness skills, and then values and action. For a sense of the second approach, you might want to look at *ACT with Love* (Harris, 2009b), my self-help book for relationship issues.

In this chapter, we're going to explore several ways of getting to and working with values, and as you read along, your mind may well imagine many different ways that clients might respond negatively. The truth is, almost anything you can imagine might go wrong…sooner or later, it probably will! So in the next chapter, "What If Nothing Matters?" we'll look at common barriers to working with values and how to overcome them.

Three Important Aspects of Values

When I describe values to my clients, I say something like "Values are our heart's deepest desires for how we want to behave; how we want to treat ourselves, other people, and the world around us. They describe what we want to stand for in life, how we want to act, what sort of person we want to be, what sort of strengths and qualities we want to develop." We often describe values as an "inner compass": they give us guidance, help us find a direction, help us stay on track, and help us find our way again when we go off track.

As you read a few books on ACT, you'll encounter several different definitions of values—and some of the more technical ones are pretty complex. Here's the one that I think is most user-friendly: values are "desired global qualities of ongoing action" (Hayes, Bond, Barnes-Holmes, & Austin, 2006, p. 16). Let's break that down into three components:

1. *Ongoing action.* Values refer to "ongoing action": how you want to behave—overtly or covertly—on an ongoing basis. For example, how do you want to behave in your relationships with loved ones? If your answer is that you want to be loving and caring, or fair and honest, or open and authentic, or mindful and compassionate, then we'd say these desired qualities are your values. And presumably, you'd want to behave with these qualities on an ongoing basis; you wouldn't want to suddenly stop acting this way tomorrow, or next week, or next month.

2. *Global qualities.* Values refer to "global qualities" of ongoing action. To illustrate, let's suppose you want to play baseball. Now clearly, playing baseball is something you can do on an

ongoing basis—it is an ongoing action, but it's not a *quality* of action. To clarify this, here are four possible qualities of that particular ongoing action: playing baseball skillfully, playing baseball enthusiastically, playing baseball passionately, playing baseball half-heartedly. So what do we mean by a *global* quality? We mean a quality that "unites" many different patterns of action. For example, if your value is "being supportive" to the other players on your team, then there are many different actions you could take with the quality of "supportiveness." And if your value is "being fair," there are many different actions you could take with the quality of "fairness."

In order to get to your values around playing baseball, I could ask you questions such as "How do you want to play baseball?" "What personal qualities or strengths do you want to model or demonstrate during the game?" "How do you want to behave in your relationships with the other players, both on your team and on the opposing team?" These questions may uncover values such as being focused, being competitive, applying yourself fully, being respectful, being cooperative with your teammates, being fair, "giving it your best," challenging yourself, and so on.

Note that these qualities of action are available to you in any moment. Even if you become paralyzed from the waist down and unable to ever play baseball again, you can still be focused, competitive, respectful, cooperative, fair; you can still apply yourself fully to whatever you're doing and "give it your best"; you can still act in ways that challenge you.

3. *Desired.* Values are "desired." They're statements about how you *want* to behave, how you *desire* to act. They're not about what you should do or have to do, or what's the "right thing" to do. (In many ACT textbooks, you'll find the word "chosen" rather than the word "desired"; this is to emphasize that you not only desire these qualities in your actions, but you also consciously choose to employ them.)

Values vs. Goals

Most of our clients are unclear as to the difference between goals and values. So we will almost always need to do some brief psychoeducation on the difference. We need to explain that goals are things you are aiming for in the future: things you want to get, have, or achieve. In contrast, values are how you want to behave right now and on an ongoing basis for the rest of your life, and how you want to behave every step of the way toward achieving your goals—whether you achieve them or not.

To help clients get this distinction, it's useful to give them a couple of examples. One of my favorites is "getting married" versus "being loving" (Hayes et al., 1999). If you want to be loving and caring, that's a value—it's ongoing, never completed; you want to behave that way for the rest of your life. And in any moment you have a choice: you can either act on that value or neglect it. But if you want to get married, that's a goal. It's something that can (potentially) be completed, achieved, "crossed off the list." And you can achieve the goal of marriage even if you completely neglect your values around being loving and caring. (Of course, your marriage might not last too long.)

Values are always available to us. In any moment, we can act on them or neglect them; the choice is ours. Not so for goals. We can't guarantee we'll ever achieve the goal we are pursuing. We can obviously do things that increase our chances of success, but we can never guarantee the outcome. For example, if we want to get married, we can't 100 percent guarantee it will happen, but in any moment, we *can* act on our values of being loving and caring. We can do this even if we don't have a partner; we can be loving and caring toward ourselves, our friends, our neighbors, our family, our environment, our pet kangaroo, and so on.

Here's another example I often give: if you want a good job, that's a goal. Once you've got it: "mission accomplished." But if you want to be helpful and reliable and honest, those are values: desired qualities of ongoing action. And in any moment, you can act on those values—even if your job sucks or if you don't currently have one.

Six Key Points About Values

There are at least six key points about values to draw out in therapy:

1. Values are here and now; goals are in the future.

2. Values never need to be justified.

3. Values often need to be prioritized.

4. Values are best held lightly.

5. Values are freely chosen.

6. Values include self and others.

Let's quickly zip through these.

Values are here and now; goals are in the future.

In any moment, you can choose to act on values or neglect them. Even if you've totally neglected a core value for years or decades, in this moment right now you can act on it. In contrast, goals are always in the future: a goal is something you're aiming for, striving for, working toward. And the moment you achieve it, it's no longer a goal.

Because of this, people who lead a very goal-focused life often find that it leads to a sense of chronic lack or frustration. Why? Because they're always looking to the future and continually striving to achieve the next goal under the illusion it will bring lasting happiness or contentment. In the values-focused life, we still have goals, but the emphasis is on living by our values in each moment;

this approach leads to a sense of fulfillment and satisfaction, as our values are always available. The metaphor of two kids in the car gets this across well (Harris, 2007). (You can find a neat animation of this on YouTube—just type in "Russ Harris Values Goals.")

Two Kids in the Car Metaphor

Therapist: Imagine there are two kids in the back of a car, and Mom's driving them to Disneyland. It's a three-hour trip to get there. Now one kid is totally goal-focused: every five minutes he's like, "Are we there yet? Are we there yet? Are we there yet?" It's a journey of sheer frustration (and bloody annoying for his mom, too). Now, the other kid has the same goal: she wants to get to Disneyland. But she's also in touch with her values of playfulness, curiosity, exploring, and having fun. So she's looking out of the window, waving at the other cars, spotting all the farm animals in the fields, singing along to the radio, and playing "I spy with my little eye." So she's actually having a fulfilling journey.

Both kids reach Disneyland at the same time, and they both have a great time when they get there. They both feel good because they both get to achieve their big goal. But the second kid also had a rewarding journey. Why? Because she wasn't just focused on the goal; she was also living her values. And on the way home, the first kid's going, "Are we home yet, are we home yet, are we home yet?" whereas the other one's enjoying the ride: looking out the window and appreciating how everything looks so different at night.

Values never need to be justified.

Values are a bit like our taste in ice cream. We don't need to justify why we like strawberry, chocolate, or maple syrup. (Indeed, we'd find it almost impossible to do so if we tried; who knows why our taste buds respond so positively to that particular flavor?) Similarly, we never need to justify our values; they are simply statements about how we want to behave. However, we may well need to justify our actions. If, for example, your value is connectedness with nature, you don't have to justify that; but if you want to move your family from the city to the countryside, you may have a lot of explaining to do.

Values often need to be prioritized.

I explain to clients that our values are like the continents on a globe of the world. No matter how fast you spin that globe, you can never see all the continents at the same time; some are always going to the back, others coming to the front. So throughout the day, the positions of your values change: as you change roles and move into different situations, some values will come to the foreground, while others recede into the background.

This means we'll often need to prioritize which values we act on in a given situation. For example, we may value being loving and caring toward our parents, but if they're continually hostile and abusive to us, we may cut off all contact with them because our values around self-protection and self-nurture take priority. But our values around being loving and caring haven't disappeared; we've just moved them to the "back of the globe" in these specific relationships. Meanwhile, in other relationships, such as with our partner or children or good friends, being loving and caring will remain "at the front of the globe."

Values are best held lightly.

In ACT we say, "Pursue your values vigorously, but hold them lightly." We want to be aware of our values and use them for guidance, but we don't want to fuse with them. If we fuse with values, they feel oppressive and restrictive, like commandments we have to obey. In other words, they change: they turn into rigid rules—*should, have to, must, ought, obligation, this is the right way, that's the wrong way, do it perfectly or not at all!* To use the compass metaphor, when you go on a journey, you don't want to clutch the compass tightly every step of the way—you want to carry it in your backpack, pull it out when you need it to find your way, then put it away again.

Values are freely chosen.

We consciously choose to bring these desired qualities to our actions. We don't have to act in this way; we choose to simply because it matters to us.

Values include self and others.

Suppose a client identifies values such as fairness, honesty, kindness, and being loving. We want to explore how she can act on these values both in her relationship with herself and in her relationships with others. In other words, we want to know what she can do to be fair, honest, kind, and loving toward herself, and what she can do to be fair, honest, kind, and loving toward others.

Bringing Values to Life

Effective conversations about values have a sense of openness, vitality, and freedom. When a client truly connects with her values, it brings a sense of liberation and expansiveness; she realizes that even in desperate situations she has choices, that she can open up her life and take it in meaningful directions.

During these conversations, your client will be very much in the present—engaging with you, sharing with you, letting you in. You'll see him "coming to life" in front of your eyes. The session will be alive, engaging, and fulfilling—and often intense emotions will arise, running the full gamut from joy and love to sadness and fear. You'll often experience a profound sense of connection as you get to see deep into the heart of a fellow human being and bear witness to the pain and the love that resides within.

Practical Tip   Some clients do not like the word "values," so make sure you have some alternative terms up your sleeve: being yourself, being true to yourself, living life your way, behaving like the sort of person you want to be, your heart's deepest desires for how you want to behave, personal qualities and strengths you want to act on/live by/bring into play, qualities you want to model for/show to/demonstrate to/inspire in/encourage in others.

How to Clarify and Contact Values

In this section, we're going to cover just a few of my favorite techniques to identify values (you'll find many more in Extra Bits). But remember, they're only a means to an end: to help our clients connect with their own humanity and find out what sort of person they really want to be, so they can live their lives with a sense of meaning and purpose. We can do these techniques in a conversational manner, or we can turn them into formal experiential exercises. If we take the latter approach, we might start off with a short mindfulness exercise (e.g., two or three minutes of dropping anchor) and then ask our client to close his eyes and silently reflect upon the question or imagine the scene. Below, you'll find three exercises I often use.

Ten Years from Now, Looking Back

Imagine that you are in the future, ten years from now, and you are looking back on your life as it is today. Complete these three sentences:

I spent too much time worrying about...

I did not spend enough time doing things such as...

If I could go back in time, what I'd do differently is...

The Video of Your Mistakenly Held Funeral

Imagine that you're a bit like Tom Hanks's character in the movie *Castaway.* You're on a plane that crashes in the ocean, and you're completely unharmed, but you get stranded on a deserted island in the middle of sea. Meanwhile, back home, everyone thinks you're dead, and they hold a funeral. A few weeks later, you get rescued, and you fly home to a happy reunion. Sometime later, you get to watch a video of that funeral. And as you're watching it, you see someone you love very much (perhaps your parent, partner, child, or best friend) walk up to the microphone at the front of the funeral parlor ... and start talking ... about you. What would you love to hear that person saying about:

the sort of person you were?

your greatest strengths and qualities?

the way you treated them?

One Year from Now

Imagine that one year from now, you are looking back at the difficulty you are facing today. Imagine that you have handled it in the best possible way, behaving like the person you really want to be, deep in your heart. From that perspective, answer these questions:

What qualities or strengths (e.g., courage, kindness, compassion, persistence, honesty, caring, support-iveness, honesty, integrity, love, commitment) did you live by or act upon in the face of this?

How did you treat yourself as you dealt with this?

How did you treat others that you care about?

Working with Values

In this next section, we'll cover interventions, forms and worksheets, and useful questions for clarifying values. Let's begin with what I like to call...

The Values Smorgasbord

There are a pentazillion ways of clarifying values, and the figure below illustrates many (but not even close to all) of them. We'll cover many of these in this book, and you can read about the others in Extra Bits.

Clarifying Values

WHAT MATTERS?
What do you really want? What matters to you in the big picture? What do you want to stand for? Is there anything in your life right now that gives you a sense of meaning, purpose, vitality?

CONFLICT AND REFLECT
Recall a time you connected well with someone you love. How are you acting in that memory?

DISAPPROVAL
What do you disapprove of, or dislike, in the actions of others? How would you act differently, if you were in their shoes?

MISSING OUT
What important areas of life have you given up or missed out on for lack of willingness?

FORMS AND WORKSHEETS
Valued Living Questionnaire
Bull's Eye
Life Compass
Valued Actions Inventory
Checklist of Common Values

CHILDHOOD DREAMS
As a child, what sort of life did you imagine for the future?

ARTISTIC METHODS
Paint, draw, or sculpt your values.

LIKES
What do you like to do?

ROLE MODELS
Who do you look up to? Who inspires you? What personal strengths or qualities do they have that you admire?

MIND-READING MACHINE
Imagine I place a mind-reading machine on your head, and I tune it into the mind of someone very important to you, so you can now hear their every thought. As you tune in, they're thinking about YOU—about what you stand for, what your strengths are, what you mean to them, and the role you play in their life. In the IDEAL world, where you have lived your life as the person you want to be, what would you hear them thinking?

MAGIC WAND
A. I wave this magic wand and you have the total approval of everyone on the planet—no matter what you do, they love, respect, and admire you—whether you become a surgeon or a serial killer. What would you then do with your life? How would you treat others?

B. I wave this magic wand, and all these painful thoughts, feelings, and memories no longer have any impact on you. What would you do with your life? What would you start, stop, do more of, or less of? How would you behave differently? If we watched you on a video, what would we see and hear that would show us magic had happened?

SPEECHES
Imagine your eightieth birthday (or twenty-first or fiftieth or retirement party, and so on). Two or three people make speeches about what you stand for, what you mean to them, the role you played in their life. In the IDEAL world, where you have lived your life as the person you want to be, what would you hear them saying?

LIFE AND DEATH
A. Imagine your own funeral: imagine what you would like to hear people saying about you.
B. Act out your own funeral—psychodrama style.
C. Write your obituary or fill in a blank tombstone.
D. Imagine you somehow know you only have twenty-four hours to live, but you can't tell anyone: who would you visit, and what would you do?

WEALTH
You inherit a fortune. What would you do with it? Who would be there to share those activities or appreciate the things you buy? How would you act toward all those people who share your new life?

EXPLORING YOUR PAIN
A. Pain as Your Ally: What does this pain tell you about what really matters, what you truly care about?
B. Pain as Your Teacher: How can this pain help you to grow or learn or develop new skills and strengths? How can it help you better relate to others?
C. From Worrying to Caring: What do your fears, worries, and anxieties show you that you care about? What do they remind you is very important?

CHARACTER STRENGTHS
What personal strengths and qualities do you already have? Which new ones would you like to develop? How would you like to apply them?

IF ... THEN ...
If you achieved that goal, then how would you change as a result? What would you do differently from there on? How you would behave differently with friends, family, colleagues, customers, and others?

Summary of Common Values Techniques

While some clients are readily able to identify and talk about their values, with many of our clients, we need to do a fair bit of work to uncover them, as you'll see in the transcript that follows. The client is a single, middle-aged woman, struggling to cope with her son's behavior. Her twenty-three-year-old son has a heroin addiction, and every few days he comes home to beg for money. If she doesn't give him the money, he becomes aggressive; he often screams and yells abusively, blames her for screwing up his childhood, accuses her of being cold and uncaring, or insists that she doesn't really love him. This has been going on for over two years. She constantly worries about him, and after his visits she feels hopeless, guilty, and remorseful. She says she knows that giving him money is "wrong" because it "just feeds his habit," but she finds it "too hard to say no."

Client: You know, to be honest, sometimes I think it'd be easier if he would just ... die. (*She bursts out crying.*)

Therapist: (*pause*) I can see you're in a lot of pain right now ... and I wonder if just for a moment we can press pause ... and take a good look at what's happening here ... I'm wondering if you could use that noticing part of yourself to take a step back and notice what's going on here ... notice how you're sitting in the chair, the position of your body ... and notice the feelings showing up inside you ... where they are in your body ... and also notice the thoughts whizzing around in your head. (*pause*) And what's your mind telling you right now?

Client: (*wiping her eyes*) I'm a monster. I mean, what sort of mother am I? How could I think something like that?

Therapist: So your mind's telling you that you're some sort of monster because you have thoughts that life would be easier if your son were dead?

Client: Yeah. I mean, he's my son. He's my son! How can I think like that?

Therapist: (*pause*) Remember we talked about how your mind is like a super-duper problem-solving machine?

Client: Yeah.

Therapist: Well, there's a big problem here, isn't there? I mean, a very big, very painful problem. Right? So quite naturally, the problem-solving machine goes into action. It starts cranking out solutions. And let's face it: one solution to any really difficult or problematic relationship is to have the other person disappear. So that thought, about your son disappearing, is just your mind doing its job: cranking out solutions to your problems. And you know what? There's no way you can stop it from doing that.

Client: But maybe David's right. Maybe I don't really love him.

Therapist: Well, that's an interesting thought. (*pause*) I'll bet your mind loves to torment you with that one.

Client: Yeah. All the time.

Therapist: Can I ask what're you feeling in your body right now?

Client: I just feel sick. Really, really sick.

Therapist: And where do you feel that most intensely in your body?

Client: Right in here. (*She places a hand on her stomach.*)

Therapist: Okay, so just notice that feeling for a moment … notice where it is … and what it's doing. (*pause*) What would you call this emotion?

Client: Oh—it's guilt. I hate it. I feel it all the time.

Therapist: Okay. So notice that guilt for a moment … Observe it … Breathe into it … Close your eyes if you'd like … and just breathe into it … and see if you can, in some way, just open up around it … give it some room.… And at the same time, see if you can tune in to your heart … Just take a moment to get in touch with what your son means to you … (*pause*) What does this feeling tell you about your son, about what he means to you?

Client: (*crying*) I just want him to be happy.

Therapist: (*pause*) So your mind says, *Maybe I don't really love him.* What does your heart say?

Client: Of course I do!

Therapist: You said it. I mean, if you didn't care about him, you'd have no guilt, right?

Client: (*teary but relieved*) Yeah.

Therapist: So tell me, you really care about David … so what sort of mom do you want to be to him?

Client: I just want him to be happy.

Therapist: Okay. So let's suppose I wave a magic wand and David is happy forever after. Then what sort of mother would you want to be?

Client: I don't know. I just want to be a good mom.

Therapist: Okay. So if you wanted to earn that title—of being a good mom—how would you be toward David? What sort of qualities would you want to have as a mother?

Client: I don't know.

Therapist: Well, suppose a miracle happens, and David sorts his life out, and a few years from now we interview him on national television, and we ask him, "David, what was your mom like when you were going through the worst of that heroin addiction?" In the ideal world, what would you like him to say?

Client: I guess I'd like to him to say that I was … um … loving … and kind … and … um … supportive.

Therapist: Anything else?

Client: That I was there for him when he needed me.

Therapist: So to be loving, kind, supportive—that's what you want to stand for as a mother?

Client: Yeah.

Therapist: Okay. So just sit with that for a moment. To be loving, kind, supportive: that's what matters to you as a mom.

Client: Yeah. (*She sits upright, nodding her head slowly.*) I want to do what's best for him. I want to do the right thing. And I know that giving him money—that's not it.

Therapist: Okay. (*pause*) So next time your son comes over, it seems like you have a choice to make. On the one hand, you can let your mind bully you—push you around and tell you what to do. And you know exactly what your mind's going to tell you—that you have to give him the money, and if you don't, you're a bad mother, and saying no is so stressful and painful, it's easier to just give him the money, and then he'll leave you alone. That's one choice. On the other hand, you could choose to let your mind say whatever it likes, but instead of buying into it, you can be the sort of mother you really want to be—loving, kind, supportive, and doing what's best for David in the long run. Which will you choose?

Client: Well, I—I want to be loving and supportive. I want to help him.

Therapist: So if you were truly acting on those values instead of being pushed around by the "can't say no" story, then how would you respond to David's requests for money?

Client: (*smiles thinly*) I'd say no.

Therapist: You'd say no?

Client: (*nods*) Uh-huh.

Therapist: What are you feeling right now, as you say that?

Client: I'm really nervous. I'm shaking.

Therapist: I can see that, and I'm sure I'd feel the same way if I were in your shoes. So the question is, are you willing to make room for these feelings of nervousness and shakiness if that's what it takes to be the sort of mom you truly want to be?

Client: Yes.

* * *

Giving her son money to "feed his habit" was actually inconsistent with this client's core values. The action was motivated by avoidance (trying to get rid of guilt and anxiety) and fusion (with thoughts like *It's too hard to say no, I can't stand to see him like this*, or *I'm a bad mother if I don't help him*), not by values. After the intervention above, the conversation turned to the many different ways in which she could act on her values: how she could be loving, kind, and supportive to David in other ways without giving him money (or things he could sell for cash).

You can see in that transcript the overlap and interplay between defusion, acceptance, and values. We call this "dancing around the hexaflex"—moving flexibly and fluidly from one process to another as required.

Forms and Worksheets

There are several forms and worksheets that can help your clients identify values. Of note are The Bull's Eye (chapter 6) and the Checklist of Common Values, which you can find at the end of this chapter. The Checklist of Common Values is especially useful when clients have absolutely no idea what their values are despite all your best efforts; they can read through the list and select the ones they relate to.

Shifting from Goals to Values: Useful Questions

Most of the time, when we first ask a client about values, he will give us goals instead. He may describe the partner, job, or body he wants to have or the things he wants to get from others, such as love, friendship, or forgiveness. Or she may say she wants fame, wealth, status, respect, beauty, a slim body, or success. Or he may give us an emotional goal: to feel happy, to have more self-confidence, or to stop feeling depressed. Or she may give us a dead person's goal: to not use heroin, to not have panic attacks, to not lose her temper, or to not feel self-conscious.

To get to the values underlying a goal, we can ask any or all of the following questions:

Let's suppose you achieve this goal. If so…

- How would you treat yourself, others, the world around you differently?

- How would you behave differently in your relationships, work life, social life, family life, and so on?

- What personal qualities or strengths would achieving this goal allow you to demonstrate?

- If people you love get to know about this, what qualities and strengths would you like it to inspire in them?

- What would achieving this goal show that you stand for or support (or stand against or oppose)?

For example, we might ask, "Suppose you have high self-esteem, or you feel happy, or you have a big car/great body/fantastic job/fame/power/success/beauty/respect…then how would you act differently? What would you say and do differently in the way that you treat your body, yourself, your partner, your friends, your family, your dog, your cat, your house, your neighbors, your work, your hobbies, and so on?"

> **Practical Tip**   If clients tell us something that they don't want to do any more, we can often get to values by asking, "What do you want to do instead?" For example, if the client says, "I want to stop fighting with my mom," we can ask, "So what would you like to do instead? How would you like to treat your mom when you spend time with her? How would you like to treat her when she does something that annoys or upsets you?"

Homework and the Next Session

Homework can involve writing about values, thinking about values, meditating on values, discussing values with loved ones, or filling in the worksheets mentioned above. A simple homework assignment is asking, "Between now and next session, would you be willing to do two things? One, notice when you're acting on your values, and two, notice what it's like to do so, what difference it makes." If you're using the choice point, you could phrase this as "Notice when you're doing towards moves and notice what that's like; what difference it makes."

I often encourage clients to experiment with "flavoring and savoring" (Harris, 2018). The spiel goes something like this:

Therapist: Each morning, before you get out of bed, pick one or two values that you want to bring into play in the day ahead. For example, you might pick, say, "loving" and "kindness." You can pick new ones each day, or you can choose the same ones every day; it's up to you. Then, throughout the day, look for opportunities to "sprinkle" those values into whatever you are saying and doing, so you give your behavior the flavor of your chosen values. And as you flavor it, savor it; notice the effects of living these values; appreciate the difference it makes.

* * *

If we don't get very far with values in a session, then in the next session, we can go on to explore them in more depth. But if we do successfully elicit core values in this session, then in the next one we can move on to values-based goal setting, problem solving, and action planning. However, if internal barriers—such as fusion and experiential avoidance—are getting in the way of living one's values, then we'd probably focus on defusion and acceptance to overcome them.

From time to time, we'll encounter a client who's already living her values and doing all the things that matter to her—going to work, looking after the kids, keeping fit, and so on—but is deeply unfulfilled. Almost always, the reason for her lack of fulfillment is that, although she's acting on her values, she's not psychologically present. Instead she's caught up in her head: lost in thoughts about all the things on her "to do" list, or fused with perfectionism, or immersed in an ongoing commentary about what's not good enough, or consumed by worrying and ruminating. With these clients, we would work on "being present": engaging, savoring, and focusing.

Extra Bits

See chapter 19 in *ACT Made Simple: The Extra Bits* (at http://www.actmindfully.com.au). There you'll discover (a) descriptions of additional values techniques; (b) the Checklist of Common Values and some other useful worksheets; (c) the issue of destructive values; (d) how to distinguish values from desires, wants, needs, feelings, virtues, morals, and ethics; (e) how to bring in values in later sessions; (f) more examples of goals versus values; and (g) how to use the ACT Companion app for values work.

Skilling Up

For this chapter, there's no homework for you. Nah, I'm just kidding! There's actually lots of it. If you haven't yet completed the aforementioned values forms, please download them and do so. Then:

- Read all the values interventions out loud, as if taking your clients through them.

- Think of other questions you might ask. Are there any other exercises you know, or ideas you have, about ways to get clients in touch with values?

- Pick two or three clients and identify what values they're out of touch with. Consider what exercises you could do to help reconnect them with their values.

- Reflect on your own values as a therapist: What matters to you, deep in your heart, about doing this work? What do you want to stand for as a therapist? What personal strengths and qualities do you want to bring into the therapy room?

- Over the next week, practice "flavoring and savoring." Pick one or two values each day, look for ways you can use them to flavor your actions, and actively savor the difference it makes in your life.

Takeaway

Technically, values are desired qualities of ongoing action. Poetically, they're our heart's deepest desires for how we want to treat ourselves, others, and the world around us during our brief time upon this planet. Metaphorically, they're like a compass: they give us direction, keep us on track, and help us find our way when we get lost.

Helping our clients to get in touch with their values can be difficult; we often encounter all sorts of misconceptions and misunderstandings, most commonly around the difference between values and goals. Furthermore, we'll frequently come up against barriers in the form of fusion and avoidance (as we'll see in the next chapter). However, with patience, kindness, and persistence, we can usually help our clients to "connect with their hearts"—and when we see that happen, it's truly magical.

Checklist of Common Values

Below are some common values. (They are not the "right ones" or "best ones," just common ones.) Please read through the list and write a letter next to each value, based on how important it is to you: V = very important, Q = quite important, and N = not so important. Of course, some values will be more important in one area of life (e.g., parenting) than in another area (e.g., work)—so this is just to get a general sense. If you wish, you can fill in one of these checklists for each major area of your life (e.g., one for work, one for relationships, etc.).

_____   Acceptance/self-acceptance: to be accepting of myself, others, life, etc.

_____   Adventure: to be adventurous; to actively explore novel or stimulating experiences

_____   Assertiveness: to respectfully stand up for my rights and request what I want

_____   Authenticity: to be authentic, genuine, and real; to be true to myself

_____   Caring/self-care: to be caring toward myself, others, the environment, etc.

_____   Compassion/self-compassion: to act kindly toward myself and others in pain

_____   Connection: to engage fully in whatever I'm doing and be fully present with others

_____   Contribution and generosity: to contribute, give, help, assist, or share

_____   Cooperation: to be cooperative and collaborative with others

_____   Courage: to be courageous or brave; to persist in the face of fear, threat, or difficulty

_____   Creativity: to be creative or innovative

_____   Curiosity: to be curious, open-minded, and interested; to explore and discover

_____   Encouragement: to encourage and reward behavior that I value in myself or others

_____   Engagement: to engage fully in what I am doing

_____   Fairness and justice: to be fair and just to myself or others

_____   Fitness: to maintain or improve or look after my physical and mental health

_____   Flexibility: to adjust and adapt readily to changing circumstances

_____   Forgiveness/self-forgiveness: to be forgiving toward myself or others

_____   Freedom and independence: to choose how I live and help others do likewise

_____   Friendliness: to be friendly, companionable, or agreeable toward others

_____   Fun and humor: to be fun-loving; to seek, create, and engage in fun-filled activities

_____   Gratitude: to be grateful for and appreciative of myself, others, and life

_____   Honesty: to be honest, truthful, and sincere with myself and others

_____   Industry: to be industrious, hardworking, and dedicated

_____   Intimacy: to open up, reveal, and share myself, emotionally or physically

_____   Kindness: to be kind, considerate, nurturing, or caring toward myself or others

_____   Love: to act lovingly or affectionately toward myself or others

_____   Mindfulness: to be open to, engaged in, and curious about the present moment

_____   Order: to be orderly and organized

_____   Persistence and commitment: to continue resolutely, despite problems or difficulties

_____   Respect/self-respect: to treat myself and others with care and consideration

_____   Responsibility: to be responsible and accountable for my actions

_____   Safety and protection: to secure, protect, or ensure my own safety or that of others

_____   Sensuality and pleasure: to create or enjoy pleasurable and sensual experiences

_____   Sexuality: to explore or express my sexuality

_____   Skillfulness: to continually practice and improve my skills and apply myself fully

_____   Supportiveness: to be supportive, helpful, and available to myself or others

_____   Trust: to be trustworthy; to be loyal, faithful, sincere, and reliable

_____   Other: _____

_____   Other: _____

CHAPTER 20

What If Nothing Matters?

Barriers to Values

It's wonderful to see our clients connect with their values. It's compulsive viewing: inspiring, heart-warming, and at times, deeply moving. However, the reality is, it often takes a fair bit of work to "get there." So in this chapter, we're going to look at common barriers to values and how to overcome them.

Experiential Avoidance

As a general rule, it's easier to do values work with high-functioning/worried-well/coaching clients than with lower-functioning clients or those with high levels of experiential avoidance. This is because the more that fusion and experiential avoidance drives us, the more we disconnect from our values. In therapy, we often see dramatic examples of this in clients with borderline personality disorder or addictions to drugs, alcohol, and gambling. Often these clients, driven by fusion and avoidance, repeatedly act in ways that are far removed from their core values: they hurt, abuse, or neglect their body, their friends, their families, their partners, and so on. And if they truly stop to acknowledge this destructive behavior—and recognize just how far removed it is from their own values—they are bound to experience a lot of emotional pain: anxiety, guilt, sadness, shame, and so on. Not surprisingly, in order to avoid this pain, these clients will resist or block working with values. Indeed, many of the barriers mentioned in this chapter function primarily as experiential avoidance: "I don't know," "Nothing matters," "I don't have any values," "I don't see the point," "I don't deserve to have a life," "This is so corny," and so on. If we know or suspect that experiential avoidance is the main barrier, we respond with dropping anchor, defusion, self-compassion, and acceptance. This might look something like this:

Client: (*in response to questions on values*) I don't know. Why are you asking this stuff? I don't have any values.

Therapist: Okay. Would it be okay if I "press pause" for a moment?

Client: If you must.

Therapist: Well look, I don't have to, if you really don't want me to. We can just plow on with the session and ignore what's happening here. But I'd prefer not to, because my sense of it is, we're both getting a bit stuck. I feel like I'm pushing you and you're kind of digging your heels in and pushing back. Is it a bit like that for you?

Client: Yeah, I feel a bit cornered.

Therapist: Yeah, so that doesn't make for a good team, right? So how about I back off, and give you some space, and we just press pause for a moment?

Client: (*smiling*) Okay.

Therapist: Cool. And thanks for letting me know you felt cornered; I really appreciate the feedback. Please let me know if I do that again. I can get overly enthusiastic about this stuff at times, and that's when I get pushy.

Client: No worries.

Therapist: So, let's just acknowledge the situation here. This is a challenging part of therapy. I'm here asking you tough questions that a lot of people struggle with. And for most people, this brings up some pretty difficult thoughts and feelings. Any of that stuff showing up for you?

(*The therapist now gets the client to do a mindful check in. The client identifies feelings of anxiety and thoughts such as* This is too hard.)

Therapist: Well, those are perfectly natural thoughts and feelings to have, in a challenging situation like this. (*Note: the therapist could, if desired, write the situation, thoughts, and feelings at the bottom of a choice point.*) And remember, your mind is a problem-solving machine. So the problem here is, I'm asking you tough questions that are triggering painful feelings. And the solution your mind comes up with to get out of this is to say *I don't know. Nothing matters. Move on. Change the topic.*

Client: I didn't think that.

Therapist: No. You didn't *consciously* think that. What I'm saying is, that's the kind of problem-solving process that your mind went through outside of your awareness. And suppose we go along with that? Suppose we give up on doing this values work, and move on to something else? What might that cost you?

Client: I'm not sure.

Therapist: Well, what has it cost you so far, going through life without an inner compass, without any sense of what really matters to you?

Client: I guess I keep f***ing up.

Therapist: Well, that's one way of saying it. On a scale of 0 to 10, how much sense of meaning and purpose and fulfillment would you say that you have in your life? Zero means life is empty, dull, and, pointless. Ten means life is rich, full, and meaningful.

Client: About a two.

Therapist: So one of our main aims with this work we're doing today is to raise that score a lot higher. Another is to help you develop a sense of inner guidance, like an inner compass to take you in the right direction, so you can do the sorts of things that will help you to build a better life.

Client: Okay. That makes sense.

Therapist: Sure. It make sense logically. But that won't stop your mind from saying things like *I've got no values.*

Client: Yeah, well that's because it's true.

Therapist: Yes, it pretty much is true, at this point. So…would you like to change that?

Client: What do you mean?

Therapist: Well there's a choice point here. We can give up on doing this work around values, and let you carry on living the way you've been going. Or we can persist with this—even though your mind will insist that it's pointless and useless and won't work—and we can keep going with it, as an experiment, and see if we can get somewhere useful. Which option do you choose?

Client: Well when you put it like that, what choice do I have?

Therapist: Whatever choice you like. It's up to you. If we give up on this values work, there are two big payoffs for you: you get to escape these uncomfortable feelings, and you get out of this awkward conversation. However, there's a big cost with that: your life doesn't change; without that inner compass to guide you forward, you keep on doing what you've been doing. On the other hand, if you choose to keep working with me on this, the big payoffs are…you're trying something new and taking your life forward. And the costs are…these uncomfortable feelings will continue. So the choice is yours; it really is up to you, not me. I don't want you to try and please me, and I certainly don't want to push you into doing something if you're not willing. It's your call.

Client: Okay, let's try.

Therapist: Thank you. I really appreciate your willingness to do this challenging work with me; I can see how hard your mind is making this for you, and it means a lot to me that you are willing to continue.

(The therapist now moves on to new, different values clarification strategies, as outlined in the section headed "I don't know.")

* * *

Now read through the transcript above a second time and note all the ACT processes that were involved. You should be able to see defusion, acceptance, flexible attention, committed action, workability, and willingness. ACT processes come into play continually throughout every session, even when addressing barriers to other processes. And if you're up for an additional challenge, imagine how the entire episode above would go if the therapist chose to write it out on a choice point; what would be written, and where? (You can find the answer in Extra Bits.)

Fusion

Many common barriers to connecting with values are due to fusion with:

- Reasons: *I can't do anything differently until I stop feeling anxious/find a job/get my kids back/ recover from this injury/win back my partner/feel better, and so on.*

- Judgments: *This is bullshit. A waste of time. What's the point in this when my life is so awful?*

- Self-concept: *Why are we spending time on this? I'm a bad person; I don't deserve a better life!*

- Past and future: *There's no point! It won't work! I've tried this sort of thing before!*

When such fusion arises, we dance across the hexaflex from values to flexible attention and defusion. We acknowledge the difficult situation—validate that the work is hard and challenging—and we notice, name, and validate the difficult thoughts and feelings showing up. We can then use any combination of the defusion strategies outlined in chapters 11 to 14, and once the client is somewhat unhooked, we can return to values.

"Nothing Matters!"

Some clients will insist that nothing matters, they have no values, they care about nothing. If this is because they are fused with hopelessness, then the first step would be to defuse from that, as in chapter 14. If not, then one simple way to respond is along these lines: "I'm curious. On the one hand, I hear you saying 'nothing matters,' and on the other hand, I see you sitting here in front of me. So I'm wondering, what matters enough that you came here to therapy?"

Some clients will answer that they came because of their partner, children, parents, or friends. If so, we can explore these relationships and find out what the client cares about and values in them. At the very least, we can tease out a value of "caring for others."

Other clients may say they came because they are sick of feeling depressed or they want to feel happy or they want to stop feeling anxious. In this case, we can reframe this as "So your mental health and well-being matter to you" and go on to label this as the value of "self-caring." Yet other clients may say they came because their doctor made them, in which case we can reframe that as "So you care enough about your health to listen to your doctor." And again, we can label this as the value of "self-caring."

Now here's a different but often very useful way to go, when the client insists "I have no values" or "I don't care about anything":

Therapist: "Yes, right now, that's pretty much how it is. You have no sense of anything guiding you from deep within your heart, no sense of this inner compass that I've been calling 'values.' Would you like to change that?"

If the client says no, then we can go back to her goals for therapy (chapter 6) and explore the idea that without values to guide or motivate her, she's likely to keep doing the same things as before therapy; her life is unlikely to change much. If, however, the client says yes, we can go on to build willingness, as outlined in the earlier section on experiential avoidance. Once the client is willing, we can move into active values clarification exercises, as outlined in the next section.

"I Don't Know"

In response to questions about values, some clients will shrug and say, "I don't know." And this may be a simple statement of fact. Sometimes the client simply has no idea what "values" are; they seem like something from another planet. It may also be a request for help: the client's basically saying, "You're asking me all these tough questions, and I'm struggling. Help me out here. Give me a clue."

If this is the case, then we do some brief psychoeducation—values as a compass, an example of values versus goals—and move on to experiential exercises as in the previous chapter. However, rather than simply asking questions, we can turn these interventions into formal exercises: take the client through two or three minutes of dropping anchor or another mindfulness practice, and then encourage her to imagine or visualize the scene or reflect upon the question(s).

Another approach is to ask the client to "sit with the question," as follows:

Therapist: So your mind's first response is *I don't know*. And that's normal. However, what we often find is…if you sit with the question a bit longer, close your eyes, and don't say anything, just silently reflect on the question, think about it…what we find is, very often, your mind starts to come up with answers. Would you be willing to do this, for a minute or two?

Often (not always), when the client does this, he will come up with good answers to the original question.

We can also pull out a pack of values cards (see appendix A), print out the Checklist of Common Values (chapter 19), or scroll through the list of values on the ACT Companion smartphone app. These tools allow the client to see examples of many different values, and he can then select the ones that personally resonate. Any of these tools are a great fallback option when all else fails, as well as a great starting point if you strongly suspect that your client will struggle with values.

Now, having said all that, the reality is that a lot of the time, the function of "I don't know" is experiential avoidance. In this case, we respond as in the above section on that issue.

"Should" and "Must" and "Have To"

When we fuse with rigid rules—*I should do this, I must do that, I have to do it this way, must get this right, that way is wrong*—we lose touch with our values. We will see this in our clients (and ourselves) repeatedly. So be alert for indicators of such fusion in your clients: a sense of heaviness or burden, inappropriate shame or guilt, perfectionistic ideas, or a sense of obligation. Look for signs of resentfulness rather than willingness, compliance rather than commitment, restriction rather than freedom.

Get into the habit of asking, "What's your mind saying about this?" And look out for key words in your client's response, such as "should," "have to," "must," "ought," "right," "wrong," "duty," "obligation," "a good person does X," "a bad person does Y," "perfect," "no mistakes," or "don't screw up." When we identify such fusion, we will of course want to help the client defuse. We might say something like this:

Therapist: Can you notice what it's like when that thought hooks you? Can you feel it constricting you, tying you up like a straightjacket? Time to pull out your unhooking skills, maybe? Your mind says you have to do this, but you and I both know that actually you don't *have to.* You have a choice. The question is, are you *willing* to do it? Is it important enough to you that you're *willing* to do it, even though it's uncomfortable?

WILLING VS. WANTING

Along the same lines, we often help clients to discriminate between willing and wanting. For example:

Therapist: We often don't *want* to do that difficult stuff that's really important. That's only to be expected. And it's absolutely fine. If you don't want to do it, acknowledge that. You don't want to do it, and you don't have to do it. The question is are you *willing* to do it, even though you don't want to and you don't have to?

DESIRE FOR APPROVAL

Some clients are so focused on gaining approval from others or so accustomed to obeying the rules of their parents, religion, or culture that they disconnect from their own core values. To help reconnect them, here's a useful question: "Suppose I have a magic wand here, and I wave it, and magic happens, and you now automatically have the love and approval of everybody whose opinion matters to you, so that whatever you do from now on, they totally approve of it and love you—whether you become a saint or a serial killer, a movie star or a dangerous criminal, a multibillionaire or a homeless person sleeping on the streets. So from now on, you never have to impress anyone or please anyone ever again—whatever you do, they'll be delighted. Then, what would you do with your life? Would you still go ahead and do this?"

Are These My Real Values?

Sometimes a client will ask, "How do I know I these are my real values?" If we're not careful, we can easily get pulled into a long intellectual discussion about this, resulting in "analysis paralysis." So a useful reply might go something like this:

Therapist: Do you know the old saying, "The proof of the pudding is in the eating"? If there's a cake or a pie on the table there, we won't know if it's any good by thinking about it or discussing it. We'll only know if we actually dig in and eat it. It's the same when it comes to values. We could spend hours discussing whether or not these really are your true values, but no matter how long we talk about it, you still won't know. If you aren't sure, the only way to know is to get out there, start actively living by these values, and carefully notice what happens. Do you get a sense of vitality, meaning, or purpose? Or a sense of behaving more like the sort of person you want to be? A sense of living life your way? Being true to yourself? Moving in the direction you want to go? If so, that tends to indicate that you've tapped into genuine values.

Extra Bits

See chapter 20 in *ACT Made Simple: The Extra Bits* (at http://www.actmindfully.com.au). There you'll find (a) how to handle other tricky issues such as values conflicts, desire for power, and difficult dilemmas and (b) an example of how to use the choice point in the scenario described under the heading "Experiential Avoidance." You can also flip back to the Checklist of Common Values in chapter 19; it's useful to print and use with clients who really struggle.

Skilling Up

Like every other part of the ACT model, if clients aren't clear on the purpose and aims—if they don't see how knowing their values is likely to help with their therapy goals—we can expect confusion and resistance. In addition, clients (like therapists) often get confused about the difference between values and goals. So if you left out the important psychoeducation on this topic that we covered in the last chapter (or if you did it but the client forgot it), then it's absolutely essential to cover this (or go over it again).

With this in mind, I once again encourage you to:

- Practice with imaginary clients, out loud or in your head, until you can quickly clarify these things.

- Practice on friends, parents, partner, children, the dog, the cat, party guests…you get the idea.

Takeaway

It's common for clients to struggle a bit with values, but if we gently persist, and remain flexible, we can usually get there. If fusion or experiential avoidance blocks the way, we can detour to work with defusion and acceptance, and then return to values later.

CHAPTER 21

Do What It Takes

What Is Committed Action?

Committed action, which includes both overt and covert behavior, happens in every session. During our session, whenever our clients do a self-compassion exercise, accept a painful feeling, get in touch with values, set goals, role-play a difficult situation, practice a new skill, willingly discuss a painful topic, or participate in formal exposure, that's committed action. And outside of sessions, when clients do any type of ACT homework—from practicing mindfulness skills to completing challenging tasks—that's committed action. In other words, whether it's overt action (e.g., what you do with your body and face and voice) or covert action (e.g., mindfulness or self-compassion), if it's flexible and guided by values, we'd class it as committed action.

Committed Action in a Nutshell

In Plain Language: *Committed action* means taking effective action, guided and motivated by values. This includes physical action (overt behavior) and psychological action (covert behavior). Committed action implies flexible action: readily adapting to the challenges of the situation and either persisting with or changing behavior as required. In other words, doing what it takes to effectively live by your values.

Aim: To translate values into ongoing, evolving, effective, dynamic patterns of overt and covert behavior.

Synonyms: Effective action, flexible action, towards moves, workable behavior.

Method: Translate values into effective patterns of physical and psychological action through the use of goal setting, action planning, problem solving, skills training, role-playing, exposure, behavioral activation, and other empirically supported behavioral interventions.

When to Use: Whenever a client needs help translating values into effective action or overcoming barriers to initiating or sustaining such action.

Skills Training for Committed Action

Under the heading of committed action, we can incorporate any and all traditional behavioral intervention: skills training, role-playing, scheduling and monitoring, exposure and response prevention, habit reversal, behavioral activation, and so on. So, for example, if we are working on relationship issues, we will often teach assertiveness skills, communication skills, negotiation skills, conflict resolution skills, self-soothing skills, and intimacy skills.

In this chapter, we will focus on what are probably the three most common skills we teach: problem solving, goal setting, and action planning.

Mindful, Values-Based Problem Solving

Problem solving is an essential cognitive skill for everyone on the planet. And many unhelpful cognitive processes such as rumination, worrying, obsessing, "analysis paralysis," and suicidal ideation are basically forms of "problem solving gone haywire." Unfortunately, many of our clients either lack problem-solving skills or fail to use them appropriately. If so, we need to actively teach these skills or encourage their appropriate use.

I assume you already know the steps of basic problem solving: identify and define the problem, brainstorm a range of solutions, evaluate the pros and cons of each option, generate an action plan, implement it, observe the results, and modify the plan as needed. (If you don't know these steps, then please learn them; it's essential basic knowledge for any mental health professional and plays an important role in the treatment of many disorders.)

The actual steps of problem solving are the same in ACT as in other models; the big difference is that we often precede these steps with mindfulness and values. So, for example, if a client is fused, struggling, and overwhelmed by emotions, we won't leap into problem solving; we'll first help him to drop anchor and unhook from unhelpful thoughts. And, depending upon his emotional state and what processes we've covered so far in therapy, we may also bring in acceptance and self-compassion. Next, we help him connect with his values: What does he want to stand for in the face of this problem? What values does he want to live by as he deals with it?

Once the client is grounded, in touch with his values, and at least a little defused, we can then take him through the nuts and bolts of problem solving. A tool I often use to help with this process is something I call "the challenge formula."

The Challenge Formula: Three Options for Any Situation

This is a simple but powerful way of helping people to realize that no matter how difficult their situation, they still have choices. (For a printable version to give your clients, see Extra Bits). For any challenging situation we face, we have three options:

1. Leave.

2. Stay and live by your values: change whatever you can to improve the situation and make room for the pain that goes with it.

3. Stay and give up acting effectively: do things that make no difference or make it worse.

Of course, option 1—*leave*—isn't always available. For example, if you're in prison, you can't just leave. But if leaving the situation *is* an option, seriously consider it. If you're in a high-conflict relationship, a meaningless job, an undesirable neighborhood, or a war-torn country, is your life likely to be richer, fuller, more meaningful if you leave the situation rather than stay?

If you can't leave, or won't leave, or don't see it as the best option available, then you are down to options 2 and 3. I say to clients that option 3 comes naturally to all of us; in challenging situations, we easily get hooked by difficult thoughts and feelings and pulled into away moves, which either keep us stuck or make things worse. So the path to a better life lies in option 2.

In chapter 10, I mentioned an ACT protocol I wrote (aided by many others) for the World Health Organization for use in refugee camps around the world. The challenge formula is a central pillar of this protocol. Now obviously, refugees can't just leave their camp, so option 1 isn't available to them. But option 2 is. Within the camp, a refugee has choices: he can leave his tent or stay inside it. If he leaves it, he can be friendly and kind toward his neighbors. Or he can ignore them or be hostile. He can join in with community activities such as singing and prayer. Or he can avoid them. And if he chooses to stay inside his tent, he can be caring and sociable with the other people in there. Or he can be uncaring and withdrawn. So the many little choices he makes throughout the day will have a significant impact on his life within the camp. And of course, anyone in a refugee camp will have many painful thoughts, feelings, and memories. Thus, the second half of option 2—*make room* for the inevitable pain—is very relevant. *Making room* includes dropping anchor, defusion, acceptance, and self-compassion.

Our clients' situations are rarely as bad as being in a refugee camp, but still, this formula is relevant. We can use it to empower our clients in any type of challenging situation: to help them see they have choices.

Goal Setting

There are two broad classes of goal setting in ACT; I'm going to call them formal and informal. The main difference is that formal goal setting follows specific steps, which I'll outline below, whereas informal goal setting does not.

INFORMAL GOAL SETTING

I think of setting behavioral goals early on in therapy (chapter 6) and encouraging clients to do things outside of session, such as "flavoring and savoring" (chapter 19), noticing their towards moves, or practicing a mindfulness skill, as "informal" goal setting. Why? Because although it is goal setting, it doesn't involve all the steps of the "formal" process outlined below.

FORMAL GOAL SETTING

Most people don't realize just how much is involved in effective goal setting. It's a complex skill. And like most new skills, it takes a while to get the hang of it. To learn how to do it, I recommend you practice on yourself, right now. So please carefully follow the three steps below and fill in each section, in sequence. (And don't you dare skip any, or I'll write your name on the naughty list! If you don't want to write in this lovely textbook, you can find a printable version of the SMART Goal-Setting worksheet in Extra Bits.)

1. *Pick a domain.*

   Choose JUST ONE life domain to work on: health, work, education, leisure, personal growth, spirituality, parenting, friends, family, intimate relationship, other.

   Domain: _____

   _____

2. *Choose your values.*

   Choose one or two values (maximum three) that you want to bring into play in your chosen life domain. These values will motivate and inspire the actions you take to pursue the goal.

   Values: _____

   _____

3. *Set a SMART behavioral goal.*

   S = Specific (Do not set a vague or poorly defined goal like "I'll be more loving." Instead, be specific: "I'll give my partner a good, long hug when I get home from work." In other words, specify the overt or covert behavior you will do. What specific psychological or physical actions will you take?)

M = Motivated by values (Double check that this goal is aligned with the values in step 2.)

A = Adaptive (Adaptive is a fancy word for "wise." Is this a wise goal to pursue? As far as you can tell, is it likely to improve your life?)

R = Realistic (Make sure the goal is realistic for the resources you have available. Necessary resources may include time, money, physical health, social support, knowledge, and skills. If these resources are unavailable, you will need to change your goal to a more realistic one. The new goal might actually be to find the missing resources: to save the money, or develop the skills, or build the social network, or improve health, and so on.)

T = Time-framed (Put a specific time frame on the goal: specify the day, date, and time—as accurately as possible—that you will take the proposed actions.)

Write your SMART behavioral goal here: _____

_____

* * *

It can take a while to run through this, so fortunately, "informal" goal setting often works just fine. Yes, you heard me right; we often don't *have to* do formal SMART goal setting. Most of us get through life reasonably well most of the time without formally setting SMART goals. Formal goal setting is most useful when we are trying to achieve something very specific and very challenging and we keep failing to make progress on it. So if your clients are not willing to set SMART goals, or don't see the benefit in doing so, then it may be best to leave it, at least for the time being, and instead focus on informal goal setting.

ASSESS THE GOAL

Whether it's a formal or informal goal, we need to consider the following questions to make sure it's an effective goal.

Is it a live person's goal? A "dead person's goal" means any goal that a corpse can achieve better than you can. If a dead body can achieve your goal better than you can, it's not much of a goal! Here's a classic example: "I'm not going to yell at the kids this week." A corpse will never yell at the kids, under any circumstances; you can't guarantee the same. A "living person's goal" is something you can do better than a corpse, for example, "When the kids are pushing my buttons this week, I'm going to drop anchor, breathe into my anger, connect with my values of being calm and patient, and speak to them in a calm, assertive manner."

Any goal that describes what you won't do is a dead person's goal. Behavioral goals describe what you *will* do—not what you won't do. So if a client ever says, "I'm not going to X," "I'm going to stop Y," or "I won't do Z," we can ask, "So what will you do instead?"

Let's say the client says, "I'm going to quit smoking!" This is a dead person's goal: a corpse will never smoke (unless you cremate it). We could then ask, "So when the craving to smoke shows up, what will you do?" From this, we can generate a live person's goal such as "When I crave a cigarette, I'll drop anchor, acknowledge and make room for the urge, and do some mindful stretching or mindfully drink some cold water, instead of smoking a cigarette."

Is it a realistic goal? It's very important that with any type of homework task, no matter how formal or informal it may be, we check with the client to ensure that it's realistic. (This is a fantastic tip that I originally picked up from a workshop with Kirk Strosahl, one of the pioneers of ACT.) Whenever a client agrees to do anything between sessions—no matter how small and simple it may seem—I recommend you ask, "On a scale of 0 to 10, where 10 equals 'this is completely realistic, I'll definitely do it, no matter what,' and 0 equals 'this is totally unrealistic, I'll never do it,' how realistic is it that you will actually do this?"

If our client scores less than a 7, then we need to modify the goal. We need to make it smaller, simpler, and easier until the client can score at least 7. If necessary, we may need to change the goal altogether.

What are the payoffs? We can enhance clients' motivation by highlighting the potential "payoffs" for their new behavior: in other words, we highlight the underlying values and consider the potential benefits. We can ask questions such as:

- Does this seem like a towards move?

- Is this stepping out of your comfort zone? Trying something new? Being more like the person you want to be?

- What values will you be living with every little step you take?

- We can't know for sure what will happen—this is an experiment—but what are some possible benefits of going ahead with this? What positive things might you gain or achieve or get out of it?

Practical Tip   It's useful to get clients to consider potential positive outcomes, as in the above question. However, we also want to warn them: "These positive outcomes might well happen, and I hope they will. But please don't start fantasizing about how wonderful life will be after you achieve your goal; research shows that fantasizing about this will actually reduce your chances of following through."

What's plan B? The best laid plans of mice and men often go awry. (A bit of trivia: this quote is attributed to the great Scottish poet, Robbie Burns, but actually, what he wrote was "The best laid schemes o' mice an' men gang aft a-gley." So there you go. Don't say you didn't learn anything in this textbook!) Sooner or later, obstacles will arise that get in the way of planned goals. If your client is naturally resourceful enough to navigate such obstacles, great. But if not, spend some time on generating a plan B. Ask, "If for one reason or another, you can't do this, what are some alternatives? What are other towards moves you could do? What are some other ways you could act on these values?"

PREPARE FOR EXTERNAL OBSTACLES

It's often useful to anticipate and prepare for possible obstacles. And it's essential with clients who come back session after session and report that they didn't follow through because unexpected problems got in their way. We can ask, "Can you think of anything that might stop you from doing this? Any obstacles, problems, or difficulties that might get in the way?"

Once we identify potential barriers to action, we can brainstorm ways to deal with them if they eventuate. And we may well need to prompt the client if we can foresee difficulties that she can't. For example, we may say, "Last week, a few things got in your way: A and B and C. I'm wondering if some of these things might crop up again; if so, how might you deal with them?"

KNOW WHAT'S IN OUR CONTROL—AND WHAT ISN'T

The more we focus on things we want to change that are NOT in our control, the more powerless and upset we feel. This can manifest as helplessness, hopelessness, anger, anxiety, guilt, sadness, rage, despair, and so on. So it's important that we learn to focus on what is in our control and to channel our energy and time into that stuff. This is at the core of self-empowerment. To help our clients understand this, we can run through a version of the…

Gun at Your Head Metaphor

Therapist: When life is difficult, we have far more control over our physical actions—what we do with our arms and legs, and what we say and how we say it—than we do over our thoughts and feelings. For example, if I hold a gun at your head and say, "Have no feelings of fear or anxiety; have no thoughts about bad things that might happen," could you do that? Of course not. No one could. But if I hold a gun at your head and demand, "Dance like a penguin and sing Happy Birthday," could you do that? For sure you could.

* * *

After using the above metaphor, we want to compassionately revisit a core ACT message: "The fact is, when life is hard, difficult thoughts and feelings show up. There's no way to avoid this; it's inevitable. But what we can do is take control of our actions and do things to make our life as good as it can be. To do this, we need to unhook ourselves from those thoughts and feelings and get clear about what we want to do in the face of this challenge, so we can behave like the sort of person we want to be."

WHEN THE GOAL IS TO CHANGE OTHERS

Many clients have goals about what they want to get from others or how they want others to behave. Here are some examples: "I want my wife/husband/mother/boss/colleague/child" to "be more cheerful/cooperative/helpful/friendly/loving/tidy/caring" or to "be less abusive/lazy/selfish/messy" or to "obey me/respect me/listen to me/help me out/show interest in me" or to "stop drinking/smoking/yelling/staying out late/swearing/playing on the computer so much/working such long hours." As you can see, these are all outcome goals—they describe the outcomes the client wants—so we need to convert them into behavioral goals: what the client wants to do (to increase the chances of these outcomes).

In these cases, we could run through what's in your control and what isn't, as outlined above, and then go on to say, "You can't control other people. Even if you hold a gun at their head, they still have a choice about whether or not they obey you. Our history books are full of heroes who chose to die with a gun at their head rather than reveal secrets to the enemy. So you can't control other people; you can only influence them. And you can influence them effectively, in ways that help you get more of what you want while building a healthy relationship, or you can influence them ineffectively, either in ways that don't work or in ways that get you what you want but damage the relationship. So can we have a look at what you've tried doing so far? So if you're doing something effective, we can look at how you can do more of it. But if you're doing something ineffective, can we look at what you can start doing differently?"

From here, we move on to behavior change 101: interpersonal effectiveness skills.

- We teach the principles of assertiveness (as opposed to being passive, aggressive, or passive-aggressive) and effective communication: how to make clear and specific requests; how to establish clear boundaries; how to ask for what you want and say no to what you don't want, in ways that respect both your own rights and the rights of others.

- We teach the client how to influence the behavior of others in ways that are healthy for the relationship, especially how to mindfully notice the behaviors she likes and reinforce them when they occur. (Sometimes this may be as simple as smiling or saying thank you.) At the same time, we encourage the client to cut back on trying to punish the behaviors she doesn't like. We emphasize the magic ratio: at least five times as much reinforcement (of the behavior you want to increase) as punishment (of the behavior you want to decrease).

- We help the client to notice strategies that may work in the short term to get her needs met (e.g., yelling, crying, blaming, lying, deceiving, acting aggressively, being passive, giving the "silent treatment," threatening, coercing) but have adverse long-term effects upon the relationship.

- We help the client to take the perspective of others, to understand how they see the world, to empathize with their needs and problems, to see things from their point of view.

I assume that any counselor, coach, or therapist reading this textbook will already know how to do all of the above. It's essential knowledge for anyone who works in such roles because so many issues stem from or are worsened by a lack of effective interpersonal skills. So if you don't know or you're somewhat rusty on assertiveness, communication, negotiation, empathy, and perspective-taking skills, please get up to speed on them, pronto. (One simple way to do this is to read my self-help book on ACT with relationship issues: *ACT with Love* [Harris, 2009b].)

Many ACT therapists like to teach these interpersonal skills through role-play in session. (This is not essential, but it's a very effective and engaging way of teaching.) During these role-plays, the therapist typically encourages the client to experiment with different ways of communicating—tone of voice, volume of voice, body posture, facial expression, and the actual words used—and gives her authentic feedback as to its impact.

In addition to the above, when teaching interpersonal skills:

- We repeatedly come back to the issue of control. The client can only influence others; he can't control them. But he can take control of his own actions, and the more effectively he does that, the better he'll be able to influence others. So let's look at what he is saying and doing to influence others and assess whether it's effective or not; and if it's not, let's look at what he can do differently.

- We help the client accept the reality that no matter how great she becomes at influencing others, there will be times she can't get what she wants; so how does she want to deal with those times? What kind of towards moves could she make when that happens?

- We repeatedly come back to values. What values does the client want to live by as she tries to achieve her goals for this relationship? What values does she want to live by (a) if she does succeed and (b) if she doesn't?

And of course, we can always use the choice point—draw it out or simply refer to it conversationally. The situation is goal setting in therapy; the thoughts and feelings are hopelessness, anxiety, "it's too hard"; and the choices are to give up or carry on.

WHEN THE GOAL IS IMPOSSIBLE

At times, clients will have impossible goals, as in this example of Alex, a forty-two-year-old former social worker on long-term disability benefits. He was referred with a history of chronic PTSD, major depression, and chronic pain syndrome. His problems had started fifteen years earlier when he had been horrifically assaulted, resulting in severe back and neck injuries that required multiple operations.

Prior to the assault, Alex had been a passionate amateur football player; now he could barely get around with a cane. When we first started to work on values and goals, Alex kept talking about how he wanted to play football again, even though many surgeons had told him it was impossible. I said to him, "Well, here's the thing, Alex. It's not my place to tell you what's possible and what's not. But can we agree that today, right now, in the next twenty-four hours, playing football is not possible?"

Alex agreed with that, so we then explored his values underlying the goal of playing football again. Initially he came up with the following: winning against other teams, getting respect, having a social life. None of these are values; they're not desired qualities of ongoing action. So I asked him, "Suppose I wave a magic wand so you instantly achieve all these goals: you play football again, you win all your games, you get lots of respect, and you have a great social life. Then, how would you act differently—toward yourself and your body and other people? As a player, what sort of personal qualities would you like to have? How would you like to behave toward the people you socialize with?"

With further exploration along these lines, we were able to get to some core values: being active, taking care of his health, contribution, cooperation, being sociable, being competitive, being a "good friend," connecting with others. I then pointed out there were many different ways he could act on these values, even though he couldn't currently play football, to which Alex protested, "But that's not the same."

Consider for a moment, before reading on: How would you have responded to Alex's comment?

* * *

What we're dealing with here is a big "reality gap": a large gap between current reality and desired reality. And the bigger that gap, the more painful the feelings that will arise. So naturally we aim to validate and normalize those feelings, to acknowledge how painful they are, and to help our client to accept them and be self-compassionate. Therefore, my response to Alex was this:

Therapist: Absolutely. It's not the same. It's not the same thing at all. Not even close. And when there's a huge gap between what you want and what you've got, that hurts. I can see how upset you are right now, and I can only begin to imagine how much you're suffering. (*pause*) And in my experience, when people are hurting the way that you are right now, it's because they're in touch with something really important; something that matters. (*pause*) So suppose I could give you a choice here. One option is that you learn how to make room for these painful feelings and how to drop the struggle with them so you can put your energy into doing something that's important, something that truly matters to you, deep in your heart—so you can stand for something in the face of this painful reality. The other option is to get all bogged down in these painful feelings and just kind of give up trying, and put your life on hold. Which option do you want to choose?

At that point, Alex experienced a huge wave of sadness, resentment, and fear, so we worked on acceptance, defusion, and self-compassion. Alex learned to accept the painful feelings related to his losses and to defuse from the thoughts that kept dragging him into bitterness and hopelessness: *I can never have the life I want, It's not fair, There's no point going on.*

Later, we returned to Alex's values and started to set small realistic goals. For example, two of his core values were "contribution" and "being sociable." Instead of a sports team, Alex started contributing to a health team: the nurses at his local "old folks'" home. He started going in on a voluntary basis to socialize with the elderly residents. He would make them cups of tea, chat about the news, and even play chess with them (acting on his value of being competitive). He found this very satisfying, even though it was a million miles from playing football.

So, to summarize, here's what to do when a goal is impossible or a long way off:

1. Validate the pain arising from the big "reality gap."

2. Respond to the pain with acceptance, defusion, and self-compassion.

3. Find the value(s) underlying the goal.

4. Set new goals based on the underlying value(s), realistic for the current life situation.

Action Planning

After setting a values-guided goal, some clients are very good at taking action to achieve it. But others will need help to break it down into a step-by-step action plan. One very useful question to ask is this: "What's the smallest, tiniest, simplest, easiest step you can take in the next twenty-four hours that will take you a little bit further in that direction?"

Learning to take small steps is important. When clients get too focused on big long-term goals, they're pulled out of living in the present; they get sucked into the mindset of "I'll be happy once I've achieved that goal." And, of course, they may never achieve it, or it may take much longer than they expected, or it may not make them happy even if they do achieve it.

So I like to remind clients of the famous saying from the Tao Te Ching: "The journey of a thousand miles begins with one step." Living our values is a never-ending journey; it continues until the moment of our final breath. And every little step we take, no matter how tiny, is a valid and meaningful part of that journey. (I also like to quote Aesop: "Little by little does the trick.")

To show you how values, goals, and actions come together, let's consider Sarah, a thirty-eight-year-old nurse, single for four years since her divorce. Sarah very much wanted to find a new partner, get married, and have children, and she was worried that she would soon be too old to conceive. Of course getting married and having kids are goals—they can (potentially) be crossed off the list, achieved, done!—but not values. So using the SMART Goal-Setting worksheet, Sarah identified two life domains as her priorities: "intimate partner" and "parenting." We then looked at her values in each domain.

Initially, Sarah said what she wanted was to be loved and appreciated. Now these are common goals; we all want to get love and appreciation from others. But they are not values; values are about *how we want to behave*, not *what we want to get*. With further exploration (and plenty of work around accepting the intense sadness that arose), Sarah identified her values in the domain of "intimate partner" as connecting, being caring, being loving, being supportive, being nurturing, being playful, being present, being emotionally intimate, and being sexually expressive. Under "parenting," her values were almost identical (except for "being sexually expressive").

Sarah recognized that marriage and kids were not realistic as immediate goals (next twenty-four hours) or short-term goals (next few days and weeks), so she wrote them down as medium- or long-term goals.

Next, she looked at short-term goals. In the domain of "intimate partner," she set goals to (a) use a smartphone dating app and go on some dates and (b) attend some mixed-sex Latin dancing classes. In the domain of "parenting," her goals were to (a) take her teenage niece out for a day trip and (b) visit a couple of friends who had young children.

In terms of immediate goals, Sarah was stumped. Here's how the session went:

Therapist: You've identified quite a few important values here. Which seems the most important?

Sarah: Um. I think, more than anything else, connecting and being intimate.

Therapist: Okay, so what's a small, simple, easy thing you could do in the next twenty-four hours, in line with those values?

Sarah: I don't know.

Therapist: No idea?

Sarah: No.

Therapist: Well, the key here is to think outside the box. If connection matters to you, there are hundreds of different ways to do it; you can connect with animals, plants, people, your body, your religion. And the same for being intimate—there are all sorts of different ways you can do that, including being intimate with yourself.

Sarah: I never thought about it that way.

After some discussion along these lines, Sarah identified an immediate goal of having a long, hot, soothing bath; this was a way of being intimate with herself and connecting with her body.

Committed Action Often Brings Discomfort

At times, it's easy to translate our values into actions. When life is going well—no major difficulties or obstacles, and we're not really stretching ourselves—it's often not that hard to behave like the sort of person we want to be, to act effectively, guided by our values. However, at other times, it's incredibly hard to do so. When we step out of our comfort zone to face our fears, to confront issues we prefer to hide away from, to learn difficult new skills that don't come naturally, and go into challenging situations with an uncertain outcome, this usually gives rise to some very uncomfortable thoughts and feelings—most commonly, anxiety. So if we're not willing to make room for the discomfort that accompanies personal growth, then we will not do what it takes for us to grow. And that is why the next chapter is about acceptance.

Extra Bits

See chapter 21 in *ACT Made Simple: The Extra Bits* (at http://www.actmindfully.com.au). There you will find (a) a description of problems arising from an excessive focus on the outcome, (b) how to handle fusion that arises while goal setting, (c) a printable version of the challenge formula with explanatory text to give to clients, (d) a printable SMART Goal-Setting worksheet, and (e) how to use the ACT Companion app for goal setting and action planning.

Skilling Up

Here are a few suggestions for you:

- Use the formal SMART goal-setting process outlined above on yourself. Do it at least three or four times to get the hang of it; then try it out with a client in session.

- Rehearse the spiels and scripts above—especially the challenge formula and the Gun at Your Head metaphor.

- Rehearse the "tiniest step" question a few times; then start regularly asking it in session.

Takeaway

Committed action means living by our values and acting effectively—overtly or covertly—to achieve our values-congruent goals. It can involve informal goal setting, such as "flavoring and savoring," or the formal setting of SMART goals. Some of our clients will have very few psychological barriers to action; simply helping them to get in touch with their values and asking about values-congruent goals will be enough to get them moving. However, the majority of our clients will have at least some barriers, and we'll look at what these are and how to overcome them in chapters 22 to 24.

CHAPTER 22

Fifty Shades of Acceptance

Acceptance of What?

As we discussed earlier, acceptance is short for "experiential acceptance." It's about actively accepting our private experiences: thoughts, feelings, memories, and so on. It is *not* about passively accepting our life situation. ACT advocates taking action to improve our situation as much as possible: acceptance and commitment! For example, if you are in a difficult intimate relationship, ACT advocates that you practice self-compassion and make room for all your painful thoughts and feelings (instead of doing self-defeating things such as drinking, smoking, overeating, ruminating, and worrying) and *at the same time*, you take action, guided by your values, to improve the relationship (or, if necessary, to leave it).

Also, sorry to keep harping on this, but it's so important, and many new practitioners get the wrong idea: we don't advocate acceptance of every single unwanted thought and feeling. We advocate acceptance if and when experiential avoidance is getting in the way of effective values-based living.

Acceptance in a Nutshell

In Plain Language: *Acceptance* means opening up to our inner experiences (thoughts, images, memories, feelings, emotions, urges, impulses, sensations) and allowing them to be as they are, regardless of whether they are pleasant or painful. We open up and make room for them, drop the struggle with them, and allow them to freely come and go, in their own good time.

Aim: To open up to unwanted inner experiences, when doing so enables us to act on our values.

Synonyms: Willingness, expansion, dropping the struggle, opening up, making room.

Method: Make full, open, undefended psychological contact with unwanted inner experiences.

When to Use: When experiential avoidance becomes a barrier to effective values-based living.

The Language of Acceptance

Clients often don't understand what we mean by "acceptance." They commonly think that accepting something means resigning yourself to it, tolerating it, putting up with it, or even liking, wanting, or approving of it. Therefore, early on in therapy, I tend to avoid the word. "Willingness" is a popular alternative term: the willingness to have your thoughts and feelings as they are, in this moment. Another term you can use is "expansion," which fits nicely with the metaphorical talk of opening up, creating space, and making room. Here are a few others to play around with:

- Allow it to be there.

- Open up and make room for it.

- Expand around it.

- Sit with it.

- Drop the struggle.

- Stop fighting it.

- Make peace with it.

- Give it some space.

- Soften up around it.

- Let it be.

- Breathe into it.

- Hold it gently/lightly/softly.

- Lean into it.

Getting to Acceptance

In many ACT protocols, acceptance follows creative hopelessness (chapter 8) and dropping the struggle (chapter 9). If that's the path you're taking, the Pushing Away Paper exercise (chapter 9) lends itself well to this transition, as we'll see below.

Therapist: So let's just do a quick recap. (*The therapist quickly recaps the Pushing Away Paper exercise and gets the client pushing it away.*) So you're pushing and pushing and pushing, and it's taking up all your time and energy. Your shoulders are tired, and you're hemmed in, and you can't do anything useful like drive a car or cook dinner or hug someone you love while you're doing this. Now let it just sit there on your lap. (*Client lays the paper on her lap.*) Now how's that? Isn't that a lot less effort?

Client: Well…yes. It's less effort. But it's still there.

Therapist: Absolutely. Not only is it still there, it's even closer to you than before. But notice the difference: now you're free to do the things that make your life work. You can hug someone you love, cook dinner, or drive a car. It's not draining you, tiring you, tying you up, closing you off. Obviously, that's just a sheet of paper, but what if you could learn how to do this with your real feelings?

Remember, there is no set sequence you must follow through the ACT core processes, so there are many other routes to get to acceptance. Here are examples of what we could say to lead into acceptance from other ACT processes:

- From defusion: "So we've looked at how to unhook from your thoughts, but what about your feelings?" or "Your mind says this feeling is horrible and unbearable. How about we check it out and see if that's the case?"

- From values: "So as you talk about these values, what feelings show up for you?"

- From committed action: "What feelings are likely to show up for you when you take this action?" or "So as you think about doing this, what are you feeling?" or "What feelings will you need to make room for in order to do this?"

- From self-as-context: "So using that part of you that notices, let's take a look at some of these feelings you've been struggling with."

Of course, the more experientially avoidant our clients, the more reluctant they'll be to accept unwanted inner experiences, so we'll need to go more slowly and gently. We'll need to do more work around creative hopelessness, and we may well have to go back to it repeatedly.

Work around values is also very important here. We need to make a clear link between acceptance and improving one's life. The client needs to recognize that accepting this discomfort is in the service of something important, meaningful, and life-enhancing. A magic wand question is often useful: "If I waved a magic wand so that these difficult feelings couldn't hold you back in any way, what would you do differently in your life?" Once we know the answer, we can say, "Okay. So if that's what you want to do with your life, let's make it possible. I don't have a magic wand, but we can learn some new ways of dealing with these feelings so they no longer hold you back."

Naturally, we want to ensure this work is safe. We want to be mindful that we don't lecture or coerce our clients; we always ask permission, always give them a choice, always let them know they can stop at any point.

The "Three As" of Acceptance

I find it helpful to think of acceptance in terms of the "three As": acknowledge, allow, accommodate. (These are not official ACT terms.) We can think of these as interweaving and overlapping phases, flowing into and out of one another, rather than discrete, well-delineated stages.

Acknowledge. The first phase in acceptance often involves the simple acknowledging of difficult inner experience: noticing it with curiosity and naming it in a nonjudgmental manner. (As you know, this is also the first step in defusion, and an important aspect of any dropping anchor exercise.)

Allow. The next phase, after acknowledging the presence of the unwanted experience, is to allow it, to give it permission to stay, to let it be. A bit of self-talk often comes in handy for this (e.g., *I don't like this feeling, but I'll allow it* or *I don't want this feeling, but I'm going to let it be*).

Accommodate. The next, and most challenging, phase is to accommodate the experience. Think of an unexpected visitor to your home: some relative you know is completely harmless but you don't particularly like. When you open the door, you acknowledge him. Then, you may decide to allow him inside. If you do allow him in, will you then go a step further and accommodate him? Offer him a seat and a cup of coffee?

"Accommodate" has three meanings in English, all of which are relevant: (a) to provide sufficient space, (b) to fit in with, and (c) to adapt to. When we accommodate unwanted thoughts, feelings, urges, sensations, or memories, we actively make room for those experiences, we give them sufficient space, we "fit in with" them, we let them stay for as long as they like, and we adapt to having them live with us.

> **Practical Tip**   In this chapter, the emphasis is on accepting emotions. However, the same principles apply to acceptance of any unwanted inner experience—thoughts, memories, urges, sensations, and so on.

The Acceptance Smorgasbord

There are a hexaflazillion ways of working with acceptance, and the following figure illustrates many (but not nearly all) of them. Some take only ten seconds, and others take up to ten minutes. We'll cover many of these in this book; the others are described in Extra Bits.

HEALING HAND
Lay a hand on the part of your body where you feel this most intensely. Imagine this is a healing hand—the hand of a loving nurse or parent or partner. Send some warmth into this area—not to get rid of the feeling, but to open up around it, make room for it, hold it gently.

PAIN AS YOUR ALLY
Use this emotion to motivate, communicate, illuminate.

ALLOWING
See if you can allow this feeling to be there. You don't have to like it or want it—just allow it.

EXPANSION
See if you can open up and expand around the feeling. It's as if, in some magical way, all this space opens up inside you.

EMOTION SURFING
Surf your feelings and urges as if they are ocean waves.

THE CURIOUS CHILD
Notice where this feeling is in your body. Zoom in on it. Observe it as if you are a curious child who has never encountered anything like this. Where are the edges? Where does it start and stop? Is it moving or still? Is it at the surface or inside you? Hot or cold? Light or heavy?

THE CHOICE TO FEEL
Suppose I could give you a choice:
A. you never have to have this feeling ever again, but it means you lose all capacity to love and care, or
B. you get to love and care, but when there's a gap between what you want and what you've got, feelings like this one show up.
Which do you choose?

DROP ANCHOR
Acknowledge the feeling, connect with your body, and engage with the world.

FEELINGS

MINDFUL NAMING
Label the feeling mindfully: *I'm noticing anxiety, Here is sadness, I'm having a feeling of anger.*

PHYSICALIZING
Imagine this feeling is an object. Is it liquid, solid, or gaseous? How big is it? Is it light or heavy? What temperature is it? Is it at the surface or inside you? What shape does it have? What color? Is it transparent or opaque? What does the surface feel like—hot or cold, rough or smooth, wet or dry?

COMPASSION
Hold this feeling gently and softly as if it's a crying baby or a scared puppy.

THE STRUGGLE SWITCH
Is the struggle switch on, off, or at the halfway point we call "tolerating it"?
If the switch was like a dial with a scale of 0 to 10, and 10 is full on struggle, and 0 no struggle at all, then right now, what level are you? Are you willing to see if we can bring it down a notch or two?

NORMALIZING
This feeling tells you that you're a normal human being who has a heart and who cares. This is what humans feel when there's a gap between what we want and what we've got.

METAPHORS
Quicksand
Passengers on the Bus
Demons on the Boat
Wade Through the Swamp
Pushing Away Paper

BREATHE INTO IT
Breathe into this feeling. It's as if your breath flows into and around it.

NOTICING
Notice where this feeling is.
Notice where it's most intense.
Notice the hot spots and cold spots.
Notice the different sensations within the feeling.

Summary of Common Acceptance Techniques

An Acceptance Tool Kit

I'm about to present a loooooong acceptance exercise, which is really a whole tool kit, so I feel the need to give you a gentle reminder (sorry): acceptance is a process, not a technique. The tools and techniques are used to help you and your clients learn the ins and outs of the process.

This exercise is actually constructed from thirteen different techniques strung together: link to values and goals, observe like a curious child, the part that notices, radio mind, notice it, name it, breathe into it, expand, allow, physicalize, normalize, be self-compassionate, and expand awareness. Yes, there's a lot to it; but don't worry—afterward I'll unpack it for you, bit by bit.

Because the exercise is so long, in early stages of therapy it may well be too challenging for many clients. However, you can easily shorten it to make it more user-friendly; you can take just one or two of the techniques and do a much briefer exercise. (And later in the chapter, we'll look at ultrabrief versions of all these methods.) You can also mix and match these techniques in any combination and any order (along with any other acceptance techniques you like)—and drop any you don't like—so you can easily create your own brief (or long) exercises.

A quick reminder: some clients do not like any exercise that focuses on the breath. One technique involves "breathing into" a feeling; most people find this very helpful for acceptance, but if you have a client who doesn't like it, just pull it out. (The same advice goes for any tool or technique in any ACT process; not one of them is essential.)

Practical Tip   When we run through these exercises in a one-to-one setting, we don't have the client sit there in silence while we talk at them. It's a dialogue, not a monologue. We keep checking in with the client, asking how it's going, getting feedback, and modifying what we do as needed.

The Acceptance of Emotions Exercise

As usual, I encourage you to read this script out loud as if talking to a client. The ellipses indicate brief pauses of two to four seconds.

Link to Values and Goals

Therapist: So we're about to do an exercise that involves learning a new way of responding to difficult feelings … and this will be challenging … so take a moment to get clear on your motivation here … what values are you living in doing this work? … And what's this in the service of? … What's it going to help you with? … What will this enable you to do differently?

Observe Like a Curious Child

Therapist: I invite you to sit upright in your chair with your back straight and your feet flat on the floor. Most people find they feel more alert and awake sitting this way, so check it out and see if this is the case for you. And either close your eyes or fix them on a spot, which-ever you prefer.

And take a moment to tap into a sense of curiosity—as if you are a curious child discov-ering something completely new—and with that sense of genuine curiosity, notice how you are sitting … notice your feet on the floor … the position of your back … where your hands are, and what they are touching … and whether your eyes are open or closed … Notice what you can see … and notice what you can hear … and smell … and taste … and notice what you are thinking … and feeling … and doing.

The Part That Notices

Therapist: So there's a part of you that notices everything … always there, always noticing. And in this exercise, you're going to use that part of you to step back and observe your difficult feelings, without getting pulled into them or swept away by them.

Radio Mind

Therapist: Let your mind chatter away like a radio playing in the background … and keep your attention on the feeling … And at any point, if your thoughts hook you and pull you out of the exercise, the moment you realize it, acknowledge it, unhook, and refocus …

Notice

Therapist: Notice where it starts and where it stops … Learn as much about it as you can …

If you drew an outline around it, what shape would it have? … Is it 2D or 3D? Is it on the surface of the body or inside you, or both? … How far inside you does it go? … Where is it most intense? … Where is it weakest? (*Pause 5 seconds.*)

And if at any moment you realize you've been hooked, simply unhook and refocus on the sensation …

Observe it with curiosity … How is it different in the center than around the edges? Is there any pulsation or vibration within it? … Is it light or heavy? … Moving or still? … What is its temperature? … Are there any hot spots or cold spots? …

Notice the different elements within it … Notice that it's not just one sensation—there are sensations within sensations … Notice the different layers. (*Pause 5 seconds.*)

Name

Therapist: Take a moment to name this feeling … What would you call it? … Okay, silently say to yourself, *I'm noticing a feeling of* X … [X = *the name that the client gave the feeling, e.g., anxiety.*]

Breathe

Therapist: And as you're noticing this feeling, breathe into it … Imagine your breath flowing into and around this feeling … Breathing into and around it …

Expand

Therapist: And it's as if, in some magical way, all this space opens up inside you … You open up around this feeling … Make space for it … Expand around it … However you make sense of that idea is just fine … Breathing into it … opening up … expanding around it …

Allow

Therapist: And see if you can just allow this feeling to be there. You don't have to like it or want it … Just allow it … Just let it be … Observe it, breathe into it, open up around it, and allow it to be as it is. (*Pause 10 seconds.*) You may feel a strong urge to fight with it or push it away. If so, just acknowledge the urge is there without acting on it. And continue observing the sensation. (*Pause 5 seconds.*) Don't try to get rid of it or alter it. If it changes by itself, that's okay. If it doesn't change, that's okay too.

Changing or getting rid of it is not the goal. Your aim is simply to allow it … to let it be. (*Pause 5 seconds.*)

Physicalize

Therapist: Imagine this feeling is a physical object … As an object, what shape does it have? … Is it liquid, solid, or gaseous? … Is it moving or still? … What color is it? … Transparent or opaque? …

If you could touch the surface, what would it feel like? … Wet or dry? … Rough or smooth? … Hot or cold? … Soft or hard? (*Pause 10 seconds.*)

Observe this object curiously, breathe into it, and open up around it … You don't have to like it or want it. Just allow it … and notice that you are bigger than this object … no matter how big it gets, it can never get bigger than you. (*Pause 10 seconds.*)

Normalize

Therapist: This feeling tells you some valuable information … It tells you that you're a normal human being with a heart … it tells you that you care … that there are things in life that matter to you … And this is what humans feel when there's a gap between what we want and what we've got … The bigger that gap, the bigger the feeling. (*Pause 5 seconds.*)

Be Self-Compassionate

Therapist: Take one of your hands and place it on this part of your body … imagine that this is a healing hand … the hand of a loving friend or parent or nurse … and feel the warmth flowing from your hand into your body … not to get rid of the feeling but to make room for it … to soften up and loosen up around it. (*Pause 10 seconds.*)

Hold it gently, as if it's a crying baby or a frightened puppy. (*Pause 10 seconds.*)

And feel free to leave your hand there, or to rest it in your lap, whichever you prefer.

Expand Awareness

Therapist: Life is like a stage show … and on that stage are all your thoughts, and all your feelings, and everything that you can see, hear, touch, taste, and smell …

And what we've been doing here is dimming the lights on the stage, and shining a spotlight on this feeling … and now it's time to bring up the rest of the lights …

So keep this feeling in the spotlight, and at the same time, bring up the lights on your body … notice your arms and legs and head and neck … and notice that you're in control of your arms and legs, regardless of what you're feeling … Just move them around a little to check that out for yourself … and now take a stretch, and notice yourself stretching …

And also bring up the lights on the room around you … Open your eyes, look around, and notice what you can see … and notice what you can hear … and notice that there's not just a feeling here; there's a feeling inside a body, inside a room, where you and I are working together on something very important … and welcome back!

In the above script, we focused on just one sensation—the most intense one. Often this is enough so that acceptance "spreads" through the whole body. But sometimes there may be other strong sensations in different parts of the body, in which case we can repeat the procedure with each one. And if the client becomes fused or overwhelmed at any point, we can segue into dropping anchor and defusion, and then return to acceptance.

> **Practical Tip**   We can work with numbness in the same way as we work with other feelings. Find the area of greatest numbness, notice it, name it, describe it, open up, make room for it, and so on. Often when we do this, numbness dissipates and other "buried" or "hidden" feelings "rise to the surface."

As we take the client through these kinds of exercises, one of two things will happen: either her feelings will change, or they won't. It doesn't matter either way. The aim is not to change or reduce feelings but to accept them—to acknowledge, allow, and accommodate them. Why? Because when we aren't investing so much time, energy, and effort in trying to control how we feel, we can invest it instead in acting on our values.

Our clients often find that when they accept a painful emotion or sensation, it reduces significantly, and sometimes disappears. When this happens, we need to clarify that (1) this is a bonus, not the goal, and (2) it won't always happen, so don't expect it. We could say, "Well, isn't that interesting? Quite often when we open up and make room for our feelings, they reduce in intensity. Sometimes they even disappear. But there's really no way to predict it. At times they will; at times they won't. So when it happens, enjoy it. But please keep in mind, it's a bonus, not the main point. If you start using these techniques to try to make these feelings go away, you'll soon be back here telling me 'it's not working.'"

If the client seems confused or disappointed by this, then it's wise to repeat the Pushing Away Paper exercise or the Struggle Switch metaphor (which you'll encounter later in this chapter) to make it really clear. I can't overemphasize the importance of this. If we don't explicitly address this issue, then, as with defusion, our clients will start doing "pseudo-acceptance"—that is, using "acceptance" techniques to try to avoid or get rid of unwanted inner experiences. And, of course, that will soon backfire, and the disappointed client will come back and complain, "It isn't working." We respond to this as we covered in chapter 16.

Unpacking the Acceptance of Emotions Exercise

Now I'll give you some pointers about these techniques. I'll also give you a ten-second version of each.

LINK TO VALUES AND GOALS

Remember, in ACT, we'd never encourage anyone to accept pain or discomfort unless it's in the service of living values and pursuing values-congruent goals. So we need to come back to this, over and over again. Without such motivation, many clients will resist acceptance.

The Ten-Second Version

Therapist: Remind me why we're doing this. What's this going to help you do differently?

OBSERVE LIKE A CURIOUS CHILD; NOTICE; NAME

The first stage in accepting a difficult inner experience is to notice it; to acknowledge it is here, right now. (This is where flexible attention overlaps with acceptance.) The metaphor of "observing like a curious child" helps to encourage openness and curiosity toward the feeling: in other words, approach instead of avoidance.

We want to also name the feeling (which clients often need help with, as we'll see in the next chapter). In everyday language, when we name our emotions, we often say things like "I am sad," which makes it sound like "I *am* the emotion." So in mindfulness-speak, we say things like "I'm noticing anxiety," "Here is a feeling of sadness," "I'm having a feeling of anger." When you name an emotion in this manner, it helps you to see that it's not who you are but an experience passing through you.

The Ten-Second Version

Therapist: Notice that feeling. Notice where it is. Notice where it's most intense.

THE PART THAT NOTICES

As in any mindfulness exercise, we can plant seeds for self-as-context. We may later water these seeds, as in chapter 25. The "noticing self" facilitates acceptance because it offers a "safe place" inside or a "safe viewpoint" from which to observe.

The Ten-Second Version

Therapist: Use that noticing part of you to really observe this.

RADIO MIND

We expect all sorts of unhelpful thoughts to pop up when doing acceptance. If we've done some work with defusion already (which I highly recommend), we can bring it in here. I'm a big fan of the simple metaphor, "Let your mind chatter away like a radio in the background."

The Ten-Second Version

Therapist: Whenever your mind hooks you, acknowledge it, unhook, and refocus.

BREATHE

Many clients—but not all—find breathing into a feeling enables them to make room for it. Slow, gentle diaphragmatic breathing seems particularly useful for a lot of people (however, it does make a small minority of people feel dizzy, light-headed, or anxious, in which case, skip it).

The Ten-Second Version

Therapist: Notice that feeling and gently breathe into it.

EXPAND

Metaphorical talk around making room, creating space, opening up, or expanding is often helpful. This takes us from the realms of "acknowledge" and "allow" into the realm of "accommodate."

The Ten-Second Version

Therapist: See if you can just open up around it—give it some space.

ALLOW

Again and again and again, we remind our clients that acceptance does not mean liking, wanting, or approving of a thought or feeling; it means allowing it, or letting it be.

The Ten-Second Version

Therapist: I know you don't want this feeling, but see if you can just let it sit there for a moment.

   You don't have to like it—just allow it.

PHYSICALIZE (OR OBJECTIFY)

Quite often our clients, especially those who are very visual, will spontaneously do this when we ask them to observe their feelings. When we imagine a feeling as a physical object, it helps us experience that this feeling is not bigger than we are; we have plenty of room for it.

In some models of therapy, you might try dissolving the object with white light or shrinking it in various ways. In ACT we would not do this, as that would reinforce the agenda of emotional control. However, as it happens, the object almost always spontaneously changes. Typically it gets smaller or softer, but sometimes it gets bigger. If the latter occurs, we might say, "No matter how big this feeling gets, it can't get bigger than you. So observe it, breathe into it, and make more room for it."

The point is, we don't need to shrink or remove the object; we just need to make room for it. With acute grief work, I often have clients leaving my office with a heavy black rock inside their stomach or a thick plank of wood on their chest. That's only to be expected. Major losses give rise to painful feelings. Let's help our clients to carry those feelings willingly, instead of getting bogged down in a struggle with them, so they can engage fully in life and do what matters.

The Ten-Second Version

Therapist: If this feeling were an object, what would it look like?

NORMALIZE

If we can recognize that it's normal and natural to have painful feelings—that this is an inevitable part of being human—we're more likely to accept them.

The Ten-Second Version

Therapist: It's completely natural and normal that you would feel this way.

BE SELF-COMPASSIONATE

Self-compassion—being kind and caring toward yourself—adds an extra element to acceptance. Presumably the warm sensations of the hand and the rich metaphor of "healing hands" contribute to the effectiveness.

The Ten-Second Version

Therapist: Just place a hand where you feel this most intensely—and see if you can hold it gently.

EXPAND AWARENESS

At times, we may want to focus intently on our emotions—such as when we're learning a mindfulness skill or grieving for a loved one. However, much of the time, focusing too intently on our feelings will get in the way of living life. At times, clients will leave your session with strong unpleasant feelings or sensations in their body. This is very likely when working with clients with chronic pain syndrome, acute grief due to a sudden loss, or anxiety about some impending major crisis or challenge. We want clients to be able to make room for their feelings and expand awareness to engage with the world around them so they can do whatever they need to do to make their life work.

This expansion of awareness is of course a big component of all dropping anchor exercises, so we may choose to explicitly mention that metaphor. If not, the Stage Show metaphor is a good alternative, and it makes it clear that this is not distraction. The feeling remains on the stage, but as the stage lights up, we get to see the whole show—and the feeling as just one part of it. This in itself facilitates acceptance: when it's just "one part of the whole show," the feeling no longer seems so big and threatening.

The Ten-Second Version

Therapist: Notice the feeling, and your body, and the room around you, and you and me working here together; there's a lot going on.

Debunking Misconceptions

Two common misconceptions about acceptance are that (a) it is all-or-nothing and (b) it is aimed at ignoring or dismissing emotions. Quite the contrary.

ACCEPTANCE IS NOT ALL-OR-NOTHING

Some ACT textbooks assert that acceptance is an all-or-nothing state: you are either accepting or you aren't; it's black or white, with no shades of gray. I find this an odd assertion. My own experience is that there are many shades of acceptance. For example, when anxiety shows up, we can acknowledge it, allow it, sit with it, make room for it, lean into it, or embrace it. For me, these terms convey different degrees of acceptance: I find it a whole lot easier to acknowledge anxiety than to embrace it. Do you get a similar sense?

I find it's often useful clinically to talk about acceptance in terms of a 0–10 scale. However, clients usually find it easier to assess their degree of struggle than their degree of acceptance, so I like to use the metaphor that follows.

The Struggle Switch

The Struggle Switch metaphor (Harris, 2007) is a powerful interactive tool for acceptance work. If clients can't do the Pushing Away Paper exercise (chapter 9) because of physical problems, then the Struggle Switch is my fallback. (I've put an animation of this metaphor on YouTube; to find it, type in "Russ Harris Struggle Switch." You can show this to clients as an alternative to delivering it yourself.)

Therapist: Imagine that at the back of our mind is a "struggle switch." When it's switched on, it means we're going to struggle against any physical or emotional pain that comes our way; whatever discomfort shows up, we'll try our best to get rid of it or avoid it.

Suppose what shows up is anxiety. (*We adapt this to the client's issue: anger, sadness, painful memories, urges to drink, and so on.*) If my struggle switch is on, then I absolutely have to get rid of that feeling! It's like, *Oh no! Here's that horrible feeling again. Why does it keep coming back? How do I get rid of it?* So now I've got anxiety about my anxiety.

In other words, my anxiety just got worse. *Oh, no! It's getting worse! Why does it do that?* Now I'm even more anxious. Then I might get angry about my anxiety: *It's not fair. Why does this keep happening?* Or I might get depressed about my anxiety: *Not again. Why do I always feel like this?* And all of these secondary emotions are useless, unpleasant, unhelpful, and a drain on my energy and vitality. And then—guess what? I get anxious or depressed about that! Spot the vicious cycle?

But now suppose my struggle switch is off. In that case, whatever feeling shows up, no matter how unpleasant, I don't struggle with it. So anxiety shows up, but this time I don't struggle. It's like, *Okay, here's a knot in my stomach. Here's tightness in my chest. Here's sweaty palms and shaking legs. Here's my mind telling me a bunch of scary stories.* And it's not that I like it or want it. It's still unpleasant. But I'm not going to waste my time and energy struggling with it. Instead I'm going to take control of my arms and legs and put my energy into doing something that's meaningful and life-enhancing.

So with the struggle switch off, our anxiety level is free to rise and fall as the situation dictates. Sometimes it'll be high, sometimes low; sometimes it will pass on by very quickly, and sometimes it will hang around. But the great thing is, we're not wasting our time and energy struggling with it. So we can put our energy into doing other things that make our lives meaningful.

But switch it on, and it's like an emotional amplifier—we can have anger about our anger, anxiety about our anxiety, depression about our depression, or guilt about our guilt. (*At this point, check in with the client: "Can you relate to this?"*)

Without struggle, we get a natural level of discomfort, which depends on who we are and what we're doing. But once we start struggling with it, our discomfort levels increase rapidly. Our emotions get bigger, and stickier, and messier, hang around longer, and have more of a negative influence over us. So if we can learn how to turn off that struggle switch, it makes a big difference. And what I'd like to do next, if you're willing, is to show you how to do that.

* * *

With the above metaphor, we introduce a simple way to measure "degrees" of acceptance (as opposed to treating it as an all-or-nothing concept). A 0 on the struggle scale correlates with maximal acceptance, whereas a 10 means maximal avoidance. A 5 is the halfway point we call tolerance, or putting up with it. The next step then is to work with a painful emotion and actively practice lowering the struggle switch. (We may not be able to turn it all the way down to zero, but even lowering it a little is a good start). The following transcript illustrates this.

The therapist has just finished asking the client to scan her body and identify where she's feeling her anxiety most intensely.

Therapist: (*summarizing*) Okay, so there's a lump in your throat, tightness in your chest, and churning in your stomach. And which of these bothers you the most?

Client: Here. (*The client touches her throat.*)

Therapist: Okay. So remember that struggle switch we talked about? (*Client nods.*) Well, right now would you say it's on or off?

Client: On!

Therapist: Okay. Suppose we turn it into a scale of 0 to 10. 10 is full on, out and out struggle—*I have to get rid of this feeling no matter what*; 0 is no struggle at all—*I don't like this feeling, but I'm not going to struggle with it*; and 5 is the halfway point, what we might call tolerance or putting up with it. On that scale, how much are you struggling with this feeling right now?

Client: About a 9.

Therapist: Okay. So a lot of struggle going on right now. Let's see if we can bring it down a couple of notches. We may or may not be able to, but let's give it a go.

(*The therapist now takes the client through several parts of the Acceptance of Emotions exercise described above: observe like a curious child, breathe into it, notice and name it, expand around it. Then he checks in with the client to see what's happening.*)

Therapist: So what's happening now with the struggle switch?

Client: Well, I feel less anxious.

Therapist: Okay, well we'll come to that in a moment. What I'm interested in now is the struggle. On a scale of 0 to 10, how much are you struggling with this feeling?

Client: Oh, about a 3.

Therapist: About a 3. Okay. Now you mentioned that your anxiety is less.

Client: Yes, it's gone down a bit.

Therapist: Interesting. Well, enjoy that when it happens; at times, when you drop the struggle with anxiety, it does reduce. But that's not what we're trying to achieve here. Our aim is to drop the struggle. Would you be willing to keep going? See if we can get the struggle switch down another notch or two?

EMOTIONS ARE IMPORTANT! WE DON'T DISMISS OR IGNORE THEM!

A common misconception—among both therapists and clients—is that we are dismissing or ignoring emotions. This isn't the case! They are a valuable source of information and guidance, so we want to make good use of them. The problem is, we can't access that valuable information and guidance from our emotions while we are busy fighting with or avoiding them; we first have to drop the struggle and make room for them. After that, we can tap into their "wisdom" and use them for guidance. In the next chapter, "Emotions as Allies," we'll look at how to do that.

Debriefing Acceptance Exercises

When we debrief these exercises, it's often good to start with open-ended questions such as "What's that like for you? Do you notice any difference?"

Often we'll get answers like "It's calming/soothing/peaceful/comforting/less effort/easier." Sometimes we'll get an answer like "strange" or "weird," in which case, we validate: "Yes, this seems weird or strange to most people at first; it's not the usual way we respond to difficult feelings." Sometimes we'll get an answer like "It's good—the feeling's gone away!", in which case we need to explain that that's a bonus, not the point. And sometimes we'll hear "It's not working"; we address this as described in chapter 16.

After these open-ended questions, we may go on to ask more leading questions, as we do when debriefing dropping anchor:

- Do you notice any difference now? Are you less hooked by these feelings; less "jerked around" by them? Do you have more self-control over your actions now? Are you in control of your body, and your words?

- Are you struggling less with these feelings? What difference does that make? Is it less tiring, less draining?

- Is it easier for you to engage with me, to be present, to focus on what I'm saying and what we are doing here?

And of course, as part of debriefing, we always want to ask, "How could this be useful for you, with XYZ?", where XYZ are the client's behavioral goals for therapy.

Common Pitfalls for Therapists

As with defusion, when working with acceptance, be alert for several common pitfalls: too much talk, not enough action; reinforcing avoidance; insensitivity; failing to link acceptance to values; and being too pushy. Let's take a quick look at each of these.

Too much talk, not enough action. Trying to explain defusion and acceptance didactically is largely a waste of time, so do it experientially. We can easily feed fusion and avoidance by getting into "analysis paralysis"—that is, discussing, analyzing, and intellectualizing instead of doing experiential work.

Reinforcing avoidance. As mentioned already, if we get excited whenever painful feelings reduce and thoughts disappear, then we reinforce avoidance (or encourage "pseudo-acceptance").

Insensitivity. If we don't validate and empathize with our clients, if we insensitively rush in with all our clever tools and techniques, we'll damage the therapeutic relationship.

Failing to link acceptance to values. If we fail to draw the connection between valued living and acceptance, our clients are likely to resist.

Being too pushy. If we push our clients into intense experiential exercises before they're ready, we're doing them a major disservice, and they may drop out of therapy.

Homework

One form of homework is to have clients formally practice a mindfulness exercise centered around acceptance of emotions. This is particularly useful for anxiety disorders and grief work. It's ideal to do such exercises in session and record them as you go, and then give your client the recording to take home. Or you can give the client a prerecorded CD or MP3 to practice with—your own or a commercially available one. (My MP3 "Mindfulness Skills: Volume 1" has a recording on track 3 very similar to the Acceptance of Emotions exercise in this chapter, and there are similar ones on the ACT Companion smartphone app.)

You can also suggest to your client, "Between now and next session, I wonder if you'd be willing to practice making room for your feelings, as we've done today. As soon as you realize you're struggling, just run through the exercise." Then, so she doesn't forget, write down the key steps you want her to practice, for example, "observe, breathe, expand" or "make it into an object and breathe into it."

A third option is this: "Over the next week, notice when you're struggling with your feelings, and notice when you're opening up and making room for them. And notice what effects it has when you respond in each way." You can also use a copy of the Struggling vs. Opening Up worksheet (see Extra Bits) and ask the client to fill it in.

Extra Bits

See chapter 22 in *ACT Made Simple: The Extra Bits* (at http://www.actmindfully.com.au). There you'll find (a) how to enhance the acceptance element of any mindfulness exercise, (b) the Struggling vs. Opening Up worksheet mentioned above, (c) additional exercises and metaphors for acceptance, including emotion surfing and urge surfing, (d) how our childhood programming sets us up to struggle with our feelings, (e) how to tackle the belief that our emotions control our actions, and (f) how to titrate acceptance so clients aren't overwhelmed.

Skilling Up

Try these techniques on yourself. Practice opening up and making room for those feelings—especially both during and after a difficult therapy session—because one of the abilities of a good therapist is being able to accept your own emotional reactions. In addition:

- Read all the exercises, metaphors, and other interventions out loud, as if you're taking a client through them.

- Review the cases of two or three clients and identify inner experiences that they are fighting with or trying to avoid. Then consider which acceptance techniques you could use with them.

Takeaway

Acceptance is the process of actively making room for unwanted private experiences. In this chapter, we've focused on emotions, but we can use the same (or slightly modified) techniques to accept thoughts, images, memories, feelings, urges, impulses, and sensations. Acceptance and defusion go hand in hand: in acceptance, as we make direct experiential contact with our private experiences, we defuse from our thoughts about them. Conversely, when we defuse and allow our thoughts to be as they are (without trying to change them or avoid them), this is an act of acceptance. Together, we can think of defusion and acceptance as "opening up." Hopefully now you're starting to see what I meant when I said the different parts of the hexaflex are all interconnected, like six facets of a diamond.

CHAPTER 23

Emotions as Allies

Emotions Matter

I occasionally bump into people who claim, "ACT is too cognitive; it doesn't deal with emotions." I usually look at them aghast and ask, "What textbook did you read? What workshop did you go to?" For sure, you could do ACT in a very cognitive way, focusing purely on thoughts and skipping over feelings—but you'd be missing out on huge chunks of the model.

There are two main themes we're going to look at in this chapter: (a) psychoeducation about the nature and purpose of emotions and (b) how to actively use our emotions.

Emotions vs. Physical Actions

Scientists have a hard time reaching a consensus on what emotions actually are. If you go searching for a good definition that everyone can agree on…well, good luck to you. However, most experts in the field of emotion do tend to agree on two things:

1. At the core of any emotion is a complex series of neurological, cardiovascular, musculoskeletal, and hormonal changes throughout the body.

2. These physical changes prepare us to take action.

We notice these physical changes as sensations, such as "butterflies" in the stomach, a "lump" in the throat, watering eyes, or clammy hands. We also notice them as urges to act in particular ways: to cry, laugh, shout, or hide, for example. The likelihood that we will act in a particular way when experiencing a particular emotion is often called an "action tendency." But notice the key word here: "tendency." A tendency means we have the inclination to do something; it doesn't mean we *have to* do it, that we have no choice. It doesn't mean we are forced to behave in a particular way and are helpless to do anything else; it just means we *tend* to act that way.

So, for example, when you're anxious about running late, you may have the *tendency* to drive above the speed limit, but you can still choose to drive legally and safely if you wish. Or when you're feeling angry with someone, you may have the *urge* or *impulse* or *desire* or *inclination* to yell at them, but you can choose to talk calmly if you wish.

In other words, we can still control our overt behavior—our physical actions—at times when we can't control how we are feeling. Again and again in ACT, we make good use of this ability; we help people to separate their physical actions from their emotions. If a client comes to us for "anger management," we can help her learn how to open up and make room for her feelings of anger and defuse from her angry thoughts, and at the same time, exert control over her voice, face, body posture, and physical actions—so she can *act* calmly, even while feeling furious. Likewise, if a client has an anxiety disorder, we can help him to open up and make room for feelings of anxiety, and at the same time, take control of his voice, face, body posture, and physical actions to act effectively in the situations that scare him—so he can *act* courageously even while feeling scared.

Practical Tip   Sometimes when I help clients to do this, they say, "Oh! You mean, fake it till you make it!" My reply to this is, "No! This isn't about being 'fake.' It's not about pretending to be something you're not. The aim is to be true to ourselves, to honestly acknowledge to ourselves what we are feeling, and to truly accept those feelings, and at the same time, to behave like the sort of person we genuinely want to be. No faking involved!"

Our ability to separate physical actions from emotions is incredibly useful. If we can control our posture, face, voice, and actions when feeling a particular strong emotion, it can enable us to act in ways that get better results.

For example, if I'm feeling furious with my son (yes, it happens) and I am able to speak in a soft, patient voice, with my arms by my side and my hands open, and explain to him assertively and patiently what the problem is and what I would like him to do…that's much healthier for our relationship than when I'm feeling furious and I yell at him (yes, it happens). As any parent knows, yelling often works in the short term to get our needs met, but in the long term it doesn't work well for a healthy relationship (nor is it good role-modeling).

What Purposes Do Our Emotions Serve?

Many clients have scant knowledge of the purposes of our emotions: why they have evolved and how they help us adapt to the world we live in. Now, we don't want to turn our sessions into long didactic seminars on these topics, but a little bit of psychoeducation can be very useful in helping clients to respond more flexibly to their emotions. If they understand how and why our painful emotions evolved, they may be able to better accept them and be more self-compassionate. And if they learn how to tune into and use their emotions, their emotional intelligence will rise, which confers a vast array of benefits. So, if we want to keep it simple, we can say our emotions can serve three main purposes: communicate, motivate, illuminate.

EMOTIONS COMMUNICATE

When we experience a particular emotion, we tend to do certain physical actions. These physical actions often communicate to others what we are feeling, without us needing to tell them. In many social situations, this is beneficial; if I see tears in your eyes, and your head downcast, and a hangdog expression on your face, I can make a good guess that you are sad; and if we have a good relationship, and I am a kind, caring person, the chances are that I will respond to you in a kind, supportive manner.

Of course, technically speaking, it's not the emotions that communicate; emotions are a private inner experience that no one else can directly know. What communicates to others are your physical actions: your facial expression, body posture, physical movement, breathing pattern, and vocalizations (as well as involuntary physical changes such as tears, pallor, or flushing). These physical actions are what we mean when we talk about "expressing your feelings"; your face, body posture, movement, and voice "express" to others the emotion that is within you.

Most of us learn from a young age how to modify such physical actions—how to change our facial expression, body posture, physical movement, breathing pattern, and vocalizations—so we can "hide our true feelings" from others. And it's a good thing that we can do this, because there are plenty of situations where that's extremely useful and adaptive.

However, there's a downside to this ability. In some situations, when we "hide our feelings" instead of appropriately "expressing" them, this is counterproductive. Why? Because it makes it harder for others to intuit what we are feeling, and if they misinterpret it, they may not respond in the manner we would wish for. For example, if you are feeling very sad but "putting on a happy face" and vocalizing that "life is great," you may not elicit the supportive, caring response from others that, deep down inside, you really want.

Likewise, suppose you are feeling sad, but your struggle switch goes on, and you react to your sadness with anger, and then you express that anger to others through your face, voice, and body posture. If so, rather than others responding to you with kindness and caring (as they might if you're expressing sadness), there's a good chance they'll back off and keep away from you, or get into conflict with you.

In such situations, we can help the client learn how to appropriately "express" the emotion she is feeling, through her facial expression, body language, and words. At the same time, we can help the client develop greater awareness of when and where and with whom it's useful to express her emotions. For example, the response you get from others if you do express your sadness will depend on who they are, what the situation is, what kind of relationship you have with them, and so on. So if you know certain other people are likely to be hostile and aggressive if you express your sadness, then usually it's best not to express it!

When we physically express our emotions in appropriate ways to caring others in suitable situations, this is what we are likely to communicate:

- Fear communicates "Watch out; there's danger!" or "I find you threatening."

- Anger communicates "This isn't fair or right" or "You're trespassing on my territory" or "I'm defending what's mine."

- Sadness communicates "I've lost something important."

- Guilt communicates "I've done something wrong and I want to put it right."

- Love communicates "I appreciate you"; "I want you to stay close."

EMOTIONS MOTIVATE

The words "emotion," "motivate," "motion," and "move" all originate from the Latin word "movere," which means "to move." Emotions prepare us to move our body in particular ways. They have evolved over countless eons to ready us for action in response to specific stimuli; they predispose us to make certain moves that are likely to be adaptive and life-enhancing.

The primitive fight-or-flight response originally evolved in fish, to help them fight off or flee from threats. In modern day humans, our fight-or-flight response gives rise to many powerful emotions: frustration, irritation, anger, and rage (fight); and concern, anxiety, fear, and panic (flight). (Note: Technically, it's the "fight, flight, or freeze" response, but this terminology can be confusing because there are three different meanings of the term "freeze." It's beyond the scope of this book to explain them, but you can go to YouTube and watch my animation "The Three Meanings of Freeze.") In contrast, social emotions, such as guilt and shame, evolved much later and are found only in mammals; they stem from the limbic center of the brain, which many people call "the mammalian brain." All the emotions we experience today incline us to act in certain ways and to do things that have been adaptive in our evolutionary past:

- Fear motivates us to run away or hide.

- Anger motivates us to stand our ground, to fight.

- Sadness motivates us to slow down, withdraw, and rest.

- Guilt motivates us to make amends, to repair social damage.

- Love motivates us to be loving, caring, and nurturing.

EMOTIONS ILLUMINATE

Our emotions illuminate what's important. They alert us that there is something going on that matters, something we need to attend to. They "shine a light" on our deepest needs and wants, as follows:

- Fear illuminates the importance of safety and protection.

- Anger illuminates the importance of defending our territory, protecting a boundary, or standing up and fighting for what is ours.

- Sadness illuminates the importance of rest and recuperation after a loss.

- Guilt illuminates the importance of how we treat others and the need to repair social bonds.

- Love illuminates the importance of connection, intimacy, bonding, caring, and sharing.

In other words, our emotions are messengers who come bearing gifts. Among other things, they can help us communicate effectively with others, take care of ourselves and our loved ones, and recognize and attend to what is important. So the more we cut off or disconnect from our emotions, the more we miss out on their benefits.

How to Gain the Wisdom of Emotions

As mentioned in chapter 22, many therapists and clients seem to get the erroneous idea that we dismiss or ignore emotions in ACT. And as you know, that is not the case. Near the end of both the Pushing Away Paper exercise and the Hands As Thoughts and Feelings metaphor, there's a line that goes, "If there's something useful you can do with these, then use them; even the most painful, unpleasant, unwanted thoughts and feelings usually have something useful to tell us." The idea is that we don't just accept our emotions; we go on to tune into them, make use of them. This idea underlies the classic ACT catchphrase: "Your pain is your ally" (Hayes et al., 1999).

Here are some questions we can ask clients to reflect on once they have accepted a difficult emotion:

- What does this emotion remind you to do in terms of caring for yourself or others?

- If this emotion could give you some words of advice, what would it say?

- If you follow that advice, will it lead you into towards or away moves?

- If you express this emotion to others *appropriately*, what might it signal?

- How might they respond to that signal in ways that could be helpful for you?

- What does this emotion tell you…

  - that you care about?

  - about what really matters to you?

  - about the sort of person you want to be?

  - about what you really want?

  - that you need to address or deal with or focus on or face up to?

  - that you need to do more of, less of, or differently?

  - that you need to do differently in the way you treat yourself or others?

Often, these explorations throw up important values, goals, needs, and desires—which we can then help the client translate into towards moves.

Harnessing the Energy of Emotions

Some emotions are extremely energizing—most obviously fear and anger. If we can defuse from unhelpful thoughts, make room for the feelings, and ground ourselves, we can often harness the energy of these emotions to take committed action. A common example is the performance anxiety that professional actors and musicians universally feel before they go out on stage in front of an audience. This can be usefully harnessed and channeled into a performance. Instead of describing their inner experience as anxiety, many performers refer to it as being "amped," "revved up," "buzzed," or having an "adrenaline rush." (For an in-depth look at this topic, see my book *The Confidence Gap* [Harris, 2011].)

What About Dissociation?

What if clients are unable to access their emotions? Some clients are so cut off from their emotions, they tell us they "don't feel anything." Technically this is known as *dissociation*, and it correlates with high levels of experiential avoidance. In fact, these clients do feel something: an unpleasant sense of numbness, which they often describe as emptiness, hollowness, or feeling dead. There is much we can do in ACT to help with this issue; I don't have space to write about it here, but I've covered it in Extra Bits.

Extra Bits

See chapter 23 in *ACT Made Simple: The Extra Bits* (at http://www.actmindfully.com.au). There you'll discover (a) how to work with dissociation, (b) how to help clients figure out when it's useful—and when it's not—to focus on their emotions, (c) links to several YouTube animations I've created about the neuroscience of emotion, and (d) emotional regulation in ACT.

Takeaway

Emotions offer a rich source of wisdom and guidance, which we can't access if we are busy avoiding them. When we work with emotions in ACT, it's not just about noticing, naming, and accepting them; it's about making active use of them. Remember the classic ACT catchphrase: your pain is your ally.

CHAPTER 24

What's Stopping You?

Change Isn't Easy

Have you ever had a client leave your office all fired up, brimming with enthusiasm, saying, "I'm going to do this, and that, and the other"? And then she comes back the next session, and she hasn't done any of it? Of course you have. But only about several thousand times, right? When my clients report such things, I immediately reply, "You are so like me!" (You should see the look of shock upon their faces.) "Yes," I continue, "Do you know how often I say I'm going to do something, but I don't actually do it?"

Typically, the stunned client says, "Oh—err—I didn't think you…"

"We're all in the same boat with this stuff," I say. "And if your mind is anything like mine, it's probably beating you up right now, telling you the 'not good enough' story." At this the client usually nods her head, so we do some work around unhooking from self-criticism, making room for anxiety and guilt, and practicing self-compassion.

After that I say, "Now before we do anything else this session, can we spend some time identifying what stopped you? Because whatever got in the way last time is also likely to get in the way this time and next time. So would it be okay if we figure out what the barriers are, and come up with a plan to address them?"

Overcoming Barriers

There are many possible barriers to change, and often therapists unwittingly reinforce them through omitting important aspects of chapter 21, such as setting SMART goals and helping clients to plan and prepare for possible obstacles. So check: Are both you and the client clear on the goal? Is it SMART: Specific? Motivated by values? Adaptive? Realistic? Time-framed? Have you identified potential obstacles and strategized how to deal with them? Have you come up with a plan B? Have you implemented all the other stuff in chapter 21?

Aside from such omissions, the four most common barriers to change compose the acronym HARD:

H—Hooked

A—Avoiding discomfort

R—Remoteness from values

D—Doubtful goals

What follows is a simple client worksheet that explains the above headings and gives the "antidotes." You'll also find a downloadable copy in Extra Bits. (This replaces the more complex From FEAR to DARE worksheets from the first edition of this book.)

What's Stopping You?

The aim of this worksheet is to clarify your own internal barriers to change—to identify what holds you back from stepping out of your comfort zone, trying new things, facing your fears, tackling your big challenges, pursuing your goals, practicing new skills, taking action to solve problems, and so on.

There are two ways to fill out this worksheet. One option is to do it for a specific domain of life (e.g., work, education, friends, partner, parenting, spirituality, hobbies, health) or a specific behavior you want to start doing (e.g., exercising, cooking, playing with your kids, studying). The other option is to do it as a broad overview of life in general.

H = HOOKED

What reasons does your mind come up with for why you can't, shouldn't, or shouldn't even have to take action? What bad things does it tell you will happen if you do take action? Please write them below.

_____

_____

_____

The antidote: If you get hooked by these thoughts, then you probably won't take action. So use your unhooking skills. You can't stop your mind from saying these things, but you can unhook from them.

A = AVOIDING DISCOMFORT

Personal growth and meaningful change means stepping out of your comfort zone. This inevitably brings up discomfort. And if you aren't willing to make room for that discomfort, you won't do the things that really matter to you. Please write below all the difficult thoughts, feelings, sensations, emotions, memories, and urges you are unwilling to have.

_____

_____

_____

The antidote: Use your "expansion" skills; practice opening up and making room for your discomfort. Before you set out to do the challenging things that matter to you, think ahead: What sort of discomfort is likely, and are you willing to make room for it?

R = REMOTENESS FROM VALUES

What values are you ignoring, neglecting, forgetting, leaving behind, or failing to act on when you opt out of doing these important things?

_____

_____

_____

The antidote: Connect with your values. Why bother to do this challenging stuff if it's not important? If it is important, then connect with what makes it meaningful. What values will you be living with every step you take?

D = DOUBTFUL GOALS

On a scale of 0–10, how realistic do your goals seem to you? (10 = totally realistic, I'll definitely do it, no matter what. 0 = completely unrealistic, I'll never do it.) If your goals seem less than a 7, it's doubtful you will follow through. Are your goals excessive? Are you trying to do too much? Trying to do it too quickly? Trying to do it perfectly? Are you trying to do things for which you lack the resources (such as time, money, energy, health, social support, or necessary skills)? Please write down your goals below, and scale them all 0–10 in terms of how realistic they seem.

_____

_____

_____

The antidote: Set more realistic goals. Make them smaller, simpler, easier, matched to your resources, until you can score at least a 7 in terms of how realistic they are.

* * *

The idea is to run through these common barriers with the client, see which ones are relevant, and come up with plans to deal with them. If the client doesn't yet have the necessary defusion or acceptance skills, we put them on the agenda for this session and actively work on them. (We don't have to use the above worksheet, of course; we can do all this through conversation without writing anything down—but the worksheet is very useful.)

Motivation: Workability and Willingness

There are many useful tools we can use to help with motivation. And my favorite (as you may have guessed) is the choice point. Suppose we have a client who recognizes a pattern of behavior as self-defeating and yet is ambivalent or hesitant about changing it. Sound familiar? Let's explore how we might help.

One option is to look at the problematic behavior in terms of...

Workability

To explore the workability of a behavior, we basically identify and validate its *payoffs* (outcomes the client wants) and compassionately and respectfully contrast them with the *costs* (outcomes the client does not want). We can highlight the payoffs of any given behavior through asking questions such as:

- What happens when (or immediately after) you do that?

- Do you feel good or better in some way: relieved, calmer, less hurt, chilled, relaxed, stronger, in the right, assertive, confident, powerful?

- Do you get to escape or avoid something you don't want, such as a difficult person, place, event, situation, interaction, task, duty, responsibility, challenge, or some difficult thoughts, feelings, or memories?

- Do you gain or get access to something you want? Do you get your needs met in some way?

Practical Tip   Remember, "payoffs" does not mean the same as "reinforcing consequences." All behavior has payoffs: the benefits, gains, rewards, or desirable outcomes of the behavior. Only if those payoffs are great enough to keep that behavior going over time would we say they are reinforcing consequences (see chapter 4).

For unworkable behavior, we aim to make the payoffs less rewarding so they no longer function as reinforcing consequences for the behavior. Unworkable behaviors may have many different reinforcing consequences, but they all boil down to some combination of these two:

- Get away from something you don't want

- Get access to something you do want

Here are some of the most common reinforcing consequences of unworkable behavior:

- Escape/avoid people, places, situations, and events (overt avoidance)

- Escape/avoid unwanted thoughts and feelings (experiential avoidance)

- Feel good

- Get your needs met

- Gain attention

- Look good (to yourself or others)

- Feel like you are right

- Feel like you are getting what you deserve

- Make sense (e.g., of life, the world, yourself, others)

Let's look at an example of validating payoffs and highlighting costs of a client's unworkable behavior. Using the choice point, the therapist first identifies and validates the payoffs of the behavior.

VALIDATE PAYOFFS

The client, a nineteen-year-old girl with trauma-related symptoms, complains of feeling numb, empty, and "dead inside." This feeling is greatest when she is alone at night. As it becomes intense, she feels increasing anxiety. These are the antecedents to the behavior, so they go at the bottom of the choice point. In response to these antecedents, she makes shallow cuts on her forearms with a razor blade. This behavior has significant payoffs: the pain, the sight of blood, and the adrenaline release combine to make her "feel more alive" and distract her from the numbness and emptiness.

The therapist validates these payoffs while writing them down. (Quick reminder: the choice point is a useful visual tool, but you don't have to use it; these same interventions can happen in a conversational manner without drawing or writing.) After this, the therapist compassionately and respectfully explores the costs. (Remember from chapter 4 that all behavior has costs: the losses, damages, deficits, energy expenditures, or undesirable outcomes of the behavior. If those costs are great enough that the behavior reduces over time, technically we would say they are *punishing consequences*.)

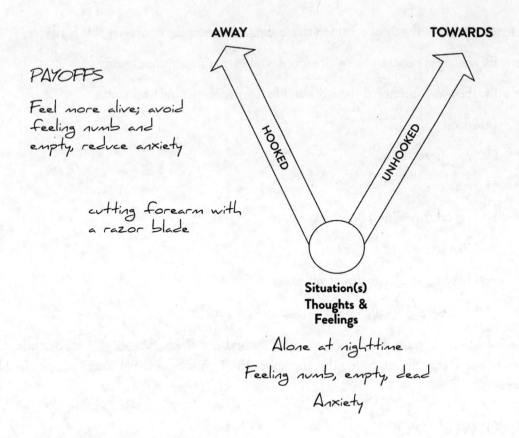

AWAY

TOWARDS

PAYOFFS

Feel more alive; avoid feeling numb and empty, reduce anxiety

HOOKED

UNHOOKED

cutting forearm with a razor blade

**Situation(s)
Thoughts &
Feelings**

Alone at nighttime

Feeling numb, empty, dead

Anxiety

Next, the therapist addresses the costs of the behavior.

HIGHLIGHT COSTS

Useful questions to elicit the costs of a behavior include:

- What do you lose or miss out on?

- What does this cost you in the long term?

- What happens as a result of this that you don't want?

- What values/goals does this pull you away from?

- What do you risk when you do this?

- What difficult thoughts, feelings, memories does this give rise to?

The therapist then writes the costs above the payoffs:

COSTS

Scarring; shame; self-
judgment; doesn't solve
issues; have to cover
arms; upsets Mom;
goes against my value
of self-care

AWAY   TOWARDS

HOOKED   UNHOOKED

PAYOFFS

Feel more alive; avoid
feeling numb and
empty; reduce anxiety

cutting forearm with
a razor blade

**Situation(s)
Thoughts &
Feelings**

Alone at nighttime

Feeling numb, empty, dead

Anxiety

What we aim to do here is diminish the influence of the payoffs by linking them to all the accompanying costs. The therapist summarizes this—with great respect and compassion—as follows: "So it's really important to acknowledge there are some real payoffs for you in doing this. When you cut yourself, it distracts you from that dead empty feeling inside and it makes you feel more alive, and this has been helpful for you. It's not surprising that you have mixed feelings about stopping it. And if you don't want to stop it, I'm not going to pressure you; our work here is about what you want for your life, not what I think you should or shouldn't be doing. But what you're telling me is, although there are some big payoffs here, there are also some pretty significant costs: scarring on your arms, feeling ashamed, covering up, upsetting your mom, and it's pulling you away from one of the main values that you've identified here: self-care."

At the same time as we are highlighting the unworkability of the current behavior, we want to enhance willingness for the new, more workable behavior.

Willingness

Willingness interventions are pretty much the flip side of workability interventions. First we identify (through working with values and goals) what the client wants to do differently. It's not enough to say "I want to stop this behavior"; we need to clarify "What will you do instead?" In other words, next time similar antecedents are present, how does the client want to respond differently in terms of effective, values-guided action?

In this case, the client—coached by the therapist—comes up with two preferable behaviors: (a) to massage skin cream onto her forearm and (b) to practice the Kind Hand self-compassion exercise (chapter 18). However, not surprisingly, she is somewhat hesitant to do this. In order to increase a client's willingness to do new more workable behaviors, we want to highlight the payoffs of the new behavior, while also compassionately acknowledging the costs of doing it. First let's look at the payoffs.

HIGHLIGHT PAYOFFS

To identify the payoffs of engaging in more workable behavior, we want to explore

A. the immediate payoffs (i.e., the instant rewards of living one's values) and

B. the potential payoffs (i.e., the likely rewards of achieving one's goals).

Useful questions to ask include:

- Would doing this seem more like being the person you want to be?

- Does this seem like moving in the direction you want to go?

- What values would you be living with every tiny step you take?

- Is this a towards move?

- What would you be standing for?

- What would doing this say about you?

- Would this be living life your way?

- If you successfully achieve this, what are the benefits likely to be?

After highlighting the payoffs, we can compassionately and respectfully explore and validate the costs involved.

VALIDATE COSTS

Useful questions to ask include:

- What difficult thoughts, feelings, or memories are likely to arise?

- What are you risking?

- What might you lose, miss out on, or need to give up?

Let's return to our example client. After eliciting the client's responses, the therapist plots this information on the other side of the choice point, as below:

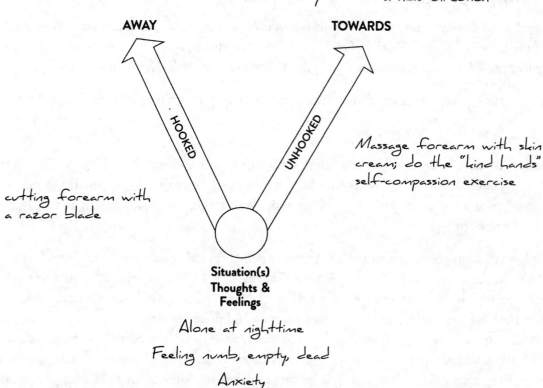

COSTS

Don't get distracted from the feeling of numbness; will have strong urges to cut; will have anxiety

PAYOFFS

Feel more alive in a more healthy way; no shame; living value of self-care; self-soothing; taking life in a new direction

AWAY

TOWARDS

HOOKED

UNHOOKED

Massage forearm with skin cream; do the "kind hands" self-compassion exercise

cutting forearm with a razor blade

**Situation(s)
Thoughts &
Feelings**

Alone at nighttime

Feeling numb, empty, dead

Anxiety

Now the therapist can explore willingness: "So next time you're alone at night, feeling numb and anxious, there's going to be a choice point for you. You can do what you usually do or you can do something different, and the choice is yours. If you choose to massage your arm and practice the 'kind hands' exercise, there are many payoffs, such as (*therapist summarizes the main benefits*). And there's also some difficult stuff that will go with it, such as (*therapist summarizes the costs*). So the big question is: are you willing to make room for all this difficult stuff, in order to go ahead with these towards moves?" (This question captures the essence of willingness.)

Of course, if the client says she *won't* be able to handle the anxiety or the urges to cut or the feeling of numbness, the therapist should take that at face value and make the session about actively working on unhooking skills: defusion, acceptance, dropping anchor, self-compassion, and so on.

The therapist may also want to look at changing the antecedent situation. If the client is spending a lot of time alone and wants to change this, then social interaction and getting out of the house will become the focus for further committed action. (Remember, we don't passively accept difficult situations such as social isolation; we commit to action to improve them.)

Breaking Commitments

Everyone breaks commitments at times. This is part of being human. Often our client will be quick to raise the issue of failure: "What if I fail?" "I've tried doing this before, but I never stick to it." And if our client doesn't raise this issue, then we'll need to raise it ourselves. Here's an example:

Therapist: It's a given that at times you aren't going to follow through on this stuff. You know why?

Client: Why?

Therapist: Because you're a real human being. You're not a Marvel Comics superhero. None of us is perfect. None of us always lives by our values or follows through on the things we say we're going to do. We can get better at doing this stuff, for sure. However, we'll never be perfect.

We have these important chats with our clients to help them unhook from "shoulds" and "musts," unrealistic expectations, and perfectionistic ideas. The reality is we can get better at staying on track, faster at catching ourselves when we go off track, and better at getting back on track again. And, at the same time, we are fallible, imperfect human beings, and there are times (many times) when we will fall back into old patterns. When we do go off track, what helps is to be self-compassionate: to be kind, caring, and accepting toward ourselves. And from there, we can reconnect with our values and get moving again. What doesn't help is beating ourselves up. I like to say to clients, "If beating yourself up were a good way to change your behavior, wouldn't you be perfect by now?" I then add, "I don't know how to stop your mind from beating you up. But what you can do is notice it and name it and unhook from it when it starts."

It's also useful to talk to clients about the two main commitment patterns:

- Pattern 1: Make a commitment, break a commitment, give up.

- Pattern 2: Make a commitment, break a commitment, lick your wounds, pick yourself up, learn from the experience, get back on track, make another commitment.

The first pattern leads to getting stuck. The second leads to continued growth. You can ask clients to identify their pattern, and if it's pattern 1, ask them to honestly assess it in terms of workability.

Basically, we want our client to build bigger and bigger patterns of valued action, extending into every area of her life. And in the process, we want her to become her own ACT therapist: identifying her own barriers and responding with core ACT processes.

If All Else Fails

If none of this helps, and the client remains stuck, then we can encourage her to:

A. Acknowledge that currently nothing is helping. In the future, this may change; right now this is reality.

B. Acknowledge her difficult thoughts and feelings and practice self-compassion.

C. Recognize that her life is so much bigger than this one issue, and shift the focus to other aspects of life where she can live her values, choose towards moves, and engage in what life has to offer.

Homework and the Next Session

For homework, hopefully your client takes the action that she committed to in the session. In the next session, we review how things turned out. Did the client follow through on her goals (or her plan B)? If so, what was that like? What difference did it make in her life? And what's the next step in this valued direction? If she didn't follow through on her goals, we explore what stopped her and take the necessary steps—as covered in this chapter—to get her moving again.

Extra Bits

See chapter 24 in *ACT Made Simple: The Extra Bits* (at http://www.actmindfully.com.au). There you'll find a HARD Barriers worksheet.

Skilling Up

A few suggestions:

- Fill in a HARD Barriers worksheet on yourself. Identify where you're getting stuck in an important area of your life and clarify what you can do to get moving again. Think of one small step you can take in a valued direction, and make a public commitment (for example, to a friend, colleague, or your partner) to follow through on it.

- If you follow through on your commitment, do it mindfully and notice what difference it makes in your life. If you don't follow through on it, identify what stopped you, in terms of HARD.

- Pick two cases where your client is stuck, and identify their probable barriers using HARD. Then write down some ideas about how you can get them moving again.

- Pick two or three cases where your client is stuck, and map the issue out on a choice point diagram, including costs and payoffs.

Takeaway

Our clients, just like us, often fail to follow through on doing things that will make life better. We want to normalize and validate this, identify what's getting in the way, and come up with effective strategies to overcome the barriers. The HARD acronym—Hooked, Avoiding discomfort, Remoteness from values, and Doubtful goals—is a good way for you and your clients to remember and identify common barriers to action.

CHAPTER 25

The Noticing Self

Warning: Tricky Concepts Ahead

Self-as-context, a.k.a. the noticing self, is without a doubt the trickiest, stickiest part of learning (and writing about) ACT. My mind is saying, *You can't do it! It's too complex. No way you're going to make this simple. You're just going to confuse everyone.* Well, thanks, mind! Now, let's have a crack at this…

Self-as-Context in a Nutshell

In Plain Language: *Self-as-context* is the part of you that does all the noticing. Metaphorically, it's like (a) a "safe place" inside you, where you can "open up" and "make room" for difficult thoughts and feelings, and (b) a "perspective" or "viewpoint" from which to "step back" and observe thoughts and feelings. We access this "psychological space" through actively noticing that we are noticing, or, in other words, through deliberately bringing awareness to our own awareness.

Aims: To enhance defusion, especially from the conceptualized self. To enhance acceptance, through accessing a safe and constant viewpoint from which to observe difficult inner experiences. To enhance flexible contact with the present moment. To experience a stable sense of self amid continual change. To experience a transcendent sense of self: that there's more to you than your body and your mind.

Synonyms: Self-as-perspective, the observing self, the noticing self, the observer self, the silent self, the transcendent self, pure awareness, the continuous you, the part of you that notices, the "I" that notices.

Method: Any ongoing mindfulness practice generally leads to an experience of self-as-context, sooner or later. We can enhance this through exercises that involve actively noticing your own noticing and metaphors that symbolize the noticing self.

When to Use: To facilitate acceptance, especially when the client is afraid of being harmed by her own inner experiences. To facilitate defusion, especially when the client is fused to self-concept. To facilitate a stable sense of self, especially when life is chaotic or involves dramatic changes. To facilitate a transcendent sense of self in response to traumatic events or as an aspect of spiritual growth.

Welcome to the Land of Confusion

Why is self-as-context is the most confusing part of the ACT model for almost everyone? Well, at least one big reason is that the term itself has two different meanings—both interconnected, yet also significantly different from each other. Most of the time, ACT textbooks use the term "self-as-context" to mean *the noticing self* (or *observer self*): that transcendent aspect of a human being that does all the mindful noticing of one's inner and outer world. You could call this experience "meta-awareness" or "pure awareness." This experience arises from the awareness of one's awareness, or the noticing of one's noticing, or the consciousness of one's consciousness. (Note: To call it a "self" or a "part" or an "aspect" is to speak metaphorically; technically, it's a repertoire of covert behavior.)

Less commonly, textbooks use the term "self-as-context" (SAC) to mean the process of *flexible perspective taking*. Flexible perspective taking underlies many ACT skills, including defusion, acceptance, contacting the present moment, self-awareness, self-reflection, empathy, compassion, theory of mind, and mental projection into the future or past. I've explored this less common meaning of SAC in my advanced textbook *Getting Unstuck in ACT* (Harris, 2013). In this book, to keep it simple, I'm mainly going to stick with the more traditional and widespread usage of the term: the noticing self or observer self; however, I will touch on the alternative meaning of SAC—flexible perspective taking—in chapter 27.

To add to the confusion, many textbooks also talk about something called "self-as-process." This term also has two meanings:

A. It describes the ongoing process of consciously noticing your thoughts, feelings, actions, and whatever you see, hear, touch, taste, and smell; arguably, a better term for this would be "self-awareness."

B. It describes the sense of self that arises from the process described above. Unfortunately, when the term is used in this way, many therapists find it hard if not impossible to distinguish it from self-as-context.

Because of such confusion, I'm not going to use the term "self-as-process" again. (Feel free to breathe a sigh of relief.)

But wait; we're not out of Confusionville just yet. We also need to talk about the *conceptualized self* or *self-concept*. This is all the beliefs, thoughts, ideas, facts, judgments, narratives, memories, and so on that interweave to form your self-concept or self-image: to describe "who you are" as a person, how you got that way, what your qualities are, what you are (and aren't) capable of doing, and so on. Fusion with self-concept shows up in therapy in a myriad of different forms: "I am broken," "I am defective," "I am worthless," "I am an addict," "I am superior," "I am inferior," "I am useless," and so on. (To add further to terminology confusion, many textbooks refer to the experience of fusion with your self-concept with terms such as "self-as-story" or "self-as-content.")

In summary, self-as-context is the locus from where noticing happens, the perspective or viewpoint from which noticing happens, the aspect of you that notices whatever it is that's being noticed.

In most textbooks and trainings, you'll find three broad classes of intervention that fall under this part of the hexaflex:

A. Metaphors for the noticing self

B. Experiential exercises that involve noticing your own noticing

C. Exercises to defuse from self-concept

We shall explore all of these shortly.

The Noticing Self Is Implicit in All Mindfulness

The basic mindfulness instruction "notice X" implies there's a locus or perspective from which X is noticed. And this locus or perspective never changes. I notice my thoughts, I notice my feelings, I notice my body, I notice the world outside my body—and I can even notice my own noticing. That which I am noticing changes continually. But the locus or perspective from which this noticing happens never changes: throughout life, everything is always noticed from a locus or perspective of I/here/now. And this unchanging locus from which we notice everything is what ACT calls *self-as-context*.

If you're struggling to make sense of this, it's not surprising, because the noticing self is an experience beyond all words. Whatever words we use to describe it, whatever images we create of it, whatever beliefs or concepts we formulate about it—they're not it! It's the nonverbal aspect of us that notices or observes all those words, images, beliefs, and concepts that we use to try and describe it. The closest we can get to this nonverbal experience in language is via metaphors, such as those that follow shortly. (Note: when you study relational frame theory, you'll discover it's not truly a nonverbal experience, but for our purposes, we can think of it that way.)

Getting to Self-as-Context

As with all six core processes, we can bring self-as-context into any session. In chapters 10 and 15, I talked about "planting seeds" of SAC throughout our sessions. If we've done this, then at any point in therapy where it seems useful, we can choose to actively "water" those seeds, using the methods in this chapter.

In most ACT protocols, self-as-context comes in after several sessions focused on defusion, acceptance, and flexible attention. We might say, "So you've been doing all this stuff that involves noticing—noticing thoughts, noticing feelings, noticing your breath, noticing your towards and away moves, and so on. And the odd thing is, this part of us that does all the noticing—well, we don't actually have a name for it in everyday language. The closest words we've got are 'consciousness' or 'awareness,' but they don't really nail it. Personally, I usually call it the 'noticing self' or 'the part of you that notices.' And the thing is, you're using this part of you all the time, in all of these different unhooking skills you've been learning. So it's kind of important. So would it be okay if we took a bit of time to explore this?"

If the client agrees, we would usually then explore SAC by first introducing a metaphor to "make sense" of SAC, and second, introducing a mindfulness exercise to actually experience it.

SAC Metaphors

There are many metaphors for SAC, but the Stage Show metaphor that follows is the simplest one I have found for easily giving clients a sense of this complex concept.

The Stage Show Metaphor

Therapist: Can I share an idea with you?

Client: Sure.

Therapist: Well, sometimes I think it's useful if we can look at life as if it's a huge stage show. Right? And it's a big stage, there's a lot of stuff going on. You've got all your thoughts and all your feelings, and everything you can see and hear and touch and taste and smell, and all the physical stuff you do with your body. And this show is changing all the time, from moment to moment. And, you know, sometimes what's up there on the stage is pretty amazing, but at other times, it's pretty dreadful, right?

Client: Uh-huh.

Therapist: And there's this part of you that can step back and watch the show. Always there, always watching. Can zoom in to any part of the show and take in the details, or zoom out and take in the big picture.

(Note: I find that most clients readily get this metaphor, and I often stop at this point. However, if we wish to tease out other transcendent qualities of SAC, such as its continuity, its unchanging presence, we could proceed as follows below.)

Therapist: And the thing is, that show is changing all the time, from moment to moment. But the part of you that watches it doesn't change. It's always there, always noticing, no matter what happens on the stage, no matter whether the show is great or awful.

* * *

We can tie this metaphor into earlier defusion and acceptance work: thoughts and feelings are like performers in the show, trying their hardest to get your full attention—and if you're not careful, they grab hold of you and pull you up onto the stage (fusion). Defusion and acceptance both involve stepping back from the stage, so you can see the performers more clearly and take in more of the show.

Two other popular metaphors are the Chessboard metaphor (Hayes et al., 1999) and the Sky and the Weather metaphor. These convey more of the spatial qualities of SAC: the sense of it as a "safe place" inside you, or a space or container for your thoughts and feelings; this makes them especially useful for enhancing acceptance. The Sky and the Weather metaphor follows below, and you'll find the Chessboard in Extra Bits.

The Sky and the Weather Metaphor

This excellent metaphor (found in Hinduism, Buddhism, and Taoism) compares the observing self to the sky. We can use this metaphor conversationally with our clients; however, I often prefer to say it at the end of a formal mindfulness exercise, as follows:

Therapist: Your noticing self is like the sky. Thoughts and feelings are like the weather. The weather changes continually, but no matter how bad it gets, it cannot harm the sky in any way. The mightiest thunderstorm, the most turbulent hurricane, the most severe winter blizzard—these things cannot hurt the sky. And no matter how bad the weather, the sky always has room for it—and sooner or later the weather always changes.

Now, sometimes we forget the sky is there, but it's still there. And sometimes we can't see the sky—it's obscured by clouds. But if we rise high enough above those clouds—even the thickest, darkest, thunderclouds—sooner or later we'll reach clear sky, stretching in all directions, boundless and pure. More and more, you can learn to access this part of you: a safe space inside from which to open up and make room for difficult thoughts and feelings; a safe viewpoint from which to step back and observe them.

Experiential Exercises: Notice Your Noticing

Almost no one will directly experience self-as-context from the metaphors mentioned above. These metaphors help us to conceptualize the noticing self and get an idea of its qualities, but they won't give us the actual experience; for that we need to do experiential exercises.

A simple way of bringing self-as-context into any mindfulness exercise is to slip in an instruction such as "And as you notice X (your breath/your thoughts/this sensation in your chest/the taste of the raisin on your tongue), be aware that you're noticing. There is X, and there's a part of you noticing X."

A variant on this might be "Recognize that there's a 'you' in there—a 'you' behind your eyes who is noticing all this."

The following exercise illustrates these kinds of instructions.

There Go Your Thoughts...

Therapist: Find a comfortable position, and close your eyes. Now notice: where are your thoughts? … Where do they seem to be located: above you, behind you, in front of you, to one side? (*Pause 10 seconds.*) And notice the form of those thoughts: are they pictures, words, or sounds? (*Pause 10 seconds.*) And notice—are they moving or still? … And if moving, what speed and what direction? (*Pause 10 seconds.*) Notice there are two separate processes going on here: there's a process of thinking—your mind is throwing up all sorts of words and pictures—and there's a process of noticing—there's a part of you noticing all those thoughts. (*Pause 10 seconds.*)

Now this gets your mind whirring, debating, and analyzing, so let's do it again.

Notice where your thoughts are located … Are they pictures or words; moving or still? (*Pause 10 seconds.*) So there go your thoughts—and there's a part of you able to notice them coming and going. Your thoughts keep changing. But the "you" that notices them does not change.

Now once again, this gets your mind whirring, debating, and analyzing, so let's just do that one last time. Notice: where are your thoughts? … Are they pictures or words; moving or still? … (*Pause 10 seconds.*) There go your thoughts—and there "you" are, observing them. Your thoughts change; the you that notices, does not.

> **Practical Tip**   There are many possible variants for the instructions in these exercises. We could say, "There's a part of you noticing," or "There you are noticing," or "Notice who is noticing," or "There's a part of you 'in there' noticing." Experiment and find what works best for you and your clients.

Talking and Listening

Here's another ultraquick exercise.

Therapist: For the next thirty seconds, silently listen in to what your mind is saying. And if your thoughts stop, just keep listening until they start again. (*Pause 30 seconds.*) So there you have it: there's a part of your mind that talks—the thinking part—and a part of your mind that listens—the noticing part.

The Continuous You

What follows is a much-shortened version of the classic Observer Self exercise from Hayes and colleagues (1999), often known as the "continuous you" exercise. The exercise seems complex, but it basically comprises five repeating instructions:

1.   Notice X.

2.   There is X—and there's a part of you noticing X.

3.   If you can notice X, you cannot be X.

4.   X is a part of you; and there's so much more to you than X.

5.   X changes; the part of you noticing X does not change.

X can include some or all of the following: your breath, your thoughts, your feelings, your physical body, the roles you play. With most clients, I run through the entire exercise in one go, which takes about fifteen minutes, but you can break it up into smaller sections and debrief each one as you go. I usually conclude this exercise with the Sky and the Weather metaphor, which has a strong impact.

Therapist: I invite you to sit up straight, with your feet flat on the floor, and either fix your eyes on a spot or close them … Notice the breath flowing in and out of your lungs … notice it coming in through the nostrils … down into the lungs … and back out again … And as you do that, be aware you're noticing … there goes your breath … and there you are noticing it. (*Pause 5 seconds.*) If you can notice your breath, you cannot be your breath. (*Pause 5 seconds.*) Your breath changes continually … sometimes shallow, sometimes deep … sometimes fast, sometimes slow … but the part of you that notices your breath does not change. (*Pause 5 seconds.*) And when you were a child, your lungs were so much smaller … but the you who could notice your breathing as a child is the same you who can notice it as an adult.

Now that gets your mind whirring, analyzing, philosophizing, debating … So take a step back and notice, where are your thoughts? … Where do they seem to be located? … Are they moving or still? … Are they pictures or words? (*Pause 5 seconds.*) And as you notice your thoughts, be aware you're noticing … there go your thoughts … and there you are noticing them. (*Pause 5 seconds.*) If you can notice your thoughts, you cannot be your thoughts. (*Pause 5 seconds.*) These thoughts are a part of you; and there's so much more to you than these thoughts. Your thoughts change continually … sometimes true, sometimes false … sometimes positive, sometimes negative … sometimes happy, sometimes sad … but the part of you that notices your thoughts does not change. (*Pause 5 seconds.*) And when you were a child, your thoughts were so very different than they are today … but the you who noticed your thoughts as a child is the same you who notices them as an adult. (*Pause 5 seconds.*)

Now, I don't expect your mind to agree to this. In fact, I expect that throughout the rest of this exercise, your mind will debate, analyze, attack, or intellectualize whatever I say, so see if you can let those thoughts come and go like passing cars, and engage in the exercise no matter how hard your mind tries to pull you out of it. (*Pause 5 seconds.*)

Now notice your body in the chair ... (*Pause 5 seconds.*) And as you do that, be aware you're noticing ... there is your body ... and there you are noticing it. (*Pause 5 seconds.*) It's not the same body you had as a baby, as a child, or as a teenager ... You may have had bits put into it or bits cut out of it ... You have scars, and wrinkles, and moles, and blemishes, and sunspots ... it's not the same skin you had in your youth, that's for sure ... But the part of you that notices your body never changes. (*Pause 5 seconds.*) As a child, when you looked in the mirror, your reflection was very different than it is today ... but the you who could notice your reflection back then is the same you that notices your reflection today. (*Pause 5 seconds.*)

Now quickly scan your body from head to toe, and notice the different feelings ... and zoom in on a feeling that captures your interest ... and observe it with curiosity ... noticing where it starts and stops ... and how deep in it goes ... and what its shape is ... and its temperature ... And as you notice this feeling ... just be aware you're noticing ... there is the feeling ... and there you are noticing it. (*Pause 5 seconds.*) If you can notice these feelings, you cannot be these feelings. (*Pause 5 seconds.*) These feelings are a part of you; and there's so much more to you than these feelings. Your feelings and sensations change continually ... sometimes you feel happy, sometimes you feel sad ... sometimes you feel healthy, sometimes you feel sick ... sometimes you feel stressed, sometimes relaxed ... but the part of you that notices your feelings does not change. (*Pause 5 seconds.*) And when you're frightened, angry, or sad in your life today ... the you who can notice those feelings is the same you that could notice your feelings as a child.

Now notice the role you're playing in this moment ... and as you do that, be aware you're noticing ... right now, you're playing the role of a client ... but your roles change continuously ... at times, you're in the role of a mother/father, son/daughter, brother/sister, friend, enemy, neighbor, rival, student, teacher, citizen, customer, worker, employer, employee, and so on.

(*Pause 5 seconds.*) And of course, there are some roles that you will never have again ... like the role of a young child ... and the role of a confused teenager (*Pause 5 seconds.*) But the you who notices your roles does not change ... It's the same you that could notice your roles—and all the things you say and do in them—even when you were very young.

We don't have a good name in everyday language for this part of you ... I'm going to call it the noticing self, but you don't have to call it that ... you can call it whatever you like ... and this noticing self is like the sky. (Finish the exercise with the Sky and the Weather metaphor.)

Longer versions of the exercise take the client back through several memories from different periods of her life and have her recognize that in each case, the noticing self was present when the memory was "recorded."

Many clients find this exercise a profoundly moving spiritual experience. However, it's better not to analyze it afterward or you run the risk of intellectualizing it.

Once you've introduced the noticing self, you can bring it into sessions as a brief intervention to enhance defusion and acceptance: "See if you can take a step back and look at this thought/feeling from the noticing self." You can see this play out in the following transcript, from a fourth session, following work on defusion, acceptance, and self-as-context. The client, a middle-aged woman, wants to tell her twenty-six-year-old son to move out of her home.

Client: (*looking pale, tense, agitated, and anxious*) I don't know if I can do it. I want to, I mean, I want him to go … I've had enough of him … but … I feel so … well, I'm his mother, aren't I? Oh, God. I can't stand this feeling.

Therapist: Take a step back for a moment and see if you can use that part of you that does all the noticing … Notice all those thoughts whizzing through your head … and all those feelings whirling around in your body … and notice your body sitting in the chair … and notice the room around you … what you can see and hear … including little old me, sitting over here … There's a whole stage show going on here—and there's a part of you in there that's able to step back and notice the show … Using that part of you, notice this feeling in your body … and recognize that it's one part of a much, much larger show … and there's a whole lot of other stuff also happening up there on that stage. Your mind says you can't stand this feeling, but when you use your noticing self to step back and look at it, is that really the case?

Client: No. It's—when I look at it like that, it's a bit easier.

Therapist: Easier to make room for it?

Client: Yeah.

The session now turns to an exploration of the mother's values. This reveals that asking her son to leave home is in the service of encouraging his independence, helping him to "grow up," and creating a home atmosphere conducive to greater intimacy with her husband. About ten minutes later, the therapist returns to the noticing self.

Therapist: For just a moment, can I get you back into contact with this noticing part? (*Client nods yes.*) Okay, so once again, just notice the thoughts passing through your mind … and notice the feelings surging through your body … and notice that the stage show has changed from a few minutes ago … but the part of you noticing the show has not changed.

The therapist goes through this brief exercise one more time near the end of the session, and then proceeds as follows.

Therapist: I wonder if you'd be willing to do this exercise two or three times a day—just take a moment to step back and notice the stage show. Notice that it changes all the time—there's a never-ending procession of new thoughts and feelings strutting their stuff on the stage. And as you do that, connect with the part of you that's noticing; see if you can really get that sense of how it's always there, always available, to help you zoom in and out of the show as need be.

Exercises to Defuse from Self-Concept

Clients will often say, "I have no self-esteem" or "I want more self-esteem." While there are different constructs of self-esteem, most of them boil down to this: self-esteem = building up a positive self-image. The majority of self-esteem programs place huge emphasis on evaluating yourself positively, focusing on your strong points, and trying to reduce or eliminate negative self-judgments. However, from an ACT perspective, fusing with your self-image is likely to create problems whether it is positive or negative. The following transcript of a defusion exercise makes this clear (I hope).

The Good Self/Bad Self Exercise

This is a simple but powerful exercise for defusion from self-concept. You'll need a paper and pen to do it.

Client: But high self-esteem is good, isn't it?

Therapist: Well, you have three young kids, right?

Client: Yeah.

Therapist: So suppose your mind tells you, *I am a wonderful mother. I do a brilliant job.* Now if you hold on tightly to that thought, there's no doubt it will give you high self-esteem. But what happens if you get completely hooked by it? Go through your day convinced you're a wonderful mom, doing a brilliant job with no need for improvement?

Client: (*chuckles*) Well, it's not true for a start.

Therapist: Okay, so one cost is you lose touch with reality. What else? What might happen to your relationship with your kids if you 100 percent believed that everything you did was wonderful?

Client: I guess I might not realize when I was doing things wrong.

Therapist:	Sure. You would lack self-awareness, and you'd probably become insensitive. And then you wouldn't grow and develop into a better mom because that only happens when you can see your mistakes and learn from them. Now let me ask you: suppose you could somehow be magically present at your own funeral—you're an angel or a friendly ghost or you're looking down from heaven—which of these would you want your kids to be saying: "Mom was really there for me when I needed her" or "Mom had a really high opinion of herself"?
Client:	(*laughs*) The first one. (*confused*) But can't self-esteem help me to be a better mom?
Therapist:	Good question. Would you be willing to do a little exercise with me, to find the answer?
Client:	Sure.
Therapist:	Cool. (*Therapist pulls out a blank sheet of paper.*) So when your mind wants to beat you up, what are some of the nastiest things it says to you?
Client:	(*sighs*) Same old stuff. I'm fat. And I'm dumb.
Therapist:	Okay. So this is the "bad self": "I'm fat" and "I'm dumb." Anything else? (*Therapist elicits a few more negative self-judgments and writes them all down on one side of the paper. He then turns the paper over.*) Now on those rare occasions when your mind is being nice to you, what are some of the nice things it says about you?
Client:	Um. I'm a good person. I'm kind to others.
Therapist:	Okay. So this is the "good self." "I'm a good person" and "I'm kind." Anything else? (*Therapist elicits a few more positive self-judgments and writes these all down on the flip side of the paper.*) This is a bit like that exercise we did a couple of sessions back. So if you're willing to, please hold the paper up in front of your face so you can read all the negative stuff. That's it—hold it right up in front of you so that's all you can see. (*Client holds the paper in front of her face, cutting off the therapist from her view.*) Hold it tightly. Get all caught up in your "bad self." Now, that's very low self-esteem, isn't it?
Client:	Yeah.
Therapist:	And imagine that directly in front of you is everything that's important in life; all the people and places and things and activities that matter to you. So while you're all caught up in these stories about yourself, what happens to the rest of your life?
Client:	It's gone.
Therapist:	Do you feel engaged, connected with the people you love and the stuff that matters?
Client:	No. I can't see it.

Therapist: Okay. Now turn the paper around, so you're looking at all those positive thoughts about yourself. That's it—and keep it up there right in front of your face. (*Client turns the paper around and continues to hold it up in front of her face.*) Now get all caught up in your "good self." Hold it tightly—let yourself get hooked with all those lovely positive thoughts. And now you've got really high self-esteem. But what's happening with the rest of your life, over here? Do you feel engaged, connected with the people you love and the stuff that matters?

Client: (*chuckling*) No.

Therapist: Okay. Now put the paper down on your lap. (*Client does so.*) Now, does that make any difference?

Client: (*Client looks at the therapist. They both grin.*) Much better.

Therapist: Easier to engage and connect with the stuff that matters?

Client: Yes.

Therapist: And notice, as long as you let it sit there in your lap, it doesn't matter which way up the paper is—good self, bad self doesn't matter—if you're not holding on to it or getting absorbed in it, it doesn't stop you from doing what you want to do. So in terms of being the sort of mom you want to be, what's more important? Trying to hold on tightly to all these thoughts about how good you are, and get away from the negative ones, or engaging and connecting with your kids and really being there for them?

Client: Being there for my kids, of course.

Who Am I?

At times, a client will ask, "Well, who am I then? If I'm not this story in my head, who am I?" If we're not careful, it's easy to get bogged down in deep, philosophical discussions at this point, and for our purposes in ACT, we don't wish to do that. We're coaches and therapists, not philosophers and gurus. So I usually reply along these lines: "That's a great question. There are many different ways we can talk about 'self,' but in everyday language, we tend to talk about it in just two ways: the physical self—our body—and the thinking self—our mind. But there's a third sense of self here that hardly ever gets mentioned: this 'noticing self,' which we can use to notice both our mind and our body. And you are all of these things: mind, body, and noticing self, all in one. So when we talk about these different 'selves' or 'parts' of you, that's just a convenient way of speaking. The reality is, you are one whole human being. There are no separate bits of you. No one has ever found a mind separate from a body, or a noticing self separate from a thinking self. These are just metaphors, ways of speaking about different aspects of being human."

Do We Have to Make Self-as-Context Explicit?

The answer to this question is no. In practice, many ACT therapists give SAC a backseat to the other five core processes and seldom mention it explicitly in therapy. One reason for this is that SAC is always implicit in any type of mindfulness practice, so as long as we're actively working with defusion, acceptance, and flexible attention, we're fostering the noticing self as a "side effect" or "by-product." Even when they do make SAC explicit, most ACT therapists don't use the terms "observing self" or "noticing self"; they're far more likely to talk about this "part of you that notices" or the "I that notices" or the "you that notices." There are five basic indications for explicitly working with SAC:

1. To enhance defusion, especially from the conceptualized self

2. To enhance acceptance of feared private experiences

3. To enhance flexible contact with the present moment

4. To access a stable sense of self

5. To access a transcendent sense of self

While it can be useful to make SAC explicit in order to achieve the first four aims, it's far from essential; these outcomes are all readily achievable through working directly on defusion, acceptance, and flexible attention skills. However, if we are aiming to achieve outcome 5, then explicit SAC work is usually necessary.

Homework and the Next Session

There are two ideas for homework in this chapter: the first involves contacting self-as-context, and the other involves defusing from self-concept. And, of course, we can make the Good Self/Bad Self exercise more specific: it could be good mother/bad mother, good therapist/bad therapist, or even good cop/bad cop.

Here's another simple option: we suggest that our client continue with any previous mindfulness practice and we add the instruction, "From now on, as you're doing that, from time to time, check in and see if you can notice that you are noticing."

You could also ask clients to practice mindfulness exercises that are explicitly oriented toward self-as-context. This is more effective if you have recorded the exercises in session or if your client has a commercial recording on a CD, MP3, or smartphone app.

Typically, we would now move on to more work with values and committed action, bringing in self-as-context experientially as needed.

Extra Bits

See chapter 25 in *ACT Made Simple: The Extra Bits* (at http://www.actmindfully.com.au). There you'll discover (a) a script for the Chessboard metaphor and a link to my YouTube animation of it, (b) a discussion of therapy versus mysticism, (c) what to do if clients ask, "Is this the soul?", and (d) what to do if clients can't access a noticing self.

Skilling Up

Don't say I didn't warn you: this is complicated stuff! But the good news is, practicing will help, so:

- Read all these exercises and metaphors out loud, and practice them as if you were working with clients.

- Pick two or three clients and for each one, identify thoughts, beliefs, judgments, and other self-descriptions that compose the conceptualized self. Consider how you could introduce self-as-context work with these clients—both brief interventions and longer ones.

- Try these exercises on yourself. In particular, pull out an index card and do the Good Self/ Bad Self exercise, and carry the card around with you for a week.

- If possible, have a friend or colleague take you through the Continuous You exercise—or record it yourself and then listen to it (or listen to my recording of it in the ACT Companion app).

Takeaway

Self-as-context has two meanings: flexible perspective taking (see chapter 27) and the noticing self. Implicit in all mindfulness, the noticing self is not really a "self" at all; rather, it is the locus or perspective from which we observe or notice everything else. Many mindfulness-based models of therapy never make self-as-context explicit; they rely on self-discovery through ongoing mindfulness meditation. However, in ACT we often like to make self-as-context explicit to enhance defusion, acceptance, and contacting the present moment, or to foster a stable or transcendent sense of self. We do this through three overlapping types of intervention: metaphors for the noticing self, experiential exercises that involve noticing your own noticing, and exercises to defuse from self-concept.

CHAPTER 26

Flexible Exposure

Exposure: A Changing Science

ACT is an exposure-based model. If you've got a degree in psychology, or you've trained in models such as eye movement desensitization and reprocessing (EMDR), cognitive behavioral therapy (CBT), dialectical behavior therapy (DBT), prolonged exposure (PE), and behavior analysis (BA), then you'll be familiar with the concept of exposure. If you don't have such a background, the concept may be completely new for you. Either way, it's important to know that exposure is at the very core of ACT; we're doing it all the time. However, exposure in ACT has significant differences from that in most other models.

What Is Exposure?

There is not one universally agreed-upon definition of exposure. However, most models of therapy that include it tend to define exposure something like this: "Organized contact with fear-evoking stimuli for the purpose of habituation." (Habituation, in everyday language, means "getting used" to the stimulus so that it is less distressing.) Fear-evoking stimuli may be external (e.g., social situations in social anxiety disorder, confined places in claustrophobia, spiders in arachnophobia) or internal (e.g., physical sensations in the body in panic disorder, traumatic memories in PTSD).

"OLD-SCHOOL" EXPOSURE

"Old-school" exposure, most commonly used in the treatment of anxiety disorders, encourages the client to stay in contact with these distressing stimuli until her distress level falls. Typically, such protocols emphasize the need for "graded exposure" via an "exposure hierarchy." This involves creating a step-by-step plan to progressively increase the degree of challenge in the exposure work. For example, suppose the issue is a spider phobia. An old-school exposure hierarchy might look like this:

Step 1. Talking about spiders

Step 2. Imagining spiders

Step 3. Looking at drawings of spiders

Step 4: Looking at photos of spiders

Step 5: Looking at videos of spiders

Step 6: Looking at real dead spiders in glass jars

Step 7: Looking at real living spiders in glass jars

Step 8: Looking at a real spider stationary on the floor or ceiling

Step 9: Looking at a real spider crawling on the floor or ceiling

While in contact with the fear-evoking stimuli, the client rates her level of distress through use of a subjective units of distress scale, or SUDS. Usually the SUDS is a scale of 0 to 10, where 10 means extremely distressed, anxious, or overwhelmed and 0 means calm, relaxed, no anxiety or distress. The therapist helps the client to remain in contact with the fear-evoking stimuli until her SUDS score drops.

Most treatment protocols consider exposure to be successful if the SUDS score drops by 50% (e.g., from an 8 out of 10 to a 4 out of 10). In other words, the primary aim of exposure in such protocols is to lower emotional distress (or the level of anxiety). If that outcome happens, exposure is considered successful. And if distress or anxiety levels don't significantly drop, exposure is deemed unsuccessful.

However, recent research based on *inhibitory learning theory* (Arch & Craske, 2011; Craske et al., 2008, Craske, Treanor, Conway, Zbozinek, & Vervliet, 2014) shows there is no correlation between the drop in distress or anxiety during exposure and the positive behavioral changes that result. In other words, clients can have no drop in distress or anxiety levels during exposure yet have significant positive behavioral changes as an outcome. Conversely, clients can have large drops in distress or anxiety levels during exposure yet have no positive behavioral change as an outcome. If this is surprising to you, please do read the papers cited above on inhibitory learning theory (which is rapidly becoming the new model of exposure in many types of CBT).

SO WHAT IS "NEW-SCHOOL" EXPOSURE?

In ACT, we define exposure somewhat differently from most other models: "Organized contact with *repertoire-narrowing* stimuli for the purpose of *increasing response flexibility.*"

"Repertoire-narrowing" basically means that behavior becomes rigid, inflexible, and limited—narrowing down to a small range of ineffective behavioral responses. (On the choice point, most if not all away moves would fit into this category.)

Our behavioral repertoires may be narrowed by all sorts of stimuli—not just by those that are fear-evoking, but also by those that evoke sadness, anger, guilt, shame, physical pain, loneliness, disgust, envy, jealousy, lust, greed, and so on. The difficult or challenging stimuli at the bottom of the choice point—situations, thoughts, and feelings—are (almost always) significantly repertoire-narrowing.

So the aim of exposure in ACT is not to reduce distress (although this frequently happens as a by-product). The aim is to increase our ability to respond more flexibly to the repertoire-narrowing stimulus. This *response flexibility* includes emotional flexibility, cognitive flexibility, and behavioral flexibility. (On the choice point, these new flexible responses are called towards moves.)

I call this "new-school" exposure because it's totally consistent with the cutting edge model of exposure that I mentioned above: *inhibitory learning theory*. (I'd love to tell you more about this theory and the research that supports it, but I don't have space, so I do strongly encourage you to read the references I mentioned above.)

Mindful, Values-Guided Exposure

In ACT, we practice mindful, values-guided exposure. In the service of our values, we take action, exposing ourselves to previously avoided or neglected people, places, situations, activities, and events. In other words, we expose ourselves to repertoire-narrowing stimuli "outside our skin."

We also practice exposing ourselves to repertoire-narrowing stimuli "inside our skin," such as difficult thoughts, memories, feelings, emotions, and sensations. We can use any or all of the four mindfulness processes—defusion, acceptance, flexible attention, and self-as-context—to facilitate this. In other words, when we consciously and deliberately turn toward difficult thoughts and feelings (repertoire-narrowing stimuli) with openness, curiosity, and flexibility (instead of a narrow, rigid behavioral repertoire), that is exposure. (Yes, acceptance is exposure!)

There are two types of exposure we practice in ACT: informal and formal.

Informal exposure. Informal exposure occurs throughout every session of ACT for every type of disorder. By informal, I mean spontaneous or unplanned exposure to the repertoire-narrowing stimuli (difficult thoughts, feelings, situations) that show up when we do ACT with anyone and everyone. Almost every intervention you've read in this book involves informal exposure. (The only exceptions are those things you do in moments when life is easy and there are no repertoire-narrowing stimuli present.)

Formal exposure. Formal exposure means planned, structured exposure routines, designed to target specific repertoire-narrowing stimuli (e.g., traumatic memories in PTSD, obsessions in obsessive-compulsive disorder, physical sensations of anxiety in panic disorder, social situations in social anxiety disorder, and painful emotions such as shame, guilt, fear, or anger in many types of clinical issues).

Rationale for Formal Exposure

The rationale for old-school exposure is to help clients lower their levels of anxiety. Obviously this rationale wouldn't fit ACT-style exposure because our aim in ACT is to increase psychological flexibility, not to avoid unwanted feelings. (Of course, anxiety levels do drop significantly with ACT, but this is a bonus, not the main aim. If you've forgotten the main aim, run through the Pushing Away Paper exercise in chapter 22 once again.)

The rationale for exposure in ACT is always to help clients live their values and act effectively. A choice point diagram can convey this very quickly. At the bottom of the choice point, we write in the repertoire-narrowing stimuli: people, places, objects, activities, thoughts, feelings, sensations, memories. Then we identify the away moves (current self-defeating narrow behavioral repertoires) and the desired towards moves (values-guided overt and covert behaviors the client would like to do instead).

Then we can summarize: "At the moment, when you encounter XYZ (repertoire-narrowing stimuli), you tend to do ABC (away moves). So our aim here is to learn a new way of responding to XYZ, so that if and when you encounter it in future, it can't push you around/run your life/hold you back/bring you down/stop you from doing what matters. This means we're going to have to spend a bit of time contacting/doing/being in the presence of XYZ, to learn this new way of responding."

Goodbye SUDS!

In old-school exposure, the emphasis on lowering distress or anxiety (through measuring drops in SUDS scores) easily reinforces the agenda of experiential avoidance. On top of that, as mentioned earlier, there is no correlation between a drop in SUDS score or anxiety levels and an outcome of effective behavioral change. Therefore, in ACT, we would not measure SUDS scores or rate anxiety levels during exposure.

Instead, we can create simple 0–10 scales to measure aspects of response flexibility, such as degree of acceptance or avoidance, degree of fusion or defusion, degree of presence/engagement, degree of control over physical actions, and degree of connection with values. A diagram that summarizes such measures follows. (However, speaking for myself as a clinician, the number one thing I want to see in my clients is not a change in numbers on a measurement scale, but the client actively living her values and engaging in life.)

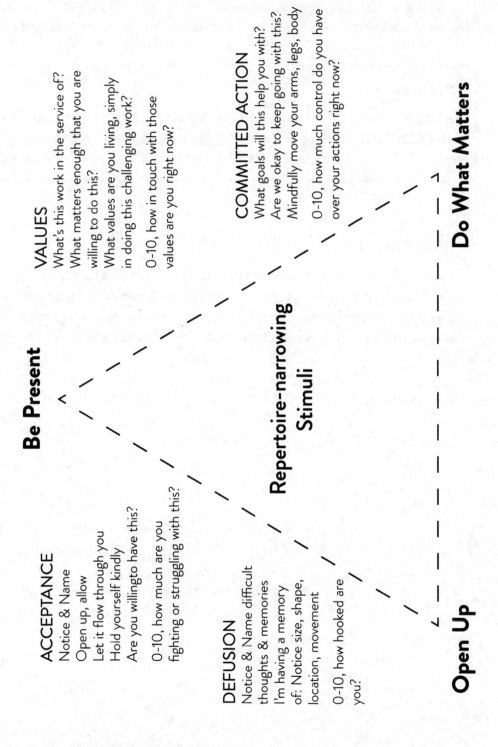

CONTACTING THE PRESENT MOMENT
Dropping anchor, Expansive awareness,
Mindful stretching, breathing, moving

0-10, how present are you right now?

Notice you and me, working together, as a team

VALUES
What's this work in the service of?
What matters enough that you are
willing to do this?
What values are you living, simply
in doing this challenging work?

0-10, how in touch with those
values are you right now?

COMMITTED ACTION
What goals will this help you with?
Are we okay to keep going with this?
Mindfully move your arms, legs, body

0-10, how much control do you have
over your actions right now?

Be Present

Do What Matters

**Repertoire-narrowing
Stimuli**

ACCEPTANCE
Notice & Name
Open up, allow
Let it flow through you
Hold yourself kindly
Are you willing to have this?

0-10, how much are you
fighting or struggling with this?

DEFUSION
Notice & Name difficult
thoughts & memories
I'm having a memory
of: Notice size, shape,
location, movement

0-10, how hooked are
you?

Open Up

Measuring Response Flexibility in Exposure

So if you wanted to combine models such as EMDR or PE with ACT, you could certainly do so, but you'd need to stop measuring SUDS and start measuring response flexibility instead.

Extra Bits

See chapter 26 in *ACT Made Simple: The Extra Bits* (at http://www.actmindfully.com.au). There you'll find (a) a printable copy of Measuring Response Flexibility in Exposure, (b) more materials on how to do formal exposure in ACT, and (c) resources for learning more about exposure.

Takeaway

Because of the way we define exposure in ACT, we can be incredibly flexible with the way we do it—arguably far more so than in any other exposure-based model. I hope you will start to recognize the ways in which you've already been doing informal exposure without even realizing it. And I hope you'll go on to learn more about it in advanced-level trainings and textbooks.

CHAPTER 27

Cognitive Flexibility

Yes, ACT Does Change Your Thinking!

One of the biggest misconceptions about ACT is that it "doesn't change your thinking." I hope and trust you can see that isn't the case. When clients (and therapists) encounter ACT, it usually dramatically changes the way they think about a vast range of topics and issues, including the nature and purpose of their own thoughts and emotions, the way they want to behave, the way they want to treat themselves and others, what they want their lives to be about, effective ways to live and act and deal with their problems, what motivates them, why they do the things they do, and so on.

However, ACT doesn't achieve this by challenging, disputing, disproving, or invalidating thoughts; nor does it help people to avoid, suppress, distract from, dismiss, or "rewrite" their thoughts or try to convert their "negative" thoughts into "positive" ones. ACT helps people to change their thinking through (a) defusing from unhelpful cognitions and cognitive processes and (b) developing new, more flexible and effective ways of thinking, *in addition* to their other cognitive patterns.

Why did I italicize the words *in addition*? Because we don't get to eliminate unhelpful cognitive repertoires. As the ACT saying goes, "There's no delete button in the brain." We can develop new ways of thinking, but that doesn't eliminate the old ones. As I say to clients, "If you learn to speak Hungarian, that won't eliminate English from your vocabulary." So again and again, we emphasize this important point to our clients in many different ways. For example: "Logically and rationally you know these thoughts aren't true—and that won't stop them from reappearing. Or: "Yes, you can see clearly that this pattern of thinking isn't helpful—and that won't stop your mind from doing it." Or: "So you know when this story hooks you, it pulls you into away moves—and knowing that won't get rid of the story; it will keep coming back."

Here are some of the main ways ACT actively fosters flexible thinking:

- Reframing

- Flexible perspective taking

- Compassion and self-compassion

- Flexible goal setting, problem solving, planning, and strategizing

- Conceiving your mind as a guide, coach, or friend

Reframing

There's a massive amount of reframing in the ACT model, most obviously *normalizing* and *validating*. Again and again we help clients to reframe their difficult, unwanted thoughts and feelings as "normal" rather than "abnormal," "valid" rather than "invalid." (Many models of therapy do this, of course, but ACT goes the extra mile.) Caveman mind metaphors reframe unhelpful cognitive processes as normal, valid, and purposeful. Defusion techniques reframe thoughts and images as nothing more or less than "words and pictures." The techniques in chapter 23 reframe emotions as allies with valuable resources rather than enemies to avoid at all costs. And values-based living powerfully reframes many popular notions of success and happiness.

Flexible Perspective Taking

You may recall that in ACT there are two meanings of the term "self-as-context" (SAC). Most commonly, SAC refers to the experience of the noticing self. Less commonly, the term refers to a wide range of behaviors collectively known as *flexible perspective taking* (FPT).

We can divide FPT interventions into two broad (but interconnected and overlapping) classes. One class includes all the mindfulness skills: defusion, acceptance, the noticing self, dropping anchor, and so on. All these skills involve flexibly changing your perspective: what you notice and how you notice it.

The other class of FPT interventions includes thinking skills that develop our ability to perceive events and understand concepts from alternative points of view—in everyday language, to "see things differently." For example, some exercises invite the client to imagine himself in the future looking back on his life today, and from that perspective, reflect on his current behavior. Others involve "inner-child" work, where the client imagines his current-day adult self going back in time to comfort and care for and instruct or support a child or adolescent version of himself.

Yet other interventions encourage clients to take the viewpoint of others:

- If your roles were reversed, how would you be feeling?

- If your roles were reversed, how would you want him to treat you?

- If you were in his shoes, what would you be thinking and feeling?

- If the same thing happened to someone you love, what would you say to them?

- What do you think she might be feeling/thinking/wanting/hoping for?

At times we may ask a client to take the perspective of her values-guided self. For example: "Right now, you're making a lot of very judgmental comments about your partner. And that's completely understandable, given all the difficulties you've been having. The problem is, when you get hooked by these thoughts, you tend to do things that make the relationship even worse, such as shouting, yelling, blaming, and name calling. So I'm just wondering—you said earlier that you want to be more loving, patient, and kind—so I'm wondering, if you were really able to be the sort of loving, patient, kind partner you want to be, how might you think about this differently? Is there another way of looking at this situation that might help you handle it better, in a way that's healthier for the relationship?"

We may even ask the client to take the perspective of parts of himself: "If this emotion could speak, what would it tell you to do?"

Compassion and Self-Compassion

ACT places great emphasis on both self-compassion and compassion for others. For many people, these are radically new ways of thinking. To consciously acknowledge suffering (our own or that of others) and remain open to it and curious about it instead of ignoring, dismissing, or turning away from it—and then respond with kindness (as opposed to judgment, hostility, or any other noncompassionate reaction)—does not come naturally or easily to most of us. Suppose we're in pain, and we say to ourselves, *This is a moment of suffering. Life is hard right now. Let's see what I can do to take care of myself.* This is obviously an extremely different way of thinking from ruminating (*Why am I feeling so bad? What's wrong with me?*) or self-criticizing (*I should be tougher than this. I'm such a pathetic loser*). Usually, we need to deliberately, actively, and regularly practice new patterns of thinking in order to develop our capacity for compassion—a difficult endeavor that many clients will actively resist.

Flexible Goal Setting, Problem Solving, Planning, and Strategizing

As we saw in chapter 21, committed action requires a lot of flexible thinking around goal setting, problem solving, action planning, and strategizing. These, in and of themselves, are new thinking skills for many clients.

When it comes to preparing for action, we may ask clients to consider:

- What's the worst thing that might happen? If it does, how will you deal with it? What can you do to reduce the likelihood of that?

- What's your plan B, if plan A falls through?

- What's the best thing that might happen? What can you do to increase the chances of that?

- What's most likely to happen? If it does, what next? If it doesn't, what next?

- What strategy are you going to use here? What will that require?

- Is there another way to think about this that might help you to handle it better?

Conceiving Your Mind as a Guide, Coach, or Friend

Last but not least, ACT often uses metaphors that compare our mind to a guide, coach, or friend. We can play with these metaphors in many ways to foster flexible thinking. Here are a few examples:

Wise Guide/Reckless Guide

Therapist: Sometimes our mind is a wise guide; it gives us great advice to help us get on in life. Other times, it's a reckless guide: encouraging us to take reckless risks or put ourselves in danger. So right now, which guide is talking?

Client: It's the reckless one.

Therapist: Okay. So what advice might the wise guide give you?

Overly Helpful Friend/Genuinely Helpful Friend

Therapist: Hmmm. Remember we talked about how our mind can sometimes be an "overly helpful friend"? Do you think that's maybe what it's doing right now? Suppose your mind wanted to be genuinely helpful, rather than overly helpful, what might it say about this?

Harsh Coach/Kind Coach

Therapist: You know, there are two types of coaches in school sports. There are harsh coaches, who yell at the kids, call them names, come down hard on every mistake, constantly judge, compare, and criticize. And there are kind coaches, who encourage the kids, build on their strengths, and give genuine feedback about mistakes in a kind and caring way. Good news is, the harsh coaches are a rapidly dying breed. Do you know why?

Client: Why?

Therapist: Because kind coaches get much better results. So right now, the way your mind is talking to you: is that harsh coach or kind coach?

Client: Harsh coach.

Therapist: So what would a kind coach say?

Extra Bits

See chapter 27 in *ACT Made Simple: The Extra Bits* (at http://www.actmindfully.com.au). There you'll find a discussion of both positive thinking and cognitive restructuring and their similarities to and differences from ACT.

Skilling Up

There are many variations on the theme of your mind as a guide, coach, or friend. We can compare the mind to an adviser, mentor, helper, assistant, or aide, and we can contrast different qualities: cautious versus careless, attentive versus inattentive, kind versus harsh, accepting versus judgmental, wise versus reckless, helpful versus unhelpful, and so on. So for practice:

- Play around with these ideas and see if you can come up with some versions of your own.

- Then think about some clients you might be able to use these with and try it out in session.

Takeaway

I hope you can see that ACT usually changes your thinking significantly. However, it doesn't do this through challenging, disputing, ignoring, dismissing, or distracting from difficult or unhelpful thoughts. It does this via (a) defusing from such thoughts, (b) accepting that they will keep recurring, and (c) at the same time, actively cultivating new, more flexible and effective ways of thinking.

CHAPTER 28

Shame, Anger, and Other "Problem" Emotions

What Makes an Emotion "Problematic"?

Therapists often ask me how to work with specific emotions, most commonly shame, guilt, and anger. I'm mostly going to focus on shame in this chapter (simply because it's the one most commonly asked about), but the principles we cover apply to any emotion.

When we work with any "difficult" emotion, we need to know specifically *how* the emotion is problematic for this client. Remember, in ACT, no emotion is inherently problematic, in and of itself. An emotion only becomes "problematic" or "difficult" when it interferes with a rich and meaningful life; and it only does this in a specific context of fusion, avoidance, and unworkable action.

So we want to ask questions to learn about the client's away moves and toward moves:

A. *Away moves:* What usually happens when this emotion hooks you and jerks you around? What do you tend to do that takes you away or pulls you out of the life you want? Does it capture your attention and take it away from more important things? Do you disengage, lose focus, get distracted?

B. *Towards moves:* If this emotion could no longer hook you and jerk you around, what would you stop doing or start doing, do more of or less of? How would you treat yourself, others, life, the world, differently? What goals would you pursue? What activities would you start or resume? What people, places, events, challenges, would you approach, face up to, deal with, handle better? What would you be better able to focus on or engage in? Who would you be more present with, focused on, or attentive to?

We can, if we wish, bring in our old friend the choice point as a visual aid to help us, and place the emotion at the very bottom. (Remember: we can do this with or without writing down all the answers on the diagram.)

Practical Tip   We often need to explain to our clients that "depression" is not an emotion. A simple way to do this is with the choice point. At the bottom, we put down the thoughts (e.g., *I'm not good enough*) and the emotions (e.g., anxiety, sadness, guilt, shame, anger). And then we map out all the away moves. We explain that the away moves are what we mean by "depression"—not the thoughts and feelings that trigger them.

Change the Context

In a context of fusion and avoidance, any emotion is problematic; this holds true for both painful emotions like shame, guilt, anger, anxiety, and sadness, and pleasant ones such as love and joy. In ACT, we aim to change such a context to one of defusion, acceptance, and values-guided action. In this new context, where the client is able to respond flexibly to the emotion (unhooking and doing towards moves), the emotion is no longer "problematic."

To help us in this work, it's often useful to deconstruct the problematic context into three elements, which we can then work with one at a time. Note that we don't do this in any specific order—we work flexibly, moment to moment, depending on what seems most relevant, useful, or likely to work for this client. In a context where any emotion has become problematic, we can expect to find all of the following elements:

1. Fusion

2. Experiential avoidance

3. Unworkable action

Let's see how this plays out in terms of shame.

Fusion and Shame

When working with shame, we expect to find fusion with:

- **The past**—especially rumination and the reliving of painful memories.

- **The future**—especially anxiety about the possibility of negative evaluation/hostility/rejection by others (particularly if these others were to discover the "truth" about the client's "shameful past").

- **Self-concept**—harsh negative self-judgment: *I am bad/broken/disgusting/unworthy/hopeless/undeserving of happiness.*

- **Reason-giving**—all the reasons why I can't or shouldn't even try to change: *Because in the past these shameful things happened, I can't change/I'm broken/I can't have relationships/I don't deserve a better life.*

Of course, we can find plenty of other types of fusion, too, but these tend to predominate in shame. With other emotions, such as anger and sadness, the cognitive content will differ, but most if not all of the six core categories of fusion (reasons, rules, judgments, past, future, self) are likely to be involved.

Experiential Avoidance and Shame

When working with shame, be aware that most clients are very keen to avoid or get rid of:

- **Unpleasant sensations or feelings of shame in the body.** These are often very similar to, or combined with, sensations/feelings of anxiety or dread (e.g., tight chest, churning stomach, or, in dissociative clients, "numbness").

- **Unpleasant cognitions**, especially harsh self-judgments, shame-evoking memories, and anxieties about negative evaluation or rejection by others.

- **Uncomfortable urges to do self-defeating actions** (e.g., to take drugs or alcohol, to self-harm, to socially isolate).

- **Other cognitions, feelings, and sensations related to other types of fusion.** For example, if fused with worthlessness, clients may notice feelings of lethargy, heaviness, or tiredness.

Again, as with any other "problematic emotion," we're likely to find that clients are trying to avoid sensations, feelings, cognitions, and urges.

Unworkable Action and Shame

Unworkable actions triggered by shame can vary enormously. Especially common are:

- Avoiding or withdrawing from important or meaningful people, places, events, activities, and situations that trigger shame

- The "usual suspects": behaviors that humans commonly do to avoid, escape, or get rid of pain (e.g., using drugs, alcohol, cigarettes, or food; addictive behaviors; distraction)

- Conflict with, criticism of, aggressiveness toward, or shaming of others

- Unconscious changes in body language (looking downward, avoiding eye contact)

- Covert behaviors such as ruminating, worrying, and disengaging

For any "problematic" emotion, we want to elicit both overt and covert patterns of unworkable action. These may vary quite a lot for different emotions; for example, with anger, we typically see lots of aggressive behavior, whereas with guilt, we often see excessive apologizing.

Important reminder: In ACT, a behavior is only considered "unworkable" in a context where it interferes with creating a rich and meaningful life. Used moderately, flexibly, and wisely, most of the strategies above are not unworkable, but when used excessively, rigidly, or inappropriately, they readily become problematic.

Shame vs. Guilt

Guilt typically refers to an uncomfortable emotion that we experience when we feel like we have DONE something bad—moved away from our core values, acted unlike the sort of person we want to be. *Shame* typically refers to an uncomfortable emotion that we experience when we feel like not only have we done something bad, but we ARE bad; so it includes a lot of fusion with harsh negative self-judgment: *I am a bad person.*

Simplistically speaking:

- Guilt = I've DONE something bad.

- Shame = I AM bad.

Many of us learn during training that "guilt is motivating—that it helps people identify what they've done wrong and motivates them to atone, amend, or get back in touch with their values and behave more congruently. At the same time we learn that shame is demotivating—it makes people "shut down" and avoid dealing effectively with their issues.

Well, there is some basis for this, but it's a gross oversimplification. After all, one of the key insights in ACT is that no emotion is good or bad in and of itself; it always depends on the context. In a context of fusion/avoidance, any emotion can be unhelpful, harmful, toxic, or life-distorting; and in a context of mindfulness and values, any emotion can be helpful or life-enhancing.

Guilt and shame are no exceptions. Guilt can be demotivating, and shame can be motivating; how the emotion functions will depend on the context. (We're right back to that functional contextualism stuff.) If we respond to shame mindfully and explore the values buried beneath it, it can be very motivating.

Learning History and Shame

We can help to foster defusion, self-acceptance, and self-compassion by looking at the client's learning history that led to such shame. For example, did the client's caregivers—or abusers or assailants—say things that fueled shame (e.g., "You deserve this," "You're a slut," "You brought this on yourself," "You should be ashamed of yourself")?

In cases of childhood abuse by a caregiver, we might discuss the following: A child unconsciously needs to maintain a positive view of her caregivers, no matter what they do wrong, because they are the child's life-support system. Consciously acknowledging that her "life support" is a source of threat and danger is terrifying for the child. Thus, when caregivers are abusive, the child's mind will often automatically and unconsciously blame the child for it: *It's my fault.* This helps protect the child from the terrifying and painful reality of her caregiver(s).

After such work, we can refer to "I am BAD" narratives as "old programming" and encourage defusion by saying, "Here's some old programming showing up."

Past Functions of Shame

It can be useful to look at how shame has functioned in the past in at least somewhat helpful or protective ways for the client (more technically, to examine the reinforcing consequences of shame). These may include:

Reducing punishment or hostility: If you look ashamed to others, then in some contexts, this will lessen their punishment, hostility, aggression, criticism, or judgment.

Eliciting support or kindness: If others know you feel ashamed, then in some contexts, this will elicit their sympathy, kindness, support, or forgiveness.

Avoiding pain: Often, in the grip of shame, people avoid people, places, situations, events, and activities that trigger difficult thoughts, feelings, and memories. So in the short term, shame helps them to escape or avoid pain. To take a common example, the downcast eyes of shame helps many clients to avoid the anxiety of eye contact with others—anxiety usually fueled by a fear of negative evaluation, rejection, or hostility.

Sense-making: Shame helps people to "make sense" of their experience: *These things happened because I am bad.* This can enable some children to make sense of abuse in a way that spares them from the terrible reality of their caregivers.

This kind of psychoeducation can play a useful role in normalizing and validating shame, which in turn promotes acceptance and helps to foster self-compassion. (Note: we don't *have to* explore past functions of shame; it's the present functions that matter. However, it can be useful to do so in the service of acceptance and self-compassion.)

Present Functions of Shame

If we've looked at past functions of shame (to normalize and validate the experience), it's important to then highlight the present functions. While shame will still often have some of the payoffs it had in the past, it clearly now also has some significant costs. Aside from the obvious—it's a very unpleasant feeling—the other detrimental functions of shame are usually easy to elicit through inquiry about away moves.

Once we have this information, we might say something like "So in the past, shame actually helped you in some ways, such as XYZ, but in the present, it's getting in the way of your being the person you want to be and doing the things you want to do, such as ABC. So would you be willing to learn some new skills here, so you can handle shame more effectively, reduce its impact on your life, take away its power, so you can start doing ABC again?"

Having established this rationale and motivation for learning ACT skills, we can frequently refer back to it, especially when the work gets challenging or the client lacks motivation.

Working with Shame (and Other "Problem" Emotions)

There are numerous approaches for working with shame (or anger, sadness, fear, guilt, anxiety, and so on). Below I will briefly touch upon many of them.

Body Posture and Shame

Shame is often (but not always) accompanied by characteristic changes in body posture. (For tips on working with posture, see Extra Bits.) These postural changes can include:

- Hanging the head down

- Limited eye-contact (e.g., looking at the floor or out of the window instead of at the therapist)

- Downcast or "hangdog" facial expression

- Slumped posture: drooping shoulders and arms, slumped spine

- Fidgeting uncomfortably when talking or thinking about anything shame related

- Covering eyes with a hand or holding head in hands

Note: In some clients, shame will at times trigger aggressive behavior, in which case we will likely see changes in body posture that typically accompany aggression.

Defusion and Shame

To help a client defuse from self-judgment, self-blame, painful memories, fear of negative evaluation or rejection by others, and so on, remember the two simple first steps for most defusion: noticing and naming. We can ask the client to notice what her mind is saying, how her mind is beating her up, how her mind is judging and blaming her, or how her mind is so quick to assume that other people will judge, criticize, or reject her.

We can also ask him to nonjudgmentally name his thoughts and feelings (e.g., *Here's shame*; *Here's my "I am BAD" schema*; *I'm having the thought that I'm BAD*; *I'm noticing self-judgment*; *I'm having thoughts that other people will judge me; Here is my mind trying to scare me; I'm having a feeling of shame; I'm noticing a feeling of shame;* or *I'm having a shameful memory*).

If we've looked at past and present functions of shame, we can use this information for defusion. The client might try noticing and naming his shame, along these lines: *Aha. Here you are again, shame. I know you're trying to help me or protect me, like you have in the past. But I don't need that sort of help anymore. Now I've got my values to help me.* Or a variant: *Aha. Here you are again, shame. Thanks for reminding me to practice self-compassion.*

Ideally, then, the client would mindfully reconnect with her values while defusing from the thoughts/memories and accepting the feelings/sensations of shame.

If we segue from noticing and naming to acceptance, the emphasis is on allowing and making room for whatever feelings and sensations the client has noticed and named. If, however, we segue more into defusion, the emphasis is on cognitions, and the aim is for the client to "see more clearly" what cognitions are: strings of words and pictures.

Note: When working with shame, it's wise to avoid zany defusion techniques like "thanking your mind" or "singing your thoughts"—at least in early sessions—because they can easily backfire and invalidate the client.

"Inner-Child" Imagery and Shame

In ACT, "inner-child" work usually takes the form of interactive experiential exercises. Typically, the therapist guides the client to vividly imagine herself, as she is today, traveling back in time to comfort and care for a childhood version of herself who is suffering. Often this is linked to an explicit memory of childhood trauma, abuse, or neglect. The therapist coaches the client—the adult self—to act compassionately toward the child self, offering comfort, solace, kindness, support, and wisdom, and to tell the child self the truth about the situation she is in (e.g., an abusive situation) so she understands that she (the child) hasn't done anything wrong; it's the adults who are at fault. The client tells the child self everything necessary for her to understand and make sense of the situation and to see that she is not to blame for what happened.

The exercises usually end with the adult self compassionately hugging or holding the child self and/or taking her to a safe place. (By the way, I'd never use the term "inner-child work" with a client because it has negative connotations for many people, especially therapy veterans. I'd simply say, "Would you be willing to do an exercise with me to help you with this issue?") You can find a script for this type of exercise in Extra Bits.

Acceptance and Shame

As you know, acceptance often begins with validation and normalization. In this case, we acknowledge that shame is a common and natural response (especially for survivors of trauma) and that the "I'm BAD" narrative is universal. From there, it's easy to segue to "noticing, naming, and allowing" the various thoughts, feelings, sensations, and memories that make up shame. Then we can use any combination of acceptance techniques we prefer. Dropping anchor is often useful, too—not to distract from shame but to discover there's a lot of other stuff here in this moment in addition to shame.

Shame as an Ally

Provided we respond mindfully, we can make good use of shame. We can use any or all of the interventions and principles in chapter 23 to turn shame into an ally.

Contacting the Present Moment and Shame

Contacting the present moment plays a major role in working with shame, including:

• Grounding and dropping anchor—essential skills to develop early in any client overwhelmed by shame or any emotion

• Fostering engagement, connection, and expansive awareness

• Noticing body posture and its effects, and experimenting with changes in body posture to promote engagement, centering, grounding, connection, communication, and vitality

• The initial noticing and acknowledging of thoughts, feelings, and memories that paves the way for defusion or acceptance

Self-Compassion and Shame

As with any painful emotion, we can respond to shame with any or all of the six building blocks of self-compassion we covered back in chapter 18:

1. Acknowledge the wound (i.e., notice the pain)

2. Be human (i.e., validate the pain)

3. Disarm the critic (i.e., defuse from harsh self-criticism)

4. Hold yourself kindly (in thoughts, words, and actions)

5. Make room for your pain (i.e., accept the pain)

6. See yourself in others (i.e., common humanity)

We can then, if desired, reframe "shame" as a reminder call to practice self-compassion.

Self-as-Context and Shame

You can use the "part of you that notices" to step back and observe the various elements of shame, including thoughts, feelings, sensations, and memories. You can notice that shame is not the essence of who you are; there is much more to you than these thoughts, feelings, sensations, and memories.

We can help clients to notice how the thoughts, feelings, sensations, and memories that together compose shame continually change over time, whereas the "part of you that notices" is unchanging.

Values and Shame

As clients become more flexible in the presence of shame—through defusion, acceptance, self-compassion, and so on—it becomes possible, and often very fruitful, to utilize their shame to explore values. We might ask:

- How would you treat, and/or what advice would you give to, a loved one who had been through similar events and felt the same way as you do?

- What does this shame tell you really matters to you that you need to address, face up to, take action on?

- What does shame remind you about the way you ideally want to treat yourself/others?

- What does shame tell you that you've lost/you need to be careful about/you want to stand up for/ you want to take a stand against/you deeply care about/you need to deal with?

- What does shame tell you about the way you'd like the world/yourself/others/life to be? What can you do to help make that happen?

From values we can readily segue to committed action.

Committed Action and Shame

Committed action involves instigating and reinforcing new, values-congruent repertoires of behavior (towards moves) as alternatives to the old "shame-driven" repertoires (away moves). This can include any or all of the following:

- Values-guided problem solving

- Values-guided goal setting and action planning

- Mindfulness skills training, practice, and application (e.g., defusion, acceptance, awareness, self-compassion, self-as-context skills) in the service of specific values and values-congruent goals

- Other relevant skills training in the service of specific values and values-congruent goals, especially training in relationship skills (e.g., communication, assertiveness, intimacy, and empathy skills).

Exposure and Shame

Many clients experience problematic narrowing of behavioral repertoires in the presence of shame. In particular, many clients' behavior becomes organized around trying to

A. avoid the thoughts, feelings, and memories that compose shame (experiential avoidance), and

B. avoid the situations, people, places, events, and activities that trigger shame (overt avoidance).

Hopefully you can see that nearly every intervention described above involves exposure. (If not, please go back and reread chapter 26.)

Acting Flexibly with Shame

It's important for the client to grasp that he can act flexibly, guided by values, in the presence of any thought, feeling, sensation, emotion, urge, image, or memory; he doesn't have to wait until it's gone. Nor does he need to let it control his actions.

This realization is usually most powerful when done as experiential work, and least effective when discussed in an intellectual or didactic manner (where it often ends with either the client insisting it's not possible or intellectually agreeing with the concept but without any idea of how to do it).

One simple experiential exercise is to have the client physically acting (e.g., taking control of her arms and legs—mindfully stretching, mindfully shifting position or changing posture, mindfully walking, mindfully eating, mindfully drinking, kind self-touching) while experiencing shame in session. The client then actually experiences that, even with shame present, she can still exert control over her actions.

Urge Surfing with Shame

Clients dealing with shame often experience urges to:

- take drugs or alcohol,

- harm themselves,

- withdraw socially,

- retreat from important but challenging situations, or

- engage in any number of self-defeating behaviors that enable short-term escape from pain.

The mindfulness exercise known as "urge surfing" (which incorporates acceptance, defusion, and contacting the present moment) is very useful for this kind of work. We can teach this to clients to help them "surf" their urges, without acting on them. They learn how to let an urge rise and fall, like a wave, without getting swept away by it. (You can download a script for urge surfing from Extra Bits.)

* * *

We can work with guilt, anger, anxiety, fear, sadness, envy, jealousy, disgust, loneliness, and so on in much the same way as we work with shame. In each case, we will identify fusion, avoidance, and unworkable action and target them with the relevant therapeutic processes. The specific thoughts, feelings, memories, sensations, urges, images, body postures, and unworkable actions will vary from emotion to emotion, but the core ACT processes we use to work with them will always be the same.

Extra Bits

See chapter 28 in *ACT Made Simple: The Extra Bits* (at http://www.actmindfully.com.au). There you'll discover (a) a script for urge surfing, (b) tips for working with anger, (c) a script for an inner-child imagery exercise, (d) "How to Work with Dissociation," and (e) tips for working with body posture.

Skilling Up

Of course, working with strong emotions takes practice:

- Think of two or three clients who are struggling with a strong emotion, such as shame or anger.

- Use the ideas in this chapter to generate at least four or five different ways you can help them handle it better.

Takeaway

Our aim in ACT is not to directly change the emotion itself but to change the context in which it arises. When the context changes from fusion and avoidance to mindfulness and values, the emotion functions differently. Of course, the emotion may still be very uncomfortable or painful, but it no longer functions in a way that is toxic, life-distorting, or self-defeating.

CHAPTER 29

Flexible Relationships

Living Well with Others

The great philosopher, Jean-Paul Sartre, famously said, "Hell is other people." However, he was only half right. Other people are also heaven. In other words, our relationships with others are a mixed bag; they bring wonder and dread, joy and fear, happiness and misery. When they're going well, relationships enrich and enhance our lives in a myriad of ways. And when they're going poorly, the pain is immense.

No surprise then that much of ACT focuses on relationships: enriching and enhancing them, dealing with the difficulties, and doing what works to build rich and meaningful connections. And remember, it's not passive acceptance therapy; we will help clients to end and leave their relationships, if that's the most effective course of action for improving their life.

In almost every client I've ever seen, with any type of issue, problem, or disorder—from trauma and addiction to depression and anxiety—relationship issues played a significant role. This makes sense. Why? Because any disorder is likely to negatively impact important close relationships, and the problems that result generally amplify the suffering. And at the same time, almost any client can significantly help herself through reaching out to supportive, caring others.

Given all this, I believe it's essential that every coach or therapist knows how to teach basic interpersonal skills. At the very least, this would include assertiveness skills, communication skills, negotiation skills, and conflict resolution skills. If clients are lacking these essential interpersonal skills, the ACT therapist would ideally teach them in session. (Personally, I like to do this through roleplay.) On the hexaflex, such skills training would come under the heading of committed action. (So if you're not up to speed in any or all of these coaching and therapy fundamentals, please do brush up on them as soon as you can; you really do need them, as do your clients.)

In this chapter, I'm going to give you some tips for applying ACT across a wide range of common interpersonal issues. For convenience, I'm going to focus on intimate partners. However, the principles we cover apply to any relationship: friends, family members, coworkers, teammates, fellow students, colleagues, employer and employee, parent and child, worker and boss, and so on. (Naturally, some of the questions and exercises would need to be modified or adapted for different relationships.)

Exploring Relationships

So what information do we need to gather, in order to help our clients improve their relationships? Let's zip through some basic lines of inquiry.

Who Matters?

Way back in chapter 6, when we looked at taking a history, we covered routine questions such as "Who are the most important people in your life?" "What are those relationships like?" "What kind of social life do you have?" "Who's there for you when you're having a hard time?" and "If this work could make a difference in just one relationship, which relationship would it be, and what would you do differently as a result?" Using such questions, we can quickly get a sense of the client's most important relationships, and the quality of them. This is a great starting point.

What's Good and Bad?

If our client wants to work on a particular relationship, we want to know both what's good and what's bad in that relationship. Useful questions include:

The Good

What do you like about your partner?

What do you see as your partner's strengths, good qualities?

What positive things does your partner say and do—in your relationship and outside of it?

Are there times when the relationship is going well (or not so badly)? When? Where? Doing what?

What things do you like doing together?

What helps you to get along better?

If I could watch you and your partner in those moments, what are the most helpful things I'd see each of you saying and doing?

The Bad

What do you dislike about your partner?

What do you see as your partner's weaknesses or poor qualities?

What negative things does your partner say and do—in your relationship and outside of it?

When is the relationship at its most challenging? What happens? What triggers it?

If I could watch you and your partner in those moments, what are the most unhelpful things I'd see each of you saying and doing?

What Do You Want?

When we focus in on any relationship, there are two important things to consider:

A. What do you want to give?

B. What do you want to get?

The first question leads to values: how you want to behave toward and treat your partner and what you want to contribute to the relationship. The second question leads to wants and needs: what you want to get from your partner and how you want her to treat you.

We want to get a picture of the sort of relationship the client wants to build and of what he's tried doing so far to try to make that happen. Useful questions include:

• If our work here is successful, how will your relationship change?

• What will you be doing differently?

• What will your partner be doing differently?

• What will you be doing less of and more of?

• What will your partner be doing less of and more of?

• How will your partner treat you differently?

• How will you treat your partner differently?

Some clients will be very focused on what they want to give the relationship and how they want to change; they are willing to work hard at living their values and behaving more like the sort of partner they want to be. Other clients are much more focused on what they want to get. They are often dissatisfied with the relationship, see their partner as the main problem, and are reluctant to look at their own role in the various ongoing issues. Needless to say, relationship work is usually a lot simpler and easier with the first scenario than with the second.

What Have You Tried, and How Has It Worked?

We want to explore all the different strategies the client has already tried to improve the relationship or deal with the difficulties and identify which ones have worked and which ones haven't. We often need to prompt the client by asking leading questions such as "Have you tried fighting, yelling, complaining, criticizing, demanding, blaming, judging, calling names, threatening? Have you tried withdrawing, going cold, going silent?"

If we identify workable strategies—that is, things the client says and does that help to build a healthier relationship in the long term—we then want to explore how the client can keep those going, and perhaps even do more of them.

Unfortunately, in most cases, we discover far more unworkable strategies than workable ones. So we want to tease this out in much the same way as we do with creative hopelessness. We help clients to recognize that many strategies that work in the short term to get their needs met don't work in the long term to build a healthy relationship. We might say, for example, "When you yell angrily at your partner and demand he does what you want, you may well get him to do it the short term, but in the long term it only fosters ill will and resentment."

Obviously, we do this exploration with the utmost of respect, empathy, and compassion, normalizing the clients' strategies and validating their painful thoughts and feelings. As clients recognize they have tried hard to improve the relationship yet many of their strategies simply make it worse in the long term, we hope they will become open to trying something new and very different.

The Challenge Formula

At this point, it's usually helpful to bring in the challenge formula (chapter 21). There are basically three options for dealing with the relationship:

1. Leave.

2. Stay and live by your values: change whatever you can to improve the situation and make room for the pain that goes with it.

3. Stay and give up acting effectively: do things that make no difference or make it worse.

We want to explore these options with the client. Sometimes leaving is the best option, for example with an abusive or narcissistic partner. If so, therapy will focus on the actions necessary to leave and how to overcome the internal and external barriers to doing so.

But if the client can't leave, won't leave, or is ambivalent about leaving, that leaves only options 2 and 3. Most clients, by this point, will readily see they've already been doing option 3 and would prefer to do option 2.

Workability

If your client says something like "It's all her fault. She's the problem. She needs to change, not me," we can validate her painful feelings, normalize her thoughts, and then compassionately bring in the concept of workability: "If you hold on tightly to those thoughts, what direction will they take you in? Will they help you try something new and different that might improve the relationship, or will they keep you doing more of the same stuff that's not working?"

Influence vs. Control

If the client is open to option 2, it's a good idea to address the issue of influence versus control.

Therapist: You know, we all get ourselves into trouble in relationships because we forget the big difference between influence and control.

Client: I'm not with you.

Therapist: Well, we can influence other people, but we can't actually control them. You know, even if you point a gun at someone's head, you don't have total control over them. Our history books are full of war heroes who chose to die rather than reveal secrets to the enemy.

Client: Okay.

Therapist: And basically, the way we influence other people is through what we say and what we do. We can influence through lying and deceiving or threatening and bullying or through being kind, fair, assertive, and honest, and you know, there are just so many different ways we can influence other people. The question is, do we want to have a good relationship with the other person? If so, then we need to focus on ways of influencing that person that are healthy for the relationship.

Client: Are you saying it's all up to me?

Therapist: I hope not. In the best of all possible worlds, both partners actively work on improving the relationship. The thing is, right now, you're the only one here. So, you know, if your partner wants to come in and work with me—or with another therapist—that'd be great. But until then, all we can really do is look at what you can do differently to influence your partner.

Client: But it's not my fault!

Therapist: Absolutely, it's not your fault. And please do let me know straight away if I ever say anything that makes you think I'm blaming you. What I'm saying is, if you want to improve the relationship, the most effective and powerful way to do that is to focus on what you have most control over, which is your words, your actions, the things that you say and do.

Client: (*unsure*) So what are you suggesting?

Therapist: I'm suggesting we look at more effective ways to influence your partner; new ways of saying and doing things that might work better both for you and for her.

At this point, some clients will come out with a bunch of reasons as to why they can't, shouldn't, or shouldn't even have to change: It's not my fault, it's hers; she should be the one to change; it won't work; I've tried before; I can't be bothered; I don't have the energy, and so on. If so, we can use the same method described in chapter 12 for defusion from barriers to therapy.

Further Exploration

Assuming that our client has chosen to stay in the relationship, important lines of inquiry include (a) how the client sees her partner and (b) what kind of partner the client wants to be.

How Do You See Your Partner?

At some point, sooner rather than later, we want to explore what happens when the client repeatedly criticizes, judges, or blames the other person. We want to validate that it's normal and natural to do so—we all have a tendency to do this—and then look at it in terms of workability.

Therapist: Do you see your partner as a rainbow or as a roadblock?

Client: What do you mean?

Therapist: Well, most of the time, do you see your partner as being like a rainbow—you know, a unique, magnificent work of nature that you can appreciate, that enriches your life—or do you tend to see him more like a roadblock—an obstacle getting in your way, stopping you from getting what you want in life?

Client: I guess I do tend to see him as a roadblock. But that's because he's always so bloody selfish!

Therapist: Look, I'm not trying to argue the point with you, I'm just wanting you to think about what effect this might have. I know that when people look at me as a roadblock, it doesn't feel good. Has anyone ever looked at you that way? Like you're just a problem, an obstacle, a barrier, getting in their way?

Client: For sure.

Therapist: And what was it like?

Client: Not good.

Therapist: So, you know, you said you're wanting to build a healthy relationship—and I'm wondering, if you keep looking at Tony like he's a roadblock, how's that going to play out?

Client: So what, I'm supposed to just ignore all his faults and worship him?

Therapist: Not at all. You want to face up to and address all those issues—but use your new influencing skills to address them in a way that's likely to get better results. And, in addition to that, I'm wondering if it might be helpful to learn how to unhook from some of these judgments and criticisms of Tony, so you're not constantly seeing him as a roadblock.

Client: But they're true!

Therapist: I hear you loud and clear. And remember, what we're interested in here is workability; if you get hooked by these thoughts, what happens? Does it pull you into towards moves that help you to build the relationship–

Client: No, it pulls me into away moves.

From here we may segue into defusion from blame, judgment, and criticism.

What Sort of Partner Do You Want to Be?

As soon as possible, we want to do some work around values, to explore "What sort of partner do you want to be?" We can use any type of values-clarification exercise for this purpose. I find the Connect and Reflect exercise (Harris, 2018) particularly useful. We ask the client to specifically recall a time when the relationship was good and she and her partner were doing something enjoyable, pleasurable, meaningful. We then get her to look at herself in that memory and identify the qualities she is bringing into the relationship.

Once we know the client's values as a partner, we can use these for motivation to change behavior and as a springboard for learning skills, setting goals, and creating action plans to build a better relationship.

Influencing Behavior 101: ACT with Love

Sessions may at this point get heavily into committed action, with a strong emphasis on learning and practicing negotiation, communication, and assertiveness skills: how to stand up for your rights, ask clearly for what you want, say no to what you don't want, set boundaries, negotiate effectively, and so on. Ideally, the therapist will role-play these skills with the client in session, so he can get in some practice before trying them out at home with his partner.

The therapist also provides essential psychoeducation about effective ways to influence the behavior of others: how to shape it gradually over time, with positive reinforcement of every step that's moving in the right direction (even if it's not exactly what you wanted). For example, if we've used the Donkeys, Carrots, and Sticks metaphor from chapter 18, we might say:

Therapist: So when you're trying to influence Tony's behavior, how much are you using the stick, and how much are you using the carrot?

Client: Mostly stick. But he deserves it.

Therapist: Well, I'm not going to debate that with you. Can I just ask you to notice that thought, and consider where it will take you, if you hold on tightly to it?

We can go on to explain that if we want a healthy relationship, we need a ratio of at least five times as many carrots as sticks. Carrots can be anything we say or do that constructively influences the other person's behavior in a way that's healthy for the relationship. Sometimes this may be as simple and basic as saying "please" instead of demanding, and "thank you" instead of taking things for granted.

Extra Bits

See chapter 29 in *ACT Made Simple: The Extra Bits* (at http://www.actmindfully.com.au). There you'll find some useful worksheets to help identify common relationship issues and conceptualize how to work with them within an ACT framework.

Skilling Up

Relationship issues affect all our clients, and there are many ways we can use ACT to help with them, including psychoeducation and skills training. Here are some important skills to have in your repertoire:

- If you don't know the four classic interpersonal skills—assertiveness, communication, negotiation, and conflict resolution—make it top priority to learn about them, pronto.

- Other relationship skills you'll want to brush up on are how to "fight fairly," make effective "repair attempts" after conflict, see things from your partner's perspective, build intimacy, give and receive constructive feedback (both positive and negative), and develop both self-compassion and compassion for your partner.

It's beyond the scope of this textbook to cover all these important topics, but you can find them all in my self-help book on common relationship issues: *ACT with Love* (Harris, 2006).

Takeaway

We encounter relationship issues all the time when working with ACT, especially when we start to explore values. The six core processes all play a major role in this work, and some clients will require active training in interpersonal skills in order to build healthier relationships.

PART 4

Wrapping Up

CHAPTER 30

I and Thou

The Therapeutic Relationship

As therapists or coaches, we aim to embody the entire ACT model in session: to be mindful, nonjudgmental, respectful, compassionate, centered, open, receptive, engaged, warm, and genuine. We regard the client as an equal: a fellow human being who, just like us, gets easily hooked by his thoughts and feelings and ends up struggling with life. In this chapter, we'll cover the key ways to create optimal therapeutic relationships.

Be Mindful

One of the greatest gifts we can give other humans is to make them the center of our attention in an atmosphere of openness, curiosity, and compassion. So we listen to our clients carefully, kindly, genuinely—with an open heart and an open mind. We listen compassionately to their struggles. We notice and validate their pain. We acknowledge how they've suffered. We ask them to be willingly vulnerable. And we create a compassionate, nonjudgmental space where all of this is possible. Through this mindful, caring interaction, we forge a strong, trusting, and open relationship.

In each and every session, we have the opportunity to bear witness to the pain and suffering of our client in a manner that perhaps no one else has ever done. We take the time to listen completely, carefully, and open-mindedly; to notice our client's body language and facial expressions; to respond genuinely and empathetically; and to validate her experience in the process. If we catch ourselves "tuning out," not paying full attention, or getting caught up in our thoughts, then the moment we realize it, we can gently acknowledge it and bring our attention back to our fellow human being. In this way, every session becomes a mindfulness practice in and of itself.

Ask Permission

"Is it okay if…?" "Could I ask you to…?" "Would you be willing to…?"—these are all useful ways to ask the client's permission. It's a key ingredient for building and maintaining rapport, especially when we're asking our clients to do exercises that are likely to bring up painful thoughts and feelings. The more painful the experience is likely to be, the more essential it is to know we have genuine permission—and not just an automatic yes response.

Say "I'm Sorry"

When we screw up, make a mistake, or offend, upset, or invalidate a client, then the moment we realize it, let's take action: acknowledge it, admit it, and give a genuine, heartfelt apology. We're modeling something very useful each time we do this; in many intimate relationships, there's a notable paucity of apologizing!

We might say something like "I'm really sorry. I've just realized what I've been doing here. I've been trying to convince you of something. You didn't come here so that I could force my belief systems on you. Can we please rewind here—go back to the point before I started trying to convince you—and start again from there?"

Be Playful

There's an ancient Zen saying: "The first sign of mental health is laughing at yourself." So let's bring some playfulness into our sessions. Playfulness, irreverence, and humor will often enhance rapport, and when laughter arises spontaneously in session, it's generally a good sign. (Of course, we need to be alert for insensitivity and invalidation. When a client is in crisis or sharing a heartbreaking story of pain and suffering, playfulness would be totally inappropriate.)

Self-Disclose, Appropriately and Wisely

We don't have to self-disclose to our clients, but ACT is very much in favor of it. ACT advocates appropriate and wise self-disclosure if and when it's likely to be beneficial to the client: to normalize and validate the client's experience, facilitate self-acceptance, model ACT for the client, or strengthen the therapeutic relationship. When our clients come into therapy, they're in a vulnerable position, which makes for a very unequal relationship. However, if we as therapists deliberately and openly share our own values and vulnerabilities, that helps to establish a powerful bond with our clients.

Obviously that doesn't mean we "dump on them" or say, "Hey, you think you've got problems—listen to mine!" We use self-disclosure judiciously—when it's likely to normalize and validate a client's experience, deepen the therapeutic alliance, or model something useful. Here are some forms of self-disclosure that could be helpful in the right context.

"I have to confess, that's thrown me…" When your client has said something that has thrown you, stunned you, or knocked you off your feet, it's often useful to admit it. You may then like to suggest a brief dropping anchor exercise so you can both ground and center yourselves.

"I feel disconnected from you," "I feel like I'm losing you," or **"It looks to me as if you're not fully here right now."** If you sense your client dissociating, disconnecting, withdrawing, detaching, disengaging, or wandering off inside her own mind, it's often helpful to draw attention to it—and to highlight what happens to your relationship with the client during these moments.

"I don't feel like we're a team here." If there is discord or tension in the relationship, we can respectfully and compassionately draw attention to it, and then go on to specify what we are noticing. For example, depending on what this tension is, we may say things like "I feel a bit like I've turned into an obstacle and you're trying to get around me," or "I feel like I'm pushing you and you're resisting," or "I could have this wrong, but I'm getting the vibe that I've upset or offended you, or you resent me for something." We can then explore the source of the discord or tension and take action to remedy any problems and repair the relationship.

"I'm noticing my mind pulling me in two different directions. On one hand, it's telling me ABC; on the other hand, it's telling me DEF. What's your take on each of those thoughts?" At times, we will have conflicting opinions about a given issue or situation. Again, in the right context, this can be useful to share.

Notice and Comment on Problematic Behavior As It Occurs

From time to time, we all have clients who behave "problematically" during the session—for example, they may endlessly rehash the same old story or continually blame everyone else for their problems without ever looking at their own role. When this happens, most of us have a tendency to grit our teeth and try and put up with it rather than openly address it.

Why do we do this? Usually because we either fuse with thoughts like *It would be rude of me to interrupt* or *She'll get upset with me*—or feelings of anxiety show up that we're not willing to have. At these times, it's very useful to explicitly model ACT. We could say something like "I'm noticing something happening here, and I want to bring it to your attention. My mind's telling me you're going to be upset or offended by what I say, and I'm noticing quite a lot of anxiety in my body, and a strong urge just to sit here and not say anything. However, I'm committed to helping you create the best life you can possibly have. And if I sit here and say nothing, then I'll be neglecting those values. So I'm going to do what matters here, even though my heart is racing—I'm going to tell you what I'm noticing."

Notice how, in doing this, we have explicitly modeled five of the six core ACT processes: defusion, acceptance, values, action, and contacting the present moment. And by now, we'll have our client's full attention! Then, with an attitude of openness and curiosity, defused from any judgments or criticisms, we describe the behavior we're noticing and point to the fact that it's preventing useful work in the session. From there, we may explore the purpose of the behavior or whether it plays out in other relationships and, if so, what are the consequences. We may also inquire about the client's thoughts and feelings in response to our observation—and do some work around acceptance and defusion if necessary.

Here's a shorter version: "I'm wanting to talk about something that I think is going on, and my mind's telling me that I'm going to come across as rude or insensitive…however, I don't want to let my mind talk me out of it because I think it's really important…so is it okay with you if I share what I think may be happening here?"

Declare Your Values

ACT advocates declaring our values to our clients. For example, we might say something like "I have one main aim in this room: to help people build a better life," or "The idea here is that you and I are a team, working together. And my aim is to help you, however I can, to turn your life around and make it better." When we declare our values genuinely, it's a powerful message that unites therapist and client in a common cause.

Slow Down and Lean In

"Slow down and lean in" is a phrase I picked up from a workshop with psychologist Robyn Walser. When we get stressed or anxious in response to what's happening in session, most of us tend to speed up—talk more, talk louder, give advice, start lecturing, and so on—or we lean back—disengage, tune out, withdraw. Obviously, this isn't helpful for the therapeutic relationship. So aim to do the very opposite: slow down and lean in! Notice your thoughts and feelings, notice your tendency to speed up and lean back. Connect with your values, and then lean in (both literally and metaphorically) and slow down. Talk less, talk slower, ask more, listen more, and pause frequently.

Defuse from Your Own Judgments

Of course we all aim to be nonjudgmental, and we may achieve that—for a while. But sooner or later, judgments will happen. Our mind is a well-oiled judgment machine; it won't stop judging for long. So when our judgments about our clients do pop up, the challenge is to recognize them and defuse from them, and to let them come and go without getting caught up in them. If we realize a judgment has hooked us, we can silently say name it—*Here's judgment!*—and gently refocus on our client.

Reveal Yourself as a Novice

When it comes to doing ACT, do you ever feel your heart racing or your stomach knotting? Do you ever have thoughts like *I don't know if I can do this* or *What if my client freaks out?* Or maybe you think, *I'll fumble my words, I'll screw it up, This is too hard,* or *I'll do it wrong.* If so, good. This shows that you're normal. Normal humans typically feel anxious whenever they move out of their comfort zone. However, if you fuse with the idea that you've got to do this stuff perfectly right from the word go or else your clients will react negatively, you're going to make life very hard for yourself. So if you're a total ACT newbie, why not take the pressure off yourself and admit it?

When I first started doing ACT, I said to each client, "Can I be totally honest with you? I'm a bit nervous about telling you this; my mind's telling me that you might lose some confidence in me. The truth is I'm a newbie to this ACT stuff. I really like the model, I've found it very helpful in my life, and obviously I think it's going to be useful for you or I wouldn't recommend it. However, because I'm a newbie, from time to time I might stumble or get a bit tongue-tied. And for some of the longer exercises, I may even need to pull out a book and use the scripts to read from. Would you be okay with that?"

As far as I can remember, no client ever reacted negatively to this spiel. Now obviously you don't have to disclose this, but many therapists find it useful to do so; we're giving ourselves permission to be imperfect, to stumble a little, to read from a script if we need to. And furthermore, we're modeling openness, authenticity, willingness, self-acceptance, and congruence.

Takeaway

Hopefully you can see that everything in this chapter follows quite naturally from applying ACT to yourself as a therapist or coach. And obviously this holds true for every relationship in your life: the more you act from a space of mindfulness and values, the healthier your relationships will be. So please don't confine ACT to the therapy room. Spend some time now reflecting on your most meaningful relationships and think about how ACT principles can enrich and enhance them. And then put it into practice and see how it works. You may be surprised!

CHAPTER 31

A Quick Guide to Getting Unstuck

Stuckness Happens

Here's my guarantee to you: As you start working with ACT, both you and your clients will get stuck. Repeatedly. I guarantee this will happen or your money back! Fortunately, ACT provides us with an incredibly powerful tool for getting unstuck: workability. Kirk Strosahl, one of the pioneers of ACT, says it this way: "When we're doing ACT, workability is our best friend."

From a stance of workability, we never need to judge, criticize, or attack a client's self-defeating behaviors; nor do we need to convince or persuade her to stop. Instead, we encourage her to look honestly and openly at her behavior and to assess whether it's a towards or an away move; in other words, is it helping her to be the sort of person she wants to be and act effectively to build the life she wants?

We always want to validate the reinforcing consequences for the behavior. For example, we might say, "What you're doing clearly has some payoffs. For example, it helps you to ABC, GHI, and PQR. So in the short term, what you're doing is useful. It's got real benefits." After this, we would go on to ask, compassionately and respectfully, questions such as:

- Is it working in the long run to make your life richer?

- Is it taking you closer to the life you really want?

- Is it helping you to be the person you want to be?

- Is it a towards move or an away move?

- Does it take you towards or away from the bull's eye?

It goes without saying, we need to be careful here: it's easy for us to start "bullying" our clients. Bullying basically means that we have already decided what will work for the client and what won't work (Strosahl, 2004). When we fuse with our own ideas about what is best or right for our client, we will impose our own agenda. Our client may then start saying the sorts of things we want to hear in order to please or appease us. If this happens, the exercise is empty because the client is not genuinely taking responsibility for his own life.

Using Workability to Get Unstuck

Strosahl warns us, "In order to use the workability strategy, you have to be relentlessly pragmatic and non-judgmental and to truly mean it. This is not a game, a trick or a form of therapeutic manipulation" (Strosahl, 2004, p. 226). Keeping this in mind, let's look at some of the many ways workability can help us.

Helping Us with Defusion

Workability enables rapid defusion, and it's particularly useful when a client insists that a thought is true. We can say, "The last thing I want to do with you is debate whether this thought is true or not. Is it okay if instead we take a look at what happens when this thought hooks you?" Then we can ask, "If you let this thought hook you and pull you around, where does it take you? What happens to your life in the long run?" or "When you're hooked by this thought, do you act like the person you want to be?" or "If you take the advice of this thought, will it help you to do the things you want to do?"

This is also useful when our clients start insisting change is impossible. For example, a client with an addiction may say, "I know this won't work for me. I've tried before. I've got no control over it." We can respond, "Okay, so your mind says, *This won't work. I've got no control.* Fair enough. That's the sort of stuff that minds say. I won't argue with that. I just want you to consider something. If we go along with that—if we let your mind dictate what happens in this room—then where do we go from here? Do we stop the session and give up?" We could then go on to say, "I fully expect your mind will keep telling you that this therapy won't work and you have no control. I don't know any way, other than major brain surgery, to stop that from happening. So can we let your mind say whatever it wants and give this a go anyway?"

This strategy also works well when clients insist that nasty negative self-judgments are true ("But it's true. I am fat/ugly/stupid/a loser"). We can say, "I don't know how to stop your mind from saying those things. My mind says similar judgmental things about me. The thing is, if you hold on tightly to these thoughts, get all caught up in them, does that help you? Does it help you to be the person you want to be, or do the things you want to do? If not, how about we practice learning to unhook from them?"

Helping Us with Clients Who Are Making Progress

Sometimes a client gets stuck because, although she has started doing something differently, the payoffs for this new behavior simply aren't enough to keep it going. To lessen this risk, if the client starts doing something "workable," we aim to amplify the reinforcing consequences for this new behavior by highlighting its very workability. For example, we could ask questions such as:

- What's it like when you act in this way?

- What happens to your life when you do this?

- What values are you living when you do this?

- Is this a towards or away move?

- Is this moving toward or away from the bull's eye?

- What happens to your sense of vitality when you do this? Are you more alive or less alive?

- Does this seem like it's aligned with ABC? (ABC = client's behavioral goals for therapy)

- So this is a different way of dealing with DEF. Does it seem better or worse than what you were doing before? (DEF = client's challenges, difficulties, problems, dilemmas)

It can also be useful to ask, "How did you do that? How did you make that happen? What did you do differently? What difficult thoughts and feelings did you need to make room for? Did your mind try to interfere? How did you unhook? So what does this tell you about what works in your life?"

Helping Us to Catch Ourselves

Because we're fallible human beings, it's inevitable that at times we'll try to persuade, convince, debate, or argue with our clients. In those moments, we obviously are not doing ACT. So whenever I catch myself doing this, I promptly apologize. I say, "I'm really sorry. I just realized what I've been doing. I've been trying to convince you/push you into something, and that's not my role here. It's not my place to impose my beliefs on you/tell you what to do with your life. We're supposed to be a team, working together, to discover what works in your life. So can we please just rewind to before I started debating with you?" Clients will almost always respond very positively to such openness.

We can then go on to ask something like "Can we bring this back to you and your experience rather than to what I think? Can I ask you to consider this question: regardless of what anyone else thinks, including me, if you keep doing what you're doing, is it working in the long run to make your life better? If it is, then by all means keep doing it, and let's focus on something else that's a problem for you. But if it's not, how about we take another look at it—but this time without me trying to convince you?"

Helping Us to Find Our Footing

When we're "lost" in a session or wondering where to go next in therapy, we can always come back to workability. We can ask, "On a scale of 0 to 10, how well is your life working? If 10 means you're spending each day behaving like the sort of person you want to be, doing the things that make your life meaningful, and 0 means you're spending each day behaving very much *unlike* the person you want to be, doing things that make your life worse rather than better, where are you on that scale?"

If a client scores highly—an 8 or a 9—then it's time to talk about wrapping up therapy. But if a client scores low—for example, a 3 or a 4—we could ask, "What would have to happen to get to a 5? What would you need to do differently? What's getting in the way of you doing that?" The client's answer will either give us information about further goals or reveal something about his psychological barriers.

Helping Us with "I've Got No Choice!"

Often, our most challenging clients will tell us they have no choice or no control over their actions. They will insist that when strong urges show up—to commit suicide, drink alcohol, take drugs, and so on—they have no choice but to "give in." Other clients may insist that they're powerless or hopeless or incapable of making change, or they may say things such as "Whenever I try to improve my life, it always goes wrong; I always fail or get hurt." We would first validate how much they have suffered: "Clearly this issue has created a lot of pain and difficulty for you. And you've tried hard, and so far nothing has worked." Then we would say, "And now you have a choice to make. One choice is to give up trying anything new, and carry on living the way you are. The other choice is to try doing something new and different, even though your mind says it's pointless and hopeless. The first choice comes with a guarantee: it's 100% guaranteed to keep your life going the way it is. The second choice doesn't have a guarantee. It's an experiment. We don't know for sure what will happen. But at least it's trying something new and different. At least it offers a chance of improving your life. So what are you going to choose?"

Helping Us with "But It Works!"

Some clients will insist that their self-defeating behavior works for them in the long run. Here are two classic examples: "Worrying helps me prepare for the worst" and "I like getting stoned. It's the only way I can relax." We need to validate that, yes, there are indeed some real benefits to these strategies, and at the same time, communicate that there are other ways to obtain those benefits that would be far more workable. To convey this, I use the following metaphor.

The Rickety Bicycle Metaphor

Therapist: You can cycle from New York to Mexico on a rickety old bicycle with bad suspension and a worn-out seat, and it will eventually get you there. But what condition will you be in by the time you arrive? There are many more effective ways to make that journey: cars, buses, trains, planes—or even a really good bicycle. So when you're… (*Name the client's behavior here, for example, getting stoned, doing all this worrying*), that's a lot like riding a rickety bicycle. Would you like to learn an alternative that will get you to your destination in a better condition?

After using the Rickety Bicycle metaphor, we teach the necessary skills (or we help the client access resources for learning them). For example, if our client wants to "prepare for the worst," we can teach him strategic planning and problem solving. If our client wants to relax, and marijuana is the only way she knows to do so, we can teach her relaxation skills (while being crystal clear about how they are radically different from mindfulness skills).

But wait…there's another big category of getting stuck: RESISTANCE.

Overcoming Resistance

In the right context, anyone would be resistant to therapy. Suppose you were being treated by a traditional healer in some foreign country. If he told you there was an evil spirit in your body and the only way to get rid of it was to eat a handful of live beetles, three times a day, would you be resistant?

Resistance in therapy generally boils down to a few key factors: treatment mismatch, reinforcing consequences, the therapeutic relationship, and the internal barriers referenced in the acronym HARD. Let's take a look at each of these now and how to prevent or overcome them.

Treatment Mismatch

Did you adequately obtain informed consent from your client for ACT? Did you explain what it involves? Was he expecting an "easy ride"? Did she just want someone to listen to her without expecting to do much work? Was he expecting something very different, such as long-term psychoanalysis? Did you clearly establish behavioral goals for therapy? Not everybody is open to ACT, and we may need to refer clients on or work with a different model. We can largely prevent this issue by (a) giving adequate information about ACT as part of informed consent (chapter 5) and (b) clearly establishing behavioral goals for therapy (chapter 6).

Reinforcing Consequences

Every problematic behavior has reinforcing consequences that maintain it. (And as you know, with clients we commonly call these "payoffs.") So what are the gains or benefits for this client (whether conscious or unconscious, intentional or not) if she continues to "stay stuck" (that is, if she keeps doing her problematic behaviors)? For example, does she get proceeds from a legal settlement; payment of disability benefits; or care, support, and attention from others while she's in the sick role? Does she get to avoid dealing with her challenges, and the inevitable anxiety that goes with them?

To address the issue of reinforcing consequences, we need to compassionately bring it into the client's awareness and gently, respectfully explore it, as we covered in chapter 24. (The choice point is often very useful for doing this.) For example, we might say, "If you keep doing this, it has benefits for you, such as X, Y, and Z. But does it work in the long run to build the life you want? What's it costing you to keep doing this?" or "I could be very wrong about this; is it okay if I tell you how I'm seeing it? Seems like, if you don't make any changes here, there are some genuine short-term benefits for you—such as A, B, and C. At the same time, there are some real long-term costs for you, such as X, Y, and Z. So, can I ask you, when you weigh up the benefits against the costs—how does it look to you?"

Therapeutic Relationship

A strong therapeutic relationship is essential for effective therapy. So is there room for improvement here? The best way to build and strengthen the therapeutic relationship is for us to embody ACT during our sessions (see chapter 30)—and look at our clients as rainbows rather than roadblocks.

The HARD Barriers to Change

In chapter 24, we discussed the HARD barriers to change: Hooked, Avoiding discomfort, Remoteness from values, Doubtful goals. Any or all of these factors play a major role in resistance. The key is to identify them and then target them with relevant ACT processes: defusion, acceptance, values, and SMART goals.

And of course, this goes for ourselves as therapists, too. We often avoid doing important aspects and elements of ACT because of our own HARD barriers: We get **Hooked** by *can't do it, won't work, client will react negatively, not important,* and so on. We **Avoid the discomfort** of experimenting with new tools, techniques, procedures, and processes. We become **Remote from our values** as a therapist, and therefore unwilling to leave our comfort zone and try new things. And we set **Doubtful goals** for ourselves as to when, where, and how much we will bring ACT into our work. So once again, a reminder: we must apply ACT to ourselves if we wish to do it well with others.

Resistance Is Fertile Ground

When our clients resist making behavioral changes, most of us tend to get frustrated or irritated, doubt our own abilities, blame the client, blame ourselves, or blame the ACT model. While this is normal, it isn't particularly helpful. A better alternative is simply to apply ACT to this issue itself.

In other words, whenever a client seems stuck, our first step is to look mindfully at what's happening, with openness and curiosity, and notice the thoughts and feelings showing up. We might say something like "Is it okay if we press pause for a moment? Take a step back and notice what's happening here?" Then we can nonjudgmentally explore the HARD factors involved.

Extra Bits

See chapter 31 in *ACT Made Simple: The Extra Bits* (at http://www.actmindfully.com.au) for the Getting Unstuck worksheet.

Skilling Up

Time for some practice:

- Play around with the concept of workability. Keep it in the back of your mind and use it as a resource for innovation in your work. Experiment with different ways of talking about it.

- Start looking at your own behavior through the lens of workability and notice what effect that has. In particular, look at what you do in your closest relationships. Instead of getting caught up in right/wrong or should/shouldn't (as we all do at times), start looking in a defused and accepting way at how workable your behavior is and whether there's any way you can improve on it.

- Think of one or two clients who seem stuck or resistant. Identify the factors that may be contributing to this and brainstorm ways you might respond. Use the Getting Unstuck worksheet from Extra bits to help you.

Takeaway

Whenever your clients seem stuck, resistant, or unmotivated, look for the HARD barriers to change and the reinforcing consequences maintaining problematic behavior, and respond with core ACT processes. Also consider the possibility of treatment mismatch or tension in the therapeutic relationship. And keep in mind, the whole ACT model rests on the concept of workability. When we rely on workability for motivation, we never have to coerce, persuade, or convince our clients to change; we simply open their eyes to the consequences of their actions and allow them to choose their own direction.

CHAPTER 32

The ACT Therapist's Journey

From Chunky and Clunky to Fluid and Flexible

When we're new to it, almost all of us do "chunky ACT." We slice up the model into six separate processes and center each session around a "chunk" of it. For example, we do a session where we mainly focus on defusion, then another focused mainly on values, and so on. That's completely natural, and a perfectly reasonable way to start our ACT journey. However, as we become more familiar with the model and we get to experience how the six core processes all interconnect and complement each other, our therapy becomes less "chunky" and more "blended." We learn to "dance around the hexaflex": to work explicitly with several or all processes in each session. Our therapy becomes more fluid, more flexible, more creative. We learn to modify and adapt our tools, techniques, and metaphors, and create new ones of our own (or borrow them from our clients).

I hope you've already started to appreciate the interconnectedness of this model. To get a better sense of it, spend some time studying the ACT hexaflex diagram (see chapter 1) and identify how each of the six components interacts with all the others. Also, as you reread this book or move on to other ACT textbooks, notice how virtually every intervention contains several overlapping core processes. For example, suppose we ask a client, "Even though your mind says you hate it, can you do an experiment? See if, even for one brief moment, you can sit with this feeling … notice where it is and what it's like … and see if you can use your noticing self to step back and look at it with a sense of curiosity." Here you have four explicit processes in one brief intervention: defusion, self-as-context, flexible attention, and acceptance. And if you look more closely, you'll see this intervention also includes values and committed action, although they are implicit, rather than explicit. Can you spot them? First, in ACT, acceptance is always in the service of values-based living, so this exercise in some way links to the client's values. Second, doing the exercise is (like any exercise) a form of committed action.

The journey from "chunky, clunky" ACT to "fluid, flexible" ACT requires time, practice, patience, persistence, and the willingness to make room for lots and lots of uncomfortable thoughts and feelings—especially anxiety and fear of failure. And the reality is, we're going to make mistakes.

Often and repeatedly. So remember the words of Sir Winston Churchill: "Success is the ability to go from failure to failure without loss of enthusiasm." For sure, we'll do things wrong. For sure, we'll screw it up. That's how we learn.

Think of any skill you take for granted today—reading, writing, walking, talking, opening doors, using a knife and fork. Whatever skill you pick, the fact is, you had to make many, many mistakes in order to learn it. And ACT is no different. It's a given you'll make mistakes, so be enthusiastic about that; turn them into opportunities for learning. Thank your mind for the "I'm a lousy therapist" story, practice self-compassion, and then reflect on the session with an attitude of openness and curiosity. Ask yourself, *What did I do that worked well? What did I do that didn't work? What did I miss? What did I fuse with? What could I do more of, less of, or differently next time around?* This is how we learn ACT.

Where to Next?

The sooner you start doing ACT, the better. After all, the only way to learn it is to do it. And I expect you'll find, like I did, that you'll immediately get positive results in your work. At the same time, I hope you'll be realistic. ACT is a big model. Let me rephrase that: ACT is a huuuuuge model. There are layers within layers within layers to this approach, and most therapists find that it takes at least a year of devoted practice, reading, and learning to get a thorough handle on ACT theory and implement it fluidly and flexibly with clients. So take your time—enjoy the journey, don't rush it. And remember Aesop's famous words: "Little by little does the trick."

In terms of further learning, I recommend that as soon as possible you attend a live ACT workshop or do some online training. It's very valuable to read books and listen to audio recordings, but this doesn't compare to attending live workshops or participating in online training. So in appendices A and C, I'll recommend a variety of resources that can take you further, and in appendix B, I'll talk about where you can find training and supervision.

Parting Words

With great reluctance, I'm going to leave you now with a few parting words.

Be Yourself

If you try to do ACT by parroting it word for word from a textbook, it's likely to come out sounding pretty stilted. So don't stick to the script. Modify and adapt; improvise; use your own words and your own style; be creative and innovative if you wish to. AND VERY IMPORTANTLY: if anything I suggest in this book doesn't suit your way of working, please either modify it or leave it out. If you read a few ACT books by different authors, or attend a few workshops with different trainers, you'll see wildly different ways of doing ACT, with many different tools, techniques, and methods. Again, this is because ACT is a process-based model, not technique-based, so the way you do ACT is likely to be somewhat different from the way others do it. (Isn't it great we can all be individuals?)

Practice, Practice, Practice

Whoever said "Practice makes perfect" was lying! But practice does lead to improvement. So if you haven't done any of the homework in this book, please take a look at what's stopping you. Have you fused with thoughts such as *Too hard*, *Too busy*, *Do it later*? Or are you trying to avoid the inevitable feelings of anxiety that come when you take risks, face challenges, or experiment with new behaviors? Have a look at your HARD barriers—and respond with the relevant ACT processes. Remember, the more you apply ACT to yourself, the better you'll be able to do it with others. (The reverse is also true: if you aren't using it on yourself, you won't do it well with others.)

Make Mistakes

I've said it before and I'll say it again: you will make mistakes and screw up. This is an inevitable part of learning. So when it happens, practice ACT on yourself. Unhook from harsh self-judgment. Open up and make room your frustration, anxiety, and disappointment. Hold yourself kindly. Then reflect on what you've done and learn from it—so that you and others can benefit from the experience.

Come Back to Your Values

Again and again and again, come back to your values. Connect with why you moved into this profession in the first place: your desire to help others, your desire to make a difference, your desire to make the world a better place. And take the time to appreciate the privilege of your work: the unique opportunity you have to see deeply into the hearts and souls of others and help them to connect with the healing forces inside them.

Acknowledgments

I'll begin with a Godzilla-sized thank you to my partner, Natasha, for all her love and support and for encouraging me to keep going when I was fused (repeatedly) with *This is all crap. It's too hard. I can't do it.*

And, as usual, I'd like to dump a zillion truckloads of gratitude on Steve Hayes, the originator of ACT—and that gratitude also extends to Kelly Wilson, Kirk Strosahl, Robyn Walser, and Hank Robb, all huge sources of inspiration for me. I also am very thankful to the entire ACT community, which is very supportive and inspirational; many ideas within these pages have arisen from discussions on the worldwide ACT Listserv and the forums of all my online courses.

Next I'd like to thank my agent, Sammie Justesen, for all her good work; and a heap of thanks to the entire team at New Harbinger—including Clancy Drake, Catherine Meyer, Jesse Burson, Michele Waters, and Matt McKay—for all the hard work, care, and attention they have invested in this book.

Editors are the unsung heroes of successful books, and so I'd like to sing my thanks to the heroic efforts of my editors on both editions of this book. Jean Blomquist truly had her work cut out with the first edition of this book, and Rona Bernstein has done a superb job in shaping and streamlining the second edition.

Thanks also to all those friends and colleagues who helped with the first edition of this book: Julian McNally, Georg Eifert, Hank Robb, Ros Lethbridge, and Carmel Harris; and also many thanks to Joe Ciarrochi and Ann Bailey, my cocreators of the earliest version of the choice point. On top of that, a truly humongous serving of thanks to Michael Brekelmans, who in the last four years has really pushed me to move in new directions and given me huge amounts of invaluable guidance along the way.

Last but not least, I want to thank my son, Max. While he is too young to help me with the book directly, he has helped enormously in a more indirect manner, simply by being in my life and filling it with so much love.

APPENDIX A

Resources

Free Resources

In addition to *ACT Made Simple: The Extra Bits*, there's a huge treasure trove of free materials—including audio recordings, eBooks, handouts and worksheets, YouTube videos, book chapters, articles, blogs, and published studies—available to you on the "Free Stuff" page of http://www.actmindfully.com.au. There you can also sign up for my quarterly newsletter, which distributes new free resources as I create them.

Books by Russ Harris

The Happiness Trap (Wollombi, NSW, Australia: Exisle Publishing, 2007)
The best-selling ACT self-help book, aimed at everyone and anyone. Over half a million copies sold; published in 30 languages.

The Reality Slap (Wollombi, NSW, Australia: Exisle Publishing, 2012)
An ACT-based self-help book for grief, loss, crisis, and trauma, with a major emphasis on self-compassion.

The Confidence Gap (Sydney, NSW, Australia: Exisle Publishing, 2011)
A self-help book that looks at confidence, success, and performance from an ACT perspective; especially suitable for life and executive coaching and sports and business performance.

ACT with Love (Oakland, CA: New Harbinger, 2009)
A popular self-help book on the use of ACT for common relationship issues. (By the way, you may have noticed my other three self-help books all have rhyming titles—*The Happiness Trap*, *The Reality Slap*, *The Confidence Gap*—but this one doesn't. I wanted to call it *The Relationship Crap*, but the publishers wouldn't let me.)

Getting Unstuck in ACT (Oakland, CA: New Harbinger, 2013)
The first advanced-level textbook on ACT. This does not cover the basics; it assumes you know them. Instead, it focuses on common sticking points for both clients and therapists.

ACT Questions & Answers (Oakland, CA: New Harbinger, 2018)
"Everything you wanted to know about ACT but were afraid to ask!" This is another advanced-level textbook, in an easy-to-read Q&A format. It covers all the tricky, sticky questions that other textbooks leave out.

Russ's Coauthored Books

The Illustrated Happiness Trap—by Russ Harris and Bev Aisbett (Boston, MA: Shambhala Publications, 2014)
A fun, comic-book version of the original—especially for teenagers and adults who are not into reading. (It's alternatively titled *The Happiness Trap Pocketbook* in the UK and Australia.)

The Weight Escape—by Joe Ciarrochi, Ann Bailey, and Russ Harris (Boston, MA: Shambhala Publications, 2014)
A self-help book on the ACT approach to fitness and weight loss.

Online Training—Public and Professional

The Happiness Trap Online: 8-Week Program

This is a personal-growth program for well-being and vitality, inspired by and adapted from the book *The Happiness Trap*. It's a beautifully filmed and very entertaining online course, developed for the general public—suitable for pretty much everyone. We've also designed a version of the program that therapists can use with clients as an adjunct to their therapy sessions. Find out more at http://www.TheHappinessTrap.com.

I'm Learning Act: Online Courses

In case you don't make it to appendix B, I want to mention this here: I have created a range of online training courses in ACT, from beginner to advanced level, covering everything from trauma to adolescents. They are available at http://www.ImLearningACT.com.

MP3s

I have three albums of MP3s that you can purchase from http://www.actmindfully.com.au: Mindfulness Skills Volume 1, Mindfulness Skills Volume 2, and Exercises and Meditations from *The Reality Slap* (a companion to the book of the same title). Sorry, the CDs are no longer available because not many people use them these days; that's modern technology for ya!

ACT Companion: Smartphone App

Australian psychologist Anthony Berrick created this app for use as an adjunct to therapy. It's loaded with cool ACT tools, including the choice point, and contains over two hours of audio recordings (some with my voice, some with Anthony's).

Values Cards

I've created a pack of full-color values cards containing simple descriptions of values accompanied by delightful cartoons. More specifically, they're "values, goals, and barriers" cards; they contain extra cards for goal setting, action planning, and dealing with barriers such as values conflicts, fusion, and so on. You can purchase these at http://www.actmindfully.com.au.

Facebook Group

The ACT Made Simple Facebook group is an online community where you can share resources, ask questions, discuss struggles and successes, get the latest updates and new free materials from me, and so much more. Just go to Facebook and search for "ACT Made Simple."

Further Training

Live Workshops

I run stacks of live workshops all around Australia, throughout the year. (Unfortunately, I rarely make it overseas because of the long travel times and horrendous jet lag, but you can attend my online trainings, described below.) My workshops include ACT for Beginners, ACT for Depression and Anxiety Disorders, ACT for Trauma, and ACT for Relationships. You can find details at http://www.actmindfully.com.au.

Online Courses

I offer a range of online courses in ACT, where you can interact with me via a forum, watch videos of therapy sessions, and access a stack of specially designed audio, visual, and text-based training materials. The scope is continually expanding; at the time of writing it includes the following six-week courses:

ACT for Beginners

ACT for Depression and Anxiety Disorders

ACT for Trauma

ACT for Adolescents

For more information go to http://www.ImLearningACT.com.

ACBS Website

The mothership organization of ACT and RFT (relational frame theory) is ACBS: the Association for Contextual Behavioral Science. The website is truly vast, and in addition to many free resources, you can find details on ACT trainings, workshops, courses, and conferences worldwide. You can also join numerous forums and special interest groups, find an ACT supervisor, find an ACT therapist, and much, much more. Go to https://www.contextualscience.org.

Further Reading on ACT and RFT

Numerous ACT textbooks and self-help books now exist, the majority of them published by New Harbinger. Visit the New Harbinger website at http://www.newharbinger.com to get a sense of the scope. The textbooks cover the application of ACT to a wide range of issues and conditions, from chronic pain and psychosis to depression and anxiety disorders. As I've already listed my own books in appendix A, I won't include them here. Instead, I'll mention two books that stand out in terms of clinical skills building:

Acceptance and Commitment Therapy: An Experiential Approach to Behavior Change by Steve Hayes, Kirk Strosahl, and Kelly Wilson (New York, NY: Guilford Press, 1999)
This is the ground-breaking theoretical and philosophical text that first introduced ACT to the world; you'll find it widely cited in every other textbook on ACT.

Learning ACT by Jason Luoma, Steve Hayes, and Robyn Walser (Oakland, CA: Context Press–New Harbinger, 2017)
This step-by-step skills-training manual for ACT therapists lives up to its description as "the most comprehensive guide to utilizing ACT in your clinical practice."

Two other books are particularly useful for learning more about relational frame theory (RFT) and other theoretical underpinnings of ACT:

The ABCs of Human Behavior: Behavioral Principles for the Practicing Clinician by Jonas Ramnerö and Niklas Törneke (Oakland, CA: New Harbinger, 2008)
This is an excellent book on the science, theory, and philosophy of functional contextualism, behavioral analysis, and RFT.

Learning RFT by Niklas Törneke (Oakland, CA: New Harbinger, 2010)
If you want to learn the nuts and bolts of RFT and how it underpins ACT, this is a great place to start.

References

American Psychiatric Association. (2013). Diagnostic and statistical manual of mental disorders (5th ed.). Washington, DC: Author.

Arch, J. J., & Craske, M. G. (2011). Addressing relapse in cognitive behavioral therapy for panic disorder: Methods for optimizing long-term treatment outcomes. *Cognitive and Behavioral Practice, 18,* 306–315.

Bach, P., & Hayes, S. C. (2002). The use of acceptance and commitment therapy to prevent the rehospitalization of psychotic patients: A randomized controlled trial. *Journal of Consulting and Clinical Psychology, 70,* 1129–1139.

Bach, P., & Moran, D. J. (2008). *ACT in practice.* Oakland, CA: New Harbinger.

Bond, F. W., & Bunce, D. (2000). Mediators of change in emotion-focused and problem-focused worksite stress management interventions. *Journal of Occupational Health Psychology, 5*(1), 156–163.

Bond, F. W., Hayes, S. C., Baer, R. A., Carpenter, K. M., Guenole, N., Orcutt, H. K.,…Zettle, R. D. (2011). Preliminary psychometric properties of the Acceptance and Action Questionnaire—II: A revised measure of psychological flexibility and experiential avoidance. *Behavior Therapy, 42,* 676–688.

Brann, P., Gopold, M., Guymer, E., Morton, J., & Snowdon, S. (2007–09). Forty-session acceptance and commitment therapy group for public-sector mental health service clients with four or more criteria of borderline personality disorder. A program of Spectrum: The Borderline Personality Disorder Service for Victoria (Melbourne, Victoria, Australia).

Branstetter, A. D., Wilson, K. G., Hildebrandt, M., & Mutch, D. (2004, November). Improving psychological adjustment among cancer patients: ACT and CBT. Paper presented at the meeting of the Association for Advancement of Behavior Therapy, New Orleans, LA.

Brown, R. A., Palm, K. M., Strong, D. R., Lejuez, C. W., Kahler, C. W., Zvolensky, M. J.,…Gifford, E. V. (2008). Distress tolerance treatment for early-lapse smokers: Rationale, program description, and preliminary findings. *Behavior Modification, 32*(3), 302–332.

Ciarrochi, J., Bailey, A., & Harris, R. (2014). *The weight escape: How to stop dieting and start living.* Boston, MA: Shambhala Publications.

Craske, M, G., Kircanski, K. Zelikowsky, M., Mystkowski, J., Chowdhury, N., & Baker, A. (2008). Optimizing inhibitory learning during exposure therapy. *Behaviour Research and Therapy, 46,* 5–27.

Craske, M. G., Treanor, M., Conway, C. C., Zbozinek, T., & Vervliet, B. (2014). Maximizing exposure therapy: An inhibitory learning approach. *Behaviour Research and Therapy, 58,* 10–23.

Dahl, J., Wilson, K. G., & Nilsson, A. (2004). Acceptance and commitment therapy and the treatment of persons at risk for long-term disability resulting from stress and pain symptoms: A preliminary randomized trial. *Behavior Therapy, 35*(4), 785–801.

Dalrymple, K. L., & Herbert, J. D. (2007). Acceptance and commitment therapy for generalized social anxiety disorder: A pilot study. *Behavior Modification, 31,* 543–568.

Eifert, G., & Forsyth, J. P. (2005). *Acceptance and commitment therapy for anxiety disorders.* Oakland, CA: New Harbinger.

Epping-Jordan, J. E., Harris, R., Brown, F., Carswell, K., Foley, C., García-Moreno, C.,...van Ommeren, M. (2016). Self-Help Plus (SH+): A new WHO stress management package. *World Psychiatry, 15*(3), 295–296.

Feldner, M., Zvolensky, M., Eifert, G., & Spira, A. (2003). Emotional avoidance: An experimental test of individual differences and response suppression using biological challenge. *Behaviour Research and Therapy, 41*(4), 403–411.

Gaudiano, B. A., & Herbert, J. D. (2006). Acute treatment of inpatients with psychotic symptoms using acceptance and commitment therapy: Pilot results. *Behaviour Research and Therapy, 44*(3), 415–437.

Gifford, E. V., Kohlenberg, B. S., Hayes, S. C., Antonuccio, D. O., Piasecki, M. M., Rasmussen-Hall, M. L., & Palm, K. M. (2004). Acceptance theory–based treatment for smoking cessation: An initial trial of acceptance and commitment therapy. *Behavior Therapy, 35*, 689–706.

Gratz, K. L., & Gunderson, J. G. (2006). Preliminary data on an acceptance-based emotion regulation group intervention for deliberate self-harm among women with borderline personality disorder. *Behavior Therapy, 37*(1), 25–35.

Gregg, J. A., Callaghan, G. M., Hayes, S. C., & Glenn-Lawson, J. L. (2007). Improving diabetes self-management through acceptance, mindfulness, and values: A randomized controlled trial. *Journal of Consulting and Clinical Psychology, 75*(2), 336–343.

Harris, R. (2007). *The happiness trap: Stop struggling, start living.* Wollombi, NSW, Australia: Exisle Publishing.

Harris, R. (2009a). ACT made simple: *An easy-to-read primer on acceptance and commitment therapy.* Oakland, CA: New Harbinger.

Harris, R. (2009b). ACT *with love: Stop struggling, reconcile differences, and strengthen your relationship with acceptance and commitment therapy.* Oakland, CA: New Harbinger.

Harris, R. (2011). *The confidence gap: A guide to overcoming fear and self-doubt.* Sydney, NSW, Australia: Penguin Books Australia.

Harris, R. (2012). *The reality slap: Finding peace and fulfillment when life hurts.* Wollombi, NSW, Australia: Exisle Publishing.

Harris, R. (2013). *Getting unstuck in ACT: A clinician's guide to overcoming common obstacles in acceptance and commitment therapy.* Oakland, CA: New Harbinger.

Harris, R. (2018). ACT *questions and answers: A practitioner's guide to 150 common sticking points in acceptance and commitment therapy.* Oakland, CA: New Harbinger.

Harris, R., & Aisbett, B. (2014). *The illustrated happiness trap: How to stop struggling and start living.* Boston, MA: Shambhala Publications.

Hayes, S. C., Bissett, R., Roget, N., Padilla, M., Kohlenberg, B. S., Fisher, G.,...Niccolls, R.. (2004). The impact of acceptance and commitment training and multicultural training on the stigmatizing attitudes and professional burnout of substance abuse counselors. *Behavior Therapy, 35*(4), 821–835.

Hayes, S. C., Bond, F. W., Barnes-Holmes, D., & Austin, J. (2006). *Acceptance and mindfulness at work.* New York, NY: The Haworth Press.

Hayes, S. C., Masuda, A., Bissett, R., Luoma, J., & Guerrero, L. F. (2004). DBT, FAP, and ACT: How empirically oriented are the new behavior therapy technologies? *Behavior Therapy, 35*, 35–54.

Hayes, S. C., Strosahl, K. D., & Wilson, K. G. (1999). *Acceptance and commitment therapy: An experiential approach to behavior change.* New York, NY: Guilford Press.

Lindsley, O. R. (1968). Training parents and teachers to precisely manage children's behavior. Paper presented at the C. S. Mott Foundation Children's Health Center, Flint, MI.

Lundgren, T., Dahl, J., Yardi, N., & Melin, J. (2008). Acceptance and commitment therapy and yoga for drug refractory epilepsy: A randomized controlled trial. *Epilepsy and Behavior, 13*(1), 102–108.

Luoma, J., Hayes, S., & Walser, R. (2017). *Learning ACT: An acceptance and commitment therapy training skills manual for therapists.* Oakland, CA: Context Press–New Harbinger.

Neff, K. (2003). The development and validation of a scale to measure self-compassion. *Journal of Self and Identity, 2*(3), 223–250.

Ossman, W. A., Wilson, K. G., Storaasli, R. D., & McNeill, J. W. (2006). A preliminary investigation of the use of acceptance and commitment therapy in group treatment for social phobia. *International Journal of Psychology and Psychological Therapy, 6,* 397–416.

Polk, K. L., & Schoendorff, B. (Eds.). (2014). *The ACT matrix: A new approach to building psychological flexibility across settings and populations.* Oakland, CA: New Harbinger.

Ramnerö, J., & N. Törneke. (2008). *The ABCs of human behavior: Behavioral principles for the practicing clinician.* Oakland, CA: New Harbinger.

Robinson, P. (2008). Integrating acceptance and commitment therapy into primary pediatric care. In L. A. Greco & S. C. Hayes (Eds.), *Acceptance and mindfulness treatments for children and adolescents* (pp. 237–261). Oakland, CA: New Harbinger.

Strosahl, K. D. (2004). ACT with the multi-problem client. In S. C. Hayes & K. D. Strosahl (Eds.), *A practical guide to acceptance and commitment therapy* (pp. 209–244). Oakland, CA: New Harbinger.

Strosahl, K. D. (2005, July). Workshop on ACT as a brief therapy. Presented at the ACT Summer Institute, Philadelphia, PA.

Strosahl, K. D., Hayes, S. C., Wilson, K. G., & Gifford, E.V. (2004). An ACT primer. In S. C. Hayes & K. D. Strosahl (Eds.), *A practical guide to acceptance and commitment therapy* (pp. 31–58). Oakland, CA: New Harbinger.

Tapper, K., Shaw, C., Ilsley, J., Hill, A. J., Bond, F. W., & Moore, L. (2009). Exploratory randomised controlled trial of a mindfulness-based weight loss intervention for women. *Appetite, 52,* 396–404.

Tirch, D., Schoendorff, B., & Silberstein, L. R. (2014). *The ACT practitioner's guide to the science of compassion: Tools for fostering psychological flexibility.* Oakland, CA: New Harbinger.

Törneke, N. (2010). *Learning RFT: An introduction to relational frame theory and its clinical application.* Oakland, CA: New Harbinger.

Twohig, M. P., Hayes, S. C., & Masuda, A. (2006). Increasing willingness to experience obsessions: Acceptance and commitment therapy as a treatment for obsessive-compulsive disorder. *Behavior Therapy, 37*(1), 3–13.

Wegner, D. M., Erber, R., & Zanakos, S. (1993). Ironic processes in the mental control of mood and mood-related thought. *Journal of Personality and Social Psychology, 65*(6), 1093–1104.

Wenzlaff, R. M., & Wegner, D. M. (2000). Thought suppression. *Annual Review of Psychology, 51,* 59–91.

Zettle, R. D. (2003). Acceptance and commitment therapy vs. systematic desensitization in treatment of mathematics anxiety. *The Psychological Record, 53*(2), 197–215.

Zettle, R. D. (2007). *ACT for depression.* Oakland, CA: New Harbinger.

Russ Harris is an internationally acclaimed acceptance and commitment therapy (ACT) trainer and author of the best-selling ACT-based self-help book *The Happiness Trap*, which has sold over 600,000 copies and been published in thirty languages. He is widely renowned for his ability to teach ACT in a way that is simple, clear, and fun—yet extremely practical.

Foreword writer **Steven C. Hayes, PhD**, is Foundation Professor of psychology at the University of Nevada, Reno, and the originator of ACT. He is author of dozens of books and scientific articles, including the successful ACT workbook *Get Out of Your Mind and Into Your Life*.

Index

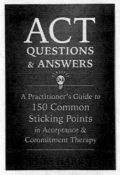
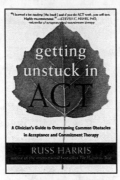
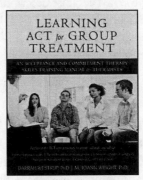
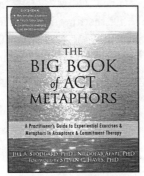
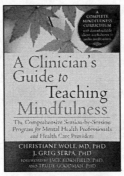
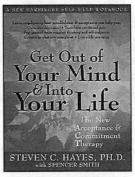
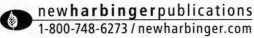